PRINCIPLES OF COMPETITIVE PROTEIN-BINDING ASSAYS

PRINCIPLES OF COMPETITIVE PROTEIN-BINDING ASSAYS

SECOND EDITION

Edited by

William D. Odell, M.D., Ph.D.
Professor of Medicine and Physiology
Chairman, Department of Medicine
University of Utah School of Medicine
Salt Lake City, Utah

Paul Franchimont, M.D., Ph.D.
Associate Professor of Medicine
Director of Radioimmunoassay Laboratory
University of Liège
Liège, Belgium

A WILEY MEDICAL PUBLICATION
JOHN WILEY & SONS
New York · Chichester · Brisbane · Toronto · Singapore

Cover design by Wanda Lubelska

Library of Congress Cataloging in Publication Data:

Main entry under title:

Principles of competitive protein-binding assays.

  (A Wiley medical publication)
  Includes index.
  1. Radioimmunoassay.   2. Protein binding.   I. Odell,
William D., 1929–   .   II. Franchimont, Paul.
III. Series.
QP519.9.R3P74   1982   616.07'57   82-10941
ISBN 0-471-08924-9

Printed in the United States of America

10 9 8 7 6 5 4 3 2 1

CONTRIBUTORS

Derek R. Bangham, M.B.
Head, Division of Hormones
National Institute for Biological Standards and Control
Holly Hill, Hampstead
London, United Kingdom

Gildon N. Beall, M.D.
UCLA School of Medicine
Los Angeles, California
Professor and Chief
Division of Allergy and Clinical Immunology
Department of Medicine
Harbor-UCLA Medical Center
Torrance, California

Jean-Pierre Bourguignon, M.D.
Assistant of the Pediatric Department and Radioimmunoassay
   Laboratory
University of Liège
Liège, Belgium

L. Arthur Campfield, Ph.D.
Assistant Professor of Physiology and Engineering Sciences
The Medical School and The Technological Institute
Northwestern University
Chicago, Illinois

Fernand Dray, M.D., Ph.D.
Institut Pasteur
Paris, France

Delbert Fisher, M.D.
Professor of Pediatrics and Medicine
UCLA School of Medicine
Los Angeles, California
Harbor–UCLA Medical Center
Torrance, California

Paul Franchimont, M.D., Ph.D.
Associate Professor of Medicine
Director of Radioimmunoassay Laboratory
University of Liège
Liège, Belgium

Pyara K. Grover, M.Sc., Ph.D.
Director, New Drugs Division
Sarabhai Research Centre
Baroda, India

Jean-Claude Hendrick, C.Sc.B., Ph.D.
Professor
Laboratoire de Radioimmunologie
University of Liège
Liège, Belgium

Ian Holdaway, M.D., B.Med.Sc.
Endocrinologist
Honorary Associate Professor of Medicine
Department of Medicine
Auckland Hospital
Auckland, New Zealand

Renzo Malvano, Ph.D.
Clinical Immunochemistry Unit SORIN Biomedica Laboratorio
  di Fisiologia
Clinica C.N.R.
Saluggia and Pisa, Italy

Jerald C. Nelson, M.D.
Associate Professor of Medicine and Pathology
Chief of Endocrinology and Metabolism
Los Angeles Campus
Loma Linda University School of Medicine
Los Angeles, California

William D. Odell, M.D., Ph.D.
Professor of Medicine and Physiology
Chairman, Department of Medicine
University of Utah School of Medicine
Salt Lake City, Utah

Aimée-Marguerite Reuter, Ph.D.
Collaborator of the University of Liège
Associate Head, R.I.A. Department
National Institute for Radioelement (I.R.E.)
Liège, Belgium

Wolfgang Seiss, M.D.
Institut Pasteur
Paris, France

Leif Wide, M.D.
Assistant Professor of Clinical Chemistry
University Hospital
Uppsala, Sweden

PREFACE

This book was conceived as a text to accompany practical workshops on competitive binding assay systems. The first workshop, sponsored by The Endocrine Society and organized by W. D. Odell, was held in 1971 at Harbor–UCLA Medical Center. The first edition resulted from that meeting; all lectures were tape-recorded and edited to form the body of the text. All proceeds from that first edition were donated by the lecturers and authors to The Endocrine Society.

In the ten years since the first edition, the text has continued to serve as a companion to workshops on immunoassays. However, methods have changed, and new ones have been developed. Accordingly, this second edition, based on the same format as the first, now offers the theoretical basis and technical data for competitive binding assay systems for the 1980s. Strictly speaking, the term "protein binding" is incomplete, since competitive binding principles are now employed using other materials in addition to proteins (e.g., nucleic acids and carbohydrates).

The authors and editors hope that this text serves the reader well in supplying generalities, theoretical bases, technical details, and practicalities of competitive binding assay systems.

We would like to thank Ms. Carole B. Tudor for her editorial assistance.

William D. Odell
Paul Franchimont

CONTENTS

1. **Introduction and General Principles** 1
    William D. Odell

2. **The Immune System in General** 15
    Gildon N. Beall

3. **Antibody Production for Immunoassay** 33
    *Paul Franchimont, Jean-Claude Hendrick,
    and Aimée-Marguerite Reuter*

4. **Conjugation Techniques—Chemistry** 55
    Pyara K. Grover

5. **Radiolabeling Techniques** 69
    William D. Odell

6. **Reference Materials and Standardization** 85
    Derek R. Bangham

7. **Separation of Bound from Free Hormone** 107
    William D. Odell

8. **Mathematical Analysis of Competitive Protein Binding
    Assays** 125
    L. Arthur Campfield

9. **Pitfalls in Peptide Radioimmunoassays** 149
    *Paul Franchimont, Jean-Claude Hendrick,
    Jean-Pierre Bourguignon, and Aimée-Marguerite Reuter*

10. **Radioimmunoassay of Steroids** 161
    Renzo Malvano

11. **Radioimmunoassay of Thyroid Hormones, Thyroid Hormone-
    Binding Inter-α-globulin, and Thyroglobulin** 205
    Delbert Fisher

12. **Radioimmunoassay of Prostanoids** **225**
     Fernand Dray and Wolfgang Seiss

13. **Noncompetitive Versus Competitive Binding Assays** **243**
     Leif Wide

14. **Principles of Radioreceptorassays** **255**
     Ian Holdaway

15. **Principles of in Vitro Bioassays** **267**
     William D. Odell

16. **Assay Performance Evaluations for Quality Control** **281**
     Jerald C. Nelson

     Index **305**

PRINCIPLES OF COMPETITIVE PROTEIN-BINDING ASSAYS

CHAPTER 1

INTRODUCTION AND GENERAL PRINCIPLES

William D. Odell

In the chapters that follow, we introduce the reader to the principles of competitive binding assay systems. To place these assay techniques in proper perspective, it is wise to have a familiarity with other assay systems and to understand the basic concepts of hormone or drug distribution and degradation in biologic fluids. This is important because in vitro assay techniques have limitations as well as advantages. Furthermore, different techniques may actually quantify different forms or portions of the molecule or molecules in question. Figure 1 illustrates the concept (1) that four assay techniques "view" differently the relation between the analyte (the substance to be measured) and the reference preparation (the yard- or meter-stick against which we measure). Although in the early days of radioimmunoassay (RIA) it was believed that validation of the technique was dependent upon demonstration that immunoassays and bioassays give similar results, this is now known to be not only unnecessary but actually not true or unlikely to be true in most instances. In fact, the in vivo bioassay is the most complex of measurement systems, involving variations and specificities of animal responses, hormone action, hormone distribution in biologic compartments, and hormone degradation. Each of these parameters may differ between reference preparation and analyte, making interpretation even more complex. It is important, then, for the assayist to know that each of these assay methods results in different information and that each method often gives different answers, *all* of which are correct. We list below the characteristics of the four viewpoints or perspectives involved in understanding an answer.

CHARACTERISTICS OF FOUR ASSAY METHODS OR PERSPECTIVES

1. *In vivo bioassays:* These bioassays vary in response with the animal species selected, as well as with the age, sex, and diet of the animals. Also,

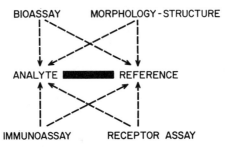

Figure 1. Schematic presentation of four viewpoints of the relation between the analyte (substance to be quantified) and the reference preparation (meterstick against which we measure). All methods usually give different "answers," yet each is "correct." [Reproduced from W. D. Odell, 1977 (1).]

these bioassays involve differences in metabolism, degradation rates, and volumes of distribution, and any of these parameters may differ in analyte and reference preparation. The in vivo bioassay is the most complex of the assay systems and is usually tedious and expensive.

2. *Radioimmunoassay:* The RIA involves the recognition of antigenic determinants with molecular weights of 600 to 800. For peptides or protein hormone preparations having molecular weights of 1,000 to 50,000 or more, this may represent only a small segment of the analyte and reference preparation. In fact, many different immunoassays having dissimilar specificities and other assay parameters may exist for the same protein analytes and reference preparations. Metabolism and distribution volumes are not involved in the same sense as in the in vivo bioassays.

3. *Radioreceptor assay:* The radioreceptor assay (RRA) involves assessment of the first step in biologic function: binding to the cellular recognition site or receptor. For such assays, the receptor is isolated from other cellular functions, that is, hormone action, and in vitro binding is quantified. The molecular structure required for binding is usually different (and usually larger) than that reacting in a RIA. As for RIA, metabolism and distribution volumes are not involved in the same sense as in the in vivo bioassays. Since after binding to a receptor a series of subsequent effects occur (e.g., internalization, linking to and generation of second messengers, and alteration of one or more cell components), receptor assays assess only one facet of hormone action.

4. *Morphology–structure or structure–function viewpoint or assay:* After binding to the recognition structure of a cell (the receptor), a variable sequence of steps proceeds, culminating in recognizable hormone action (e.g., steroid synthesis and secretion). The structure of the molecule required for completion of hormone action may be different from that required simply for binding to the receptor. Similarly, analytes reacting in a RIA via a particular structure may show no binding to the receptor and pos-

sess no bioactivity. Analysis of structure–function relations is complex and often involves measurements in the first three assay systems and a common fourth, the in vitro bioassay. For example, pro-ACTH possesses full or nearly full RIA activity and little or no RRA activity; however, it may possess some in vivo bioactivity (because of conversion to ACTH). The thyroid-stimulating immunoglobulins possess excellent in vivo thyroid-stimulating activity; they show no reaction in human thyroid-stimulating hormone (TSH) RIAs but do show good activity in TSH RRA systems.

In summary, the four viewpoints (in vivo bioassay, RIA, RRA, and morphology–structure analysis) result in the analysis or quantification of different aspects of the relation between analyte and reference preparation. All may, at times, give different but still correct answers.

HISTORY OF COMPETITIVE BINDING ASSAYS

The assay techniques involving in vitro competitive binding had their historical origins in the laboratory of Solomon Berson and Rosalyn Yalow at the Bronx Veterans Administration Hospital in New York City. Tracing these origins is of interest and may help the beginning assayist understand the principles as explicated herein.

During the years 1953–1956, two groups [Berson and Yalow (2–4) and Welsh et al. (5)] were studying the metabolism of ^{131}I-labeled insulin in humans with and without diabetes. These studies were being carried out for a different purpose than assay development. It had been postulated by Mirsky (6) that non-insulin-dependent diabetes (referred to at the time as maturity-onset diabetes mellitus) was not due to a deficiency of insulin secretion but was caused by increased degradation of insulin by an enzyme complex called hepatic insulinase. Surprisingly, both groups [Berson et al. (4) and Welsh et al. (5)] discovered, as part of these studies, that all insulin-treated diabetics had serum substances that bound insulin. Both suggested that these were antibodies to insulin produced by insulin treatment. However, only Berson and Yalow characterized these substances adequately to prove they were antibodies. Further, Berson and Yalow showed that, when unlabeled insulin was added in vitro to a fixed dilution of these antisera, the amount of ^{131}I-labeled insulin bound to antibodies decreased.

It was Berson and Yalow who recognized the potential of developing an assay system from such data (7). They followed up their observations on human antibodies to insulin by immunizing guinea pigs with insulin to prepare larger quantities of antiserum containing antibodies with higher affinity capable of being used for sensitive assay development (8,9). They further undertook studies of the kinetics and specificity of the binding of insulin to antibodies. These very important studies (10) were probably the first employment of the law of mass action and its mathematical expression for antigen–antibody interaction.

Interestingly, starting from a different base within approximately the same time frame, Roger Ekins in London arrived at a similar principle for hormone assay. As a house officer, he began to study the binding of thyroxine to thyroxine-binding globulin (TBG) at about the same time that Berson and Yalow and Welsh et al. were studying the metabolism of ^{131}I-labeled insulin. Ekins also recognized that one could quantify thyroxine using TBG as a binding protein. As so often occurs in science, his publication in 1960 on this thyroxine assay method (11) postdated the first insulin RIA publication of Yalow and Berson in 1959 (8–10). However, his analysis and methods had been derived independently during the preceding years, possibly at about the same time as those of Berson and Yalow. In the years to follow, Ekins and Berson and Yalow frequently differed (12–15) on conclusions from mathematical analysis of these binding assay principles. A common ingredient in these disagreements stemmed from differences in the consideration of experimental errors in the separation of bound and free hormone, and of counting rates and specific activity of the labeled hormone.

Two other groups published important studies during these early years of assay development. Unger et al. (16), benefiting from direct early communication with Berson and Yalow, in 1959 reported the development of an immunoassay for glucagon. Grodsky and Forsham (17) also reported a RIA for insulin in 1960.

In Chapter 8 Campfield reviews the mathematical analysis of these assay systems, so this subject will not be discussed here. However, the components of the assay and some of their properties will now be reviewed. As indicated earlier, there are at least four different assay approaches (Fig. 1). RIA is discussed first and in more detail in this book.

RADIOIMMUNOASSAY

RIAs are composed of four components:

1. The antiserum (antianalyte, e.g., guinea pig antiserum against insulin).
2. The labeled analyte (usually radioiodinated) (e.g., ^{125}I-labeled insulin), frequently called the *label*.
3. The reference preparation (e.g., unlabeled, purified insulin), frequently called the *standard*.

4. A method of separating antibody-bound labeled analyte (bound) and non-antibody-bound labeled analyte (free).

Each of these components has its own properties, and each must have these properties optimized for the best assay performance.

THE ANTISERUM

Antisera are generally prepared by immunization of animals with the analyte in purified or fairly purified form. For peptides or proteins of greater than 6,000 molecular weight, the protein is usually administered in its native form with complete Freund's adjuvant. For peptides having a lower molecular weight, covalent conjugation to a larger carrier protein (e.g., thyroglobulin or albumin) is generally performed and the conjugate injected. For steroids, thyronines, and drugs, covalent conjugation to carrier proteins is also performed. The chemistry and techniques of various methods of conjugation are reviewed by Grover in Chapter 4. Methods of immunization are also reviewed by Franchimont in Chapter 3.

A variety of animal species have been used to prepare antisera, generally guinea pigs and rabbits but also goats, sheep, donkeys, chickens, and many others. The properties of this antiserum (often called the first antibody, because one kind of method for the separation of bound and free involves another antiserum—the second antibody) include its (1) titer, (2) specificity, and (3) affinity of association or dissociation. In addition to a variety of animal species used to prepare antiserum, so-called monoclonal antibodies may be produced in vitro by myeloma cell lines (11). This technique involving the fusion of an antibody-producing cell with a myeloma cell has been successfully performed with mouse cells. It will probably be expanded to other species of cells and theoretically could result in the production of large quantities of homogeneous antibodies with known specificity and affinity (18,19). In future years, it is likely that this technique will become the usual source of antisera.

Titer, simply stated, is the dilution of antiserum binding a given amount or percentage of labeled analyte; for example, the dilution binding 30% of the label. It is determined by incubating serially diluted amounts of antiserum with a small amount (trace) of label.

Figure 2 shows a typical dilution curve for a RIA. Titers in use in immunoassays vary, but often range from 100,000 to 1,000,000 or more. It is important for the assayist to use constant terminology in discussions. Frequently, the terms *initial* and *final* titer are used. If not specifically defined, assay instructions often result in considerable error or confusion. *Final titer* refers to titer in the completed assay tube, and *initial titer* is the titer added to the tube. Thus, if 100 μl of 1:100,000 dilution (the initial titer) is added to an assay tube containing a total volume of 1000 μl, the final titer will be

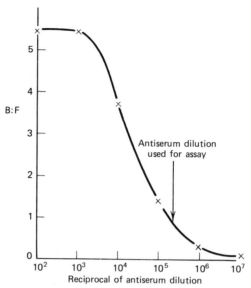

Figure 2. Dilution of antihuman TSH antiserum to determine titer. The arrow indicates the final titer used in the assay (1:200,000 dilution) for this example. The actual titer used in assays may be adjusted lower or higher, depending on the purposes for which the assay will be used. [Reproduced with permission from Raud and Odell, 1969 (20).]

1:1,000,000. If a different final total assay volume is used (e.g., 500 μl), the final titer will differ.

Specificity of the antiserum is generally determined by assessing the antiserum under assay conditions for reaction with potentially cross-reacting or interfering antigens. Although monoclonal antibodies (containing only a single population of antibodies with identical characteristics) are desirable, a specific RIA is not dependent on the existence of such an antibody or an antiserum containing only these antibodies. If other antibodies exist in the antiserum that do not bind the labeled analyte or the reference preparation, no interference with the assay exists. Figures 3a and b illustrate this

(a) $Ab_1 + a_1 \rightleftharpoons Ab_1 \cdot a_1$ (b) $Ab_1 + a_1 \rightleftharpoons Ab_1 \cdot a_1$

       $Ab_2 + a_2 \rightleftharpoons Ab_2 \cdot a_2$ $Ab_1 + a_2 \rightleftharpoons Ab_1 \cdot a_2$

       $Ab_3 + a_3 \rightleftharpoons Ab_3 \cdot a_3$ $Ab_1 + a_3 \rightleftharpoons Ab_1 \cdot a_3$

Figure 3. (a) Illustration that multiple antibodies in an antiserum could permit a specific radioimmunoassay. (b) Alternatively, a monoclonal or monovalent antibody may still result in a nonspecific assay. Ab_1, Ab_2, and Ab_3, indicate three antibody populations; a_1, a_2 and a_3 indicate three analytes. See text for details.

$$(a) \quad Ab_1 + a_1 \underset{K_2}{\overset{K_1}{\rightleftharpoons}} Ab_1 \cdot a_1$$

$$(b) \quad \frac{[Ab_1 \cdot a_1]}{[Ab_1] \cdot [a_1]} = \frac{K_1}{K_2} = K_{eq}$$

Figure 4. (a) K_1 is the rate of forward reaction (i.e., formation of the complex $Ab_1 \cdot a_1$); K_2 + the rate of backward reaction (i.e., dissociation of $Ab_1 \cdot a_1$) (b) $[Ab_1]$ and $[a_1]$ are the concentrations in moles per liter of each form.

point. In Figure 3a, if each antibody reacts only with its respective analyte, each assay system could be specific. If analyte a_2 were labeled with ^{125}I, then unlabeled a_2 could be quantified because a_2 does not react with Ab_1 or Ab_3. In contrast, if Ab_2 reacts with a_2 and a_3, as shown in Figure 3b, a nonspecific assay results, even though a monovalent or monoclonal antiserum is available. Notice, however (in Fig. 3b), that if a purification method were available to separate a_1, a_2, and a_3 before assay, the nonspecific assay could still be used for quantificaton of a_2. This latter principle is often employed in steroid RIAs.

As stated previously, the reader should be cognizant that the specificity of RIA relates to the reaction of a structural portion of the analyte (an antigenic determinant of MW 600–800) and has nothing to do with the biologic function of the analyte. Thus, substances with very different biologic properties or no biologic action may share an 8- to 10-amino-acid sequence in common and still react in the same RIA.

Affinity may be defined as the avidity with which an antibody reacts with its antigen—the tightness of binding, so to speak. It may be estimated experimentally from the mass action law illustrated in one form in Figure 3. This is shown in a slightly different manner in Figure 4. When the reaction is in equilibrium, $k_1 = k_2$, and the expression in Figure 4b holds. The numerical values of this affinity of association (K_a) range between approximately 1 10^9 and 10^{11} liters/mole for most antisera in good RIAs.

THE LABELED ANALYTE

This analyte is also called a *label* or a *tracer* in slang terminology. For peptides or proteins, this usually means "tagged" with ^{125}I. However, other isotopes such as ^{131}I and ^{35}S have also been used. Generally, ^{14}C has too long a half-life and does not result in adequate counting rates for RIAs requiring sensitivity of 10^{-9}–10^{-12} moles/liter, the concentrations in which most hormones are found in biological fluids. For steroids, ^3H with C-3 and C-4 substitutions in the molecule give adequate counting rates. For drugs and antibiotics occurring in molar concentrations 100 to 10,000 times higher than hormones, both ^{14}C and ^{3}H can be used.

The label also has several properties:

1. *Purity:* The labeled analyte should be as pure as possible. It is obvious that, if an assay is designed to quantify one hormone and the analyte to be labeled contains a high fraction or contamination of other analytes, an error in specificity or in identifying bound and free hormone may result. If antibodies against the contaminating analyte are present in the antiserum, this contaminating analyte will react in the assay and become difficult or impossible to distinguish from the analyte the assay is intended to quantify. If no antibodies against the contaminating analyte exist in the antiserum, this portion of label will be identified as free, not antibody-bound. This error in assignment can be magnified if, for various possible reasons, the contaminant is preferentially labeled by whatever procedure is chosen.

2. *Purity after iodination:* All labeling procedures are followed by a purification step. Optimally, this step also removes nonimmunoactive or "damaged" (Berson and Yalow's terminology) hormone. The maximal degree of immunoreactivity can be identified by incubation with excess first antibody and generally should be over 90% of the label. It is worth stressing that immunoreactivity with excess antibody may not distinguish a fairly good label from an outstanding label. Affinity of the label could be low for a fairly good label and still show high immunoreactivity *with excess* antiserum. Differences in assay characteristics with two such different labels would result.

3. *Stability:* Once labeled and purified, the label is unstable. It undergoes a variety of damaging events, such as radiation inactivation (which is greatly accelerated in water solutions) and oxidation of the analyte. Immunoreactivity must be assessed at frequent intervals, the exact frequency of which varies with each hormone. This ranges from every 48 hours for ^{125}I-labeled ACTH to every 1–2 months for ^{3}H-labeled steroids.

THE REFERENCE PREPARATION

Bangham amplifies the consideration of reference preparations in Chapter 6. The working standard may be defined as the reference preparation used in each assay and may or may not be identical to a laboratory, national, or international reference preparation. A good deal of confusion exists concerning the relation of reference purity to assay performance. Figure 5 illustrates that, no matter how pure the standard or reference, it will not make a nonspecific assay into a specific one. Conversely, a specific assay can

(a) Ab_1 a_2*

   $Ab_2 + a_1 + a_2 + a_3 \rightleftharpoons Ab_2 \cdot a_2 + Ab_2 \cdot a_2* + a_2*$

   Ab_3

(b) a_2*

   $Ab_2 + a_1 \cdot a_2 \cdot a_3 \rightleftharpoons Ab_2 \cdot a_1 + Ab_2 \cdot a_2 + Ab_2 \cdot a_3 + Ab_2 \cdot a_2*$

Figure 5. Ab_1, Ab_2, and Ab_3 indicate populations of antibodies each with their own specificity and affinity. a_1, a_2, and a_3 are three different analytes: a_2* indicates analyte 2, labeled. (a) The reaction between Ab_2 and a_2 and a_2* is specific; a_1 and a_3 cannot compete. Thus, their presence in the reference preparation may dilute a_2 but does not otherwise influence the assay. Similarly, a_1 and a_2 in the sample to be assayed (e.g., serum) will not interfere with the assay. (b) The reaction between Ab_2 and a_2 is not specific; competition from a_1, a_2, and a_3 all occur. Purifying the reference only clouds the issue, for unknown samples, for example, serum, may contain a_1 and a_3. Thus, the assay remains nonspecific.

easily employ a crude reference preparation. For protein or peptide analytes, the reference is commonly defined in terms of units arbitrarily assigned to a large, stable pool or batch of the material. If the structure is known, as for some small peptides (e.g., vasopressin and gonadotropin-releasing hormone), a purified reference might be used and quantities stated in mass (e.g., picograms or nanograms) or, more preferably, in moles per liter. For easily obtainable, stable preparations of known structure such as steroids and thyronines, reference preparations are usually defined in mass or in moles per liter.

SEPARATION OF BOUND AND FREE

Of all the assay components, this step or component of the RIA is probably the greatest source of error. A variety of methods exists but, as is discussed in a later chapter, each has some inherent problem. As Ekins has discussed (12,13,15), if the method of separation of bound and free were perfect (i.e., no existing errors of classification, all bound identified as bound, and all free identified as free), the most sensitive and precise assay would be one in which the antiserum is infinitely dilute and a tiny fraction of bound hormone is present. However, all separation methods do "misclassify" (Ekins terminology). Each separation method (as does the entire assay system) has its own precision, specificity, and sensitivity. Thus, optimization of the separation method, maximizing its precision and its "ruggedness" (Ekins terminology), is essential. Ruggedness may be defined as freedom from alteration or freedom from the introduction of errors in repeated use in different laboratories, in different environments, and by different personnel.

THE COMPLETE RADIOIMMUNOASSAY

As indicated, the properties of each assay component affect the total assay when assembled. In addition, a number of other factors affect the assay. The affinity of antibodies for antigens is affected by the pH and osmolality of the environment in which the reaction occurs. Since osmolality or pH may vary from assay tube to assay tube, when many unknowns are introduced into an assay, artifactual results can occur based on pH or osmolality. Separate from these two parameters, the amount or concentration of protein affects assay results, possibly by influencing separation methods or in other poorly understood ways.

The rate of achieving equilibrium in antibody–antigen reactions with very small concentrations, such as those in RIAs, is relatively slow. This rate is modified by the temperature and concentration of each reagent. Because many commercial assays are now nonequilibrium assays or have short incubation times to minimize the turnaround time (time required to complete the obtaining of data), any modification of this "rate toward equilibrium" from tube to tube produces artifactual results. Since, as has been stressed repeatedly, one is comparing a reference preparation to an unknown analyte, and each frequently occurs in different degrees of purity, in different fluids, at different initial temperatures, at different protein concentrations,

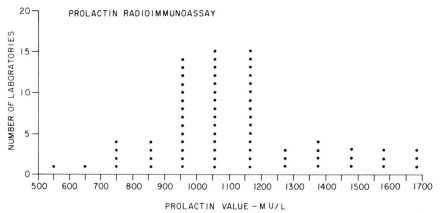

Figure 6. Determination of the prolactin value in a single sample distributed to 80 laboratories located in many parts of the world. All laboratories used the same reagents (label, antiserum, standards, and methods). (Reproduced with permission from WHO matched reagents program.)

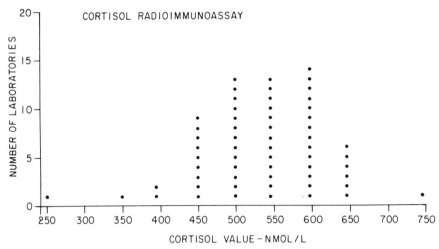

Figure 7. Determination of the cortisol content of a single sample distributed to 60 laboratories throughout the world. All laboratories used the same reagents (label, antiserum, and standards). (Reproduced with permission from WHO matched reagents program.)

or at different pH values, a variety of errors are easily introduced. This also means that a RIA established for plasma may not be suitable for urine, for cerebrospinal fluid, or for tissue extracts or buffer solutions of analyte.

Finally, the assay is the sum of all these components and is influenced when assembled by all the qualities of each component. All errors or adverse parameters of each component are additive. Thus, the sum of all errors frequently results in large assay error.

As will be discussed in later chapters, each RIA is in essence a chemical type of method and, unlike bioassays, has an estimable precision which is surprisingly small. However, quite independent assays performed at different times by different personnel produce results that are surprisingly varied, even when the same reference and analyte are used. The range of potency estimates for a given analyte developed by different laboratories, even with identical reagents, is not too different for RIA than it is for good in vivo bioassays. As an example, see Figures 6 and 7, which illustrate RIA determination of the hormone content of a single sample distributed to a large number of laboratories throughout the world. Almost all these laboratories used exactly the same reagents (i.e., antiserum, standards, label, and separation reagents) and an identical assay protocol. In spite of this, variation in hormone value in the sample is considerable.

In the pages to follow, we analyze many aspects of RIA and of other in vitro assay systems. However, the assayist, no matter how accomplished, should always be cautious.

REFERENCES

1. Odell WD: We don't look at hormones the way we used to. *Radioimmunoassay and Related Procedures in Medicine, First International Symposium on Radioimmunoassays and Related Procedures in Medicine, 1977.* Vienna, International Atomic Energy Agency, 1978, p 3.

2. Berson SA, Yalow RS, Schreiber SS, et al: Tracer experiments with I^{131} labeled human serum albumin: Distribution and degradation studies. *J Clin Invest* 32:746, 1953.

3. Berson SA, Yalow RS: The distribution of I^{131} labeled human serum albumin introduced into ascitic fluid: Analysis of the kinetics of a three compartment catenary transfer system in man and speculations on possible sites of degradation. *J Clin Invest* 33:377, 1954.

4. Berson SA, Yalow RS, Bauman A, et al: Insulin-I^{131} metabolism in human subjects: Demonstration of insulin binding globulin in the circulation of insulin-treated subjects. *J Clin Invest* 35:170, 1956.

5. Welsh GW, Henley ED, Williams RH, et al: Insulin I-^{131} metabolism in man: Plasma-binding, distribution and degradation. *Am J Med* 21:324, 1956.

6. Mirsky IA: The etiology of diabetes mellitus in man. *Rec Prog Horm Res* 7:437, 1952.

7. Berson SA, Yalow RS: Isotopic tracers in the study of diabetes. *Adv Biol Med Phys* 6:349, 1958.

8. Berson SA, Yalow RS: Recent studies on insulin-binding antibodies. *Ann NY Acad Sci* 82:338, 1959.

9. Yalow RS, Berson SA: Assay of plasma insulin in human subjects by immunological methods. *Nature* 184:1648, 1959.

10. Berson SA, Yalow RS: Species-specificity of human antibeef, pork insulin serum. *J Clin Invest* 38:2017, 1959.

11. Ekins, RP: The estimation of thyroxine in human plasma by an electrophoretic technique. *Clin Chim Acta 5:453, 1960.*

12. Ekins R, Newman B: Theoretical aspects of saturation analysis, in Diczfalusy E (ed): *Steroid Assay by Protein Binding.* Stockholm, 2nd Karolinska Symposia on Research Methods in Reproductive Endocrinology, 1970, p 11.

13. Ekins RP, Newman GB, O'Riordan JLH: Saturation assays, in McArthur JS, Colton T (eds): *Statistics in Endocrinology.* Cambridge, MIT Press, 1970, p 345.

14. Yalow RS, Berson SA: Introduction and general considerations in Odell WD, Daughaday WH (eds): *Principles of Competitive Protein-Binding Assays,* ed 1. Philadelphia, J. B. Lippincott Co, 1971, p 1.

15. Ekins RP: Problems of sensitivity with special reference to optimal conditions, in Margoulis M (ed): *Protein and Polypeptide Hormones,* Part 3, International Symposium Liège, 1968. Amsterdam, Excerpta Medica Foundation ICS 161, 1969, p 672.

16. Unger RH, Eisentraut AM, McCall MS, et al: Glucagon antibodies and their use for immunoassay for glucagon. *Pro Soc Exp Biol Med* 102:621, 1959.

17. Grodsky GM, Forsham PH: An immunochemical assay of total extractable insulin in man. *J Clin Invest* 39:1070, 1960.

18. Kohler G, Milstein C: Continuous cultures of fused cells secreting antibody of predefined specificity. *Nature* 256:495, 1975.

19. Kohler G, Milstein C: Derivation of specific antibody-producing tissue culture and tumor lines by cell fusion. *Eur J Immunol* 6:511, 1976.

20. Raud HR, Odell WD: The radioimmunoassay of human thyrotropin. *Br J Hosp Med*, Immunoassay-6, August 1969.

CHAPTER 2
THE IMMUNE SYSTEM IN GENERAL

Gildon N. Beall

The extraordinary specificity of responses by the immune system in higher vertebrates, presumably evolving as an adaptation to changing challenges from a hostile environment, has provided a highly effective defense mechanism. This same specificity of response has made possible the development of assays useful for quantitating numerous substances of biologic interest. Those who would use the immune response to develop reagents or other materials for immunoassay are well advised, however, to keep in mind the functions of the immune system. Successful parasites are themselves capable of adaptation to a host's defense mechanisms, so that a single line of defense is insufficient. Antigens can be mutated or deleted, enzymes controlling vital functions of the parasite can adapt, and genetic information can be passed from one organism to another. The host's defenses will be most effective if they are multiple, overlapping, and capable of modification as the battle proceeds. It should not be surprising then to find that immunologic responses are always heterogeneous. Most antigens contain many different antigenic determinants, each stimulating antibodies of several immunoglobulin types, together with several types of cellular responses. As helpful as this heterogeneity of response may be in host defense, it is usually not helpful in developing a specific immunoassay procedure.

Immune responses are often associated with hypersensitivity phenomena which may be relatively independent of the protective effects of immunization. Hypersensitivity phenomena are generally due to the activation of effector mechanisms in blood or tissue. Such activation, too, may have unwanted effects in the development of antisera or immunoassays. For instance, antigen–antibody interaction ordinarily activates the proteolytic enzymes of the complement system, resulting in the lysis of bacteria or cells. It is possible, although not usual, for these proteolytic enzymes to act upon the antigens used in a serologic system. Complement proteins also deposit with and add to the weight of an antigen–antibody precipitate. Mediators released from lymphocytes, mast cells, or platelets may also conceivably interfere with serologic systems if such cells are included in the system.

These examples illustrate the importance of an understanding of the immune system if one is to use it in immunoassay work. In this chapter we will attempt to provide such a basic, although admittedly superficial, view of the immune system.

ANTIGENS

Antigens are substances that can both elicit antibody formation and react specifically with the antibody produced. Combination with antibody requires the specific chemical structure of the immunizing antigen, but these specific structures may be present on compounds that cannot stimulate antibody formation. Such substances are called *haptens,* and those capable of eliciting antibody formation are called *immunogens.* A complete antigen has both functional activities. Haptens can be rendered immunogenic if they are strongly coupled, by covalent bonds, to an immunogenic carrier molecule.

Chemical structure and molecular size are known to be important in determining immunogenicity. Proteins, carbohydrates, and lipopolysaccharides may all be immunogenic, whereas most lipids and nucleic acids are not, but special treatment of the latter may allow antibody formation. Simple chains of amino acids, such as polylysine, are characteristically nonimmunogenic regardless of molecular size. Proteins, carbohydrates, or other materials with a molecular weight of 5,000 or less are usually not immunogenic and require coupling to a carrier. Polypeptides as small as 1,000 in molecular weight have been successfully used for immunization, but it is likely that the antibody formation that sometimes follows immunization with such low-molecular-weight materials is due to binding of these substances to carrier molecules in the immunized animal.

In addition to chemical structure and molecular size, immunogenicity is dependent on several other factors. The antigen must be foreign to the recipient animal, and it must be given physical access to immunologically competent cells. Since the most effective carriers for haptens seem to be molecules with the most immunogenicity, one is led to the conclusion that carrier function involves the participation of multiple antigenic determinants and the recruitment of several antibody responses.

Haptens, unable to stimulate antibody formation but capable of bonding to antibody, have given a great deal of information about the specificity of the immune response. Haptens that consist of a single chemical grouping, univalent haptens, can be considered analogous to antigenic determinants on complete antigens. Most substances that act as immunogens have many antigenic determinant sites and consequently give rise to antibodies with multiple specificities. Univalent haptens, on the other hand, are capable of stimulating a much more homogeneous antibody response. The study of haptens has also produced information about the requirements for binding to antibodies, information that can be extrapolated to antigenic determinants. Since the time of Landsteiner, it has been known that simple organic chemicals such as picryl chloride and dinitrobenzene are highly effective as specific haptens, binding strongly and specifically to the antibodies elicited by immunization with these haptens bound to carrier molecules. Most antigenic determinants and their complementary antibody-combining sites, however, are larger than these simple chemicals. Evidence indicates that an antigenic determinant of a dextran molecule consists of several dextrose residues and that that of a polypeptide chain resides in several amino acids.

ANTIBODY

Antibodies are proteins with gamma or beta electrophoretic mobility. Five different classes, IgG, IgA, IgM, IgD, and IgE, have been demonstrated in humans and in most mammals. The following discussion will emphasize human immunoglobulins, but the general picture is valid for all mammalian species. Numerous subclasses of immunoglobulins have been discovered, many with unique antigenic and functional characteristics. The pattern of these immunoglobulin subclasses and their functional characteristics vary greatly in different animal species. In all species, however, over 80% of the antibody protein manufactured by the animal is composed of IgG. The immunoassayist interested in producing large amounts of specific, high-affinity antibody is usually interested in this IgG antibody. High-titered antibodies of the IgM class have been stimulated by immunization, but it has been difficult to obtain large amounts of antibody from other immunoglobulin classes. This restriction has now been lifted, since it is now possible to develop monoclonal antibodies of any desired antibody class or subclass by fusing an appropriate antibody-forming cell with a myeloma cell so as to produce an antibody-forming hybridoma, a process that will be discussed in more detail in a subsequent section.

The structure of IgG molecules has been intensively studied and, fortunately, can serve as a model for understanding the other immunoglobulins as well (Fig. 1). The IgG molecule is composed of four polypeptide chains, two light chains of approximately 20,000 daltons and two heavy chains (γ chains) of approximately 60,000 daltons. The chains are held together by interchain disulfide bonds, and intrachain disulfide bonds maintain the folding of the protein. One of only two types of light chains (κ or λ) is found in all immunoglobulins. The heavy chains, however, are unique for each immunoglobulin class, and they are designated by the appropriate Greek letters: IgG, γ; IgM, μ; IgA, α; IgD, δ; and IgE, ϵ.

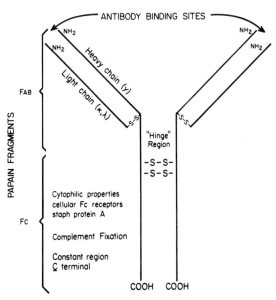

Figure 1. Schematic diagram of an immunoglobulin molecule. The molecule is composed of paired heavy (γ) chains and light (κ or λ) chains. Only two of the interchain disulfide bonds are shown. Although arranged differently in the various immunoglobulin classes and subclasses, these bonds are located near a region of molecular flexibility, the hinge region. The Fab and Fc portions of the molecule, recognized as a result of papain fragmentation, have differing but important functional properties, as shown in the diagram.

The site at which antibody combines with antigen is localized to the portion of the heavy and light chains nearer the N-terminal amino acid; both heavy and light chains participate in the site. Consistent with this functional role, the N-terminal portions of the chains contain most of the variability in amino acid sequence that distinguishes one antibody (or myeloma protein) from another. Most of this variability of the polypeptide chains is in fact confined to three or four hypervariable regions of 8 to 10 amino acids each. The heavy and light chains appear to be folded so as to bring these hypervariable regions together at the antibody-combining site of which there are two for each IgG molecule. The C-terminal portions of the heavy and light chains are referred to as the *constant regions,* since great homology in amino acid sequence is found among immunoglobulins of the same class in this region. At the position in the molecule where heavy and light chains are joined there is some flexibility, so this has been called the *hinge region.* A small amount of carbohydrate, more in IgA and IgE than in IgG, is attached in this area.

Exposure of IgG molecules to papain results in cleavage, so that three fragments are produced, two containing antibody-combining sites (Fab) and one the C-terminal end of the molecule (Fc). The Fc portion of the IgG molecule is responsible for many of the functions of the antibody. Specific receptors for Fc of IgG exist on many cells, including monocytes and macrophages, polymorphonuclear leukocytes, and some B cells. Some tumor cells also have this ability to bind IgG through Fc receptors. Placenta has IgG Fc receptors that may have some function in transplacental passage of IgG. In some instances, binding of IgG Fc by such receptors is not restricted to the species from which the cells are derived, and IgG of other species may be bound as well, a possibly important factor in some immunoassay work, particularly if tissue receptors are involved. The Fc fragment of the IgG molecule is also responsible for complement fixation and the mediation of many allergic reactions. When whole IgG is used as an immunizing antigen, antibodies are developed to many portions of the IgG molecule, but most of them are related to antigenic determinants in the Fc fragment.

Like IgG, both IgD and IgE exist as four-chain units, each with two antigenic combining sites. IgD is found on the surface of most B cells, where it appears to exist in combination with IgM. The concentration of IgD in the serum, however, is small, and few functions have been found for it. The serum concentration of IgE is even less, but IgE function is well established. The ϵ chains of IgE, slightly larger than γ chains, bind specifically to IgE Fc sites on basophils and mast cells. When such cell-bound IgE is cross-linked with antigen, mast cells release mediators which produce allergic reactions. IgA and IgM ordinarily exist as polymers of the basic four-chain structure. IgM consists of five of these units bound together by a J chain with a total molecular weight of 900,000. Serum IgA often exists as a single four-chain unit, but secretory IgA on mucous membranes is combined with a special protein, a secretory portion, and two four-chain units are linked together with a J chain.

CELLS OF THE IMMUNE SYSTEM

The lymphocyte is the central cell of the immune system. These deceptively simple appearing cells harbor a number of functionally distinct subpopulations. Even some of the nonlymphocytic cellular contributions to the immune system imitate lymphocytes in their morphologic appearance. There are two main types of lymphocytes, each with a number of subpopulations. First, the B cells are lymphocytes that have a potential for forming immunoglobulin. This subpopulation of lymphocytes was first found associated with, and acquired their appellation from, an avian lymphoid organ, the bursa of Fabricius. In mammals, B cells appear to arise from the bone marrow. Only about 10% of the circulating mononuclear cells of the peripheral blood are B lymphocytes, but B cells may comprise nearly 50% of the mononuclear cells found in the spleen and almost as many in lymph nodes and the gut-associated lymphoid tissue, such as Peyer's patches. A distinctive characteristic of mature B lymphocytes is their possession of immunoglobulin integrally incorporated into the plasma membrane. When detected with fluorescence-labeled anti-immunoglobulin (anti-Ig), this property has become the usual means for quantitation and separation of B cells. Some B cells and many other mononuclear cells also have receptors on their surface for the Fc fragment of IgG. Since serum IgG binds to these Fc receptors and the bound IgG can be detected with fluorescent anti-Ig, this has caused much confusion, leading to the erroneous conclusion that many B cells possess membrane IgG and falsely identifying as B cells other mononuclear cells with Fc receptors. The membrane immunoglobulin of most B cells is a type of IgM, apparently existing only as a single unit of two light chains and two heavy (μ) chains with added m components which insert into the membrane. This membrane immunoglobulin is in a dynamic state, so that antibodies to the immunoglobulin are capable of coalescing it into patches which can then be capped off and removed from the B cell. The functional consequences of this phenomenon are not entirely clear, but this alteration, too, can lead to difficulty in identifying a B cell by removing its most distinctive characteristic. It now appears that in most adult animals B cells also possess membrane IgD. The functional role of membrane immunoglobulin, particularly IgM, unquestionably is to serve as an antigen receptor.

B cells with membrane immunoglobulin are antigen-sensitive and capable of a proliferative response to antigenic stimulation (Fig. 2). Evidence in mice suggests that membrane IgD is utilized for thymus-dependent antigens, antigens for which an immunologic response requires both T and B cells (1). A few B cells (probably less than 1% of peripheral blood lymphocytes) are IgG-bearing cells. Small numbers of IgE- and IgA-bearing B cells have also been described. In vitro evidence indicates that antigenic stimulation not only induces proliferation of IgM-bearing cells, which manufacture IgM antibody, but also that some of these cells transform into IgG-bearing cells, which may manufacture IgG antibody.

Most (60–80%) of the mononuclear cells in normal peripheral blood are T cells. There are also large numbers in the lymph nodes and spleen, and almost all the lymphocytes in the normal thymus are T cells. The letter "T," of course, is derived from the known necessity for thymic endothelium either for processing directly or providing the thymic hormone that ensures maturation of T cells to their immunocompetent status in adult animals. The absence of an epithelial thymus leads to gross deficiencies in T-cell number and function. Human T cells are easily recognized by their ability to form rosettes with sheep red blood cells because, for unknown reasons, they possess receptors for these red cells. Nonspecific markers of

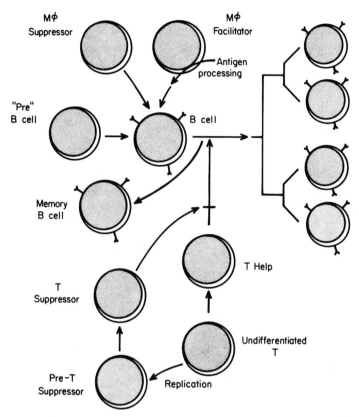

Figure 2. Cellular interaction in antibody formation. Pre-B cells which have no surface immunoglobulin develop to antigen-sensitive B cells with surface immunoglobulin. Macrophages (Mφ) may enhance antibody formation, possibly through processing of antigen, or they may suppress antibody formation, possibly as a result of prostaglandin secretion. T cells have both helper and suppressor activities for antibody formation. Suppresssion is expressed as a result of an effect of undifferentiated T cells, promoting replication of presuppressor cells to form T suppressors. Helper and suppressor T cells may secrete soluble factors, may act directly on B cells, or both. Antigen-sensitive B cells proliferate under the influence of antigen to form antibody-forming B cells. Some B cells remain as antigen-sensitive memory cells available for the anamnestic response.

this sort are not available for all other species, but specific T-cell antigens have been identified and specific antisera for T-cell typing are available for many species.

T cells have been divided into several subsets by both their functional activity and certain unique cellular markers. The functional activities of some of these subsets of T cells will be discussed in this chapter's section on immunoregulation. It is sufficient to note here that T cells can both help and suppress antibody formation. These functional activities are associated with surface antigen markers. Preparation of monoclonal antibodies to these markers now allows identification and separation of functional T cell subsets in mice and men.

T cells are required for most antibody synthesis. They play an important role in regulating the immune response in both antibody formation and cell-mediated immunity. In addition, T cells have important effector functions in cell-mediated immune responses.

The third essential cell of the immune system, the monocyte–macrophage, traces it lineage to a different stem cell than does the lymphocyte. In peripheral blood 20–40% of the mononuclear cells are monocytes, and there are large numbers of macrophages and monocytes in all the lymphoid organs. In the peripheral blood many of these monocytes are morphologically indistinct from lymphocytes, but they can be recognized by their electron microscopic appearance or by histochemical procedures, including nonspecific esterase staining. Monocytes and macrophages show a marked tendency to adhere to glass or plastic surfaces, and they can often be partially separated from other mononuclear cells by adherence to dishes, beads, or tubes. It is likely that the fixed tissue macrophages in lymph nodes and the spleen may have important relationships to in vivo immune responses similar to those shown with monocytes in vitro. Monocytes make important contributions to the immune response and its regulation, both of which will be discussed in subsequent sections. These cells also play important roles in mediating host defense and hypersensitivity phenomena. It is appropriate to point out that monocytes have important nonimmunologic functions such as microbicidal activity, scavenging of dead tissue, and roles in erythro- and granulopoeisis.

IMMUNOGLOBULIN FUNCTIONS

The primary purpose of the immunologic system is to provide protection against parasitism of various kinds. Therefore, it is all the more remarkable to note the tremendous range of functional effects observable with immunoglobulin antibodies. Antibodies may stimulate growth or promote cytotoxicity. They can inhibit hormone effects or mimic and promote such effects. Although in most instances these functions of immunoglobulins are a consequence of their ability to bind to a specific antigen, immunoglobulins can also bind in a relatively specific manner to immunoglobulin Fc receptors on many types of cells. This capacity allows an exception to the general rule that the functional activities of immunoglobulins proceed from their activity as antibodies. Nonimmunologic aggregates of IgG can imitate antigen–antibody complexes by binding to Fc receptors or complement C1q molecules..

The combination of antigen and antibody is reversible. The bonding forces are thought to involve coulombic (charge) attractions and, most importantly, hydrogen bonding and van der Waals forces. These antigen–antibody bonds are usually maximal near physiologic pH and ionic strength, and the interactions can usually be dissociated with low pH or high pH (<3 or >12) or increased salt concentrations. Which of these is most appropriate in dissociating a given antigen–antibody complex depends upon the stability of the antigen and antibody as well as the characteristics of the bond. The affinity of the antigen–antibody interaction varies widely. Association constants of 10^5 to 10^{12} have been described.

When an antigen has enzymatic, toxic, or humoral activity, combination with antibody will neutralize this activity if the active site is at or near the antibody-combining site. If the antigenic determinants that bind antibody are located at a distance from the active site of the antigenic molecule, the effects on the antigen can be quite variable. An immune complex may be formed which, by promoting clearance from the circulation, might localize the toxic or hormonal effect of the antigen to some tissue, rather than allowing its effect to be exerted in the circulation. The reaction with the antigen on occasion produces secondary changes in the antigen, resulting in either increased or decreased activity of a distant active site. It is also possible for antibody to combine with antigen so as to block another immunologic reaction.

Simple combinations of antigen with antibody are called *primary immunologic reactions.* The effects of such reactions will be observable only if some activity of the antigen can be assayed, as in the examples just cited. Since it is often desirable to study these interactions, special means for their detection have been developed. One or the other of the materials, antigen or antibody, must be purified and labeled and a means devised to detect the amount of the constituents that is bound versus the amount that is free. In practice, purification of antigen has often been more easily accomplished. Most means for antibody purification rely, in turn, on preliminary purification of antigen. Antigen may be intrinsically labeled by virtue of unique chemical or physical qualities, or artificially labeled with a radioactive or fluorescent indicator. A common technique is to use radioactively labeled antigen of a size small enough to pass through a cellophane dialysis membrane. Mixtures dialyzed to equilibrium can then be assayed for the amount of antigen bound to antibody inside the bag versus the amount free outside the dialysis bag. Another means for studying primary antigen–antibody interactions is the Farr technique. This procedure takes advantage of the fact that globulins are precipitated by 50% saturated ammonium sulfate (AS), whereas albumin and many smaller antigenic molecules are in a 50% AS supernatant. Labeled (usually iodinated) antigens, such as albumin, bound to specific antibody are found in a washed AS precipitate, whereas free antigen is found in the supernatant. Coprecipitation of labeled antigen–antibody complexes by an anti-immunoglobulin serum is another common means for separating bound from free antigen.

Secondary immunologic reactions include phenomena induced by combinations of antigen and antibody that require the participation of other mediators or further combinations of antigen and antibody for their expression. These include most of the commonly used methods for the detection of antibody, such as precipitation, bacterial or particle agglutination, opsonification, and complement fixation.

Precipitation of antigen by antibody is an important secondary immunologic reaction which, since precipitation is so widely used in immunoassay procedures, we will consider in further detail. Some antibodies are more useful for precipitation than others. IgG antibodies from rabbits, horses, goats, and sheep are usually effective precipitating antibodies. Precipitation requires extensive combinaton of antigen and antibody to form a large lattice. Time is required, and the antigen molecule must have several antigenic determinants, such as the six or seven antigenic determinants usually found on each molecule of protein or carbohydrate antigens. Monovalent haptens, of course, do not form precipitates, since they can combine with only one antibody-combining site and, therefore, will inhibit precipitation.

If one places equal amounts of antibody in each of a number of tubes to which serial increases in concentration of antigen are made, it will be found after incubation that the tubes containing only small amounts of antigen have little or no precipitate. In such tubes antigen combines with antibody in antibody excess. Soluble immune complexes such as Ab_2Ag and Ab_5Ag_2 predominate, remaining in the supernatant, and a lattice cannot be formed. The supernatant in such tubes contains free antibody as well as antigen–antibody complexes. In tubes to which larger amounts of antigen are added, a zone of optimal proportions is found in which maximal precipitation occurs. At maximal precipitation all the antigen and all the antibody are involved in the precipitate, and the supernatant fluid contains neither reactant. Addition of still larger amounts of antigen to antibody results in the formation of soluble immune complexes in antigen excess, with structures such as $AbAg_2$ and Ab_2Ag_3. The amount of precipitate is small, because antibody sites are not available to form a complete lattice. The supernatant fluid contains free antigen as well as the soluble immune complexes. From experiments of this sort it is possible to estimate the molar ratios of antigen and antibody needed for maximal precipitation at the zone of optimal proportions. Although these ratios vary with different antigen–antibody systems, they approximate 4:1 or 5:1 for many common serum protein antigens. The immunoassayist should recall this phenomenon when he or she uses IgG or a portion of IgG as an antigen. Complete precipitation of 1 mg of IgG (the approximate amount in 0.1 ml of human serum) requires at least 5 mg of IgG antibody to IgG. The exact amounts needed must be determined experimentally.

IMMUNIZATION

Many types of antigenic exposure to the immunologic system result in immunization. Injection of antigen intravenously or into the skin or subcutaneous tissues, as is done in experimental studies, usually stimulates both IgM and IgG antibodies. Absorption of antigen through the mucosa of the respiratory, gastrointestinal, or urinary tract preferentially stimulates IgA and IgE antibody formation, since mucosal surfaces are rich in B cells with these capabilities. In either situation, the initial event in immunization is the ingestion of antigen by phagocytic cells. Particulate antigens are usually cleared from blood or lymph by cells of the reticuloendothelial system, whereas soluble antigens may be ingested by circulating monocytes. Processing of antigen by phagocytes renders the antigen more immunogenic in a manner that is not completely understood. Another function of phagocytic cells in immunization is to localize and concentrate antigen so as to allow antigen-sensitive cells to contact the antigen. The architecture of the lymphoid organs, such as the spleen and lymph nodes, probably contributes to the cellular interactions necessary for this process. The necessity for this concentration of antigen is readily understood if one contemplates the relatively small number of antigen-sensitive B cells available for each antigen. These cells, present in the nonimmunized animal, are capable of both binding antigen and being stimulated to proliferate by this antigen, each cell giving rise to 100 or more descendents in a few days, ultimately to form a clone of antibody-producing cells. The number of these cells sensitive to each antigen is thought to be extremely limited to allow for the enormous diversity of antigenic responses that are possible, since antigen-sensitive B cells are assumed to exist for each conceivable antigenic determinant. The antigen-sensitive B cells have antigen-binding immunoglobulin receptors on their plasma membrane. Although no complete inventory of B cells has been made, antigen-binding cells in virgin, unimmunized animals have been regularly found, although the numbers reported are larger than would be anticipated from the considerations noted above, an unresolved problem.

In the primary immune response to an injected antigen most of these antibody-forming cells manufacture IgM antibody which peaks in amount in 7–10 days. These antibody-forming cells are no longer antigen-sensitive, and some differentiate into plasma cells that lack membrane immunoglobulin. A certain number of stimulated antigen-sensitive cells give rise to antigen-sensitive memory cells which, persisting after the death of the original antibody-forming cells, are responsible for the anamnestic response. When antigen again reaches the immunologic system, the large number of memory cells present gives rise to a rapid (less than a week) increase in antibody formation which is mostly IgG. Such IgG antibody is secreted in larger amounts for a longer period of time than during the primary antibody response.

As pointed out earlier, the route of administration of antigen significantly alters the nature of the immune response. Immunization by injection into the skin appears to give a modest repository effect, so that antigen continues to be absorbed over a period of time and there is a longer duration of antigenic stimulus. Intracutaneous injection directs the immune response slightly toward cell-mediated immunity rather than toward humoral antibody responses. Injections into the skin, subcutaneous tissue, or muscles lead to antibody response primarily in the draining lymph nodes, while intravenous or intraperitoneal injections result in the localization of antigen in the spleen and abdominal lymph nodes, thereby stimulating the central immunologic organs, with resulting higher circulating titers of both IgM and IgG antibodies.

Adjuvants can have an important role in regulating the immune response. Insoluble carriers such as alumina, charcoal, calcium alginate, and bentonite probably serve largely to delay absorption of the antigen. Mineral oils of various types are also frequently used to produce a repository antigen effect. Antigen absorption from such depots depends on the quality of the emulsion produced. Since antigen release tends to be delayed and continuous, injection of antigen in such an adjuvant results in a primary response immediately followed by a secondary response. IgG responses are greater than IgM responses. The effects of adjuvant, of course, may be more subtle. Weigle and co-workers (2) demonstrated that injection of autologous thyroglobulin in mineral oil resulted in an intense local inflammatory reaction which partially denatured the thyroglobulin, thereby making it antigenic to an otherwise tolerant animal.

Freund's adjuvant is a mixture of two mineral oils and mycobacteria. The effects of the mycobacteria are not completely understood and certainly exceed repository effects from the mineral oil alone (incomplete Freund's adjuvant). This material has been shown to be extremely potent in stimulating production of both IgG antibody and cell-mediated immunity.

Antisera produced by antigen injection are invariably heterogeneous in terms of antibody class, specificity, and affinity. The immune system is capable of recognizing multiple antigenic determinants with all but the most simple chemical structures. Even simple haptens may expose two or three facets to antigen-sensitive cells. As immunization proceeds either through continued release of antigen from adjuvant depots or continued injection of antigen, there are continual changes in the quality of the antibody produced. Antibody affinity, in particular, tends to gradually increase with time, although there may be dramatic shifts with apparent losses of some clones of antibody-producing cells and their replacement by others.

PRACTICAL ASPECTS OF IMMUNIZATION: The Immunization of Animals in the Production of Antisera for Immunoassays

A number of practical points about immunization can be made. Some of these are logical consequences of the principles just outlined. Others are the product of experience.

Antigens should be as highly purified as possible, but one must beware of the possibility that preparatory steps may cause the denaturation of desired antigenic determinants, appearance of new antigenic determinants, or loss of the antigen itself.

The amounts of antigen used for immunization should not be too great. Amounts on the order of 1 mg protein per 2 to 4-kg rabbit are appropriate.* Much greater amounts of antigen may decrease the affinity of the antibody that is stimulated. In many instances, Freund's adjuvant is selected to accompany the antigen or hapten–carrier conjugate. If antigen is in short supply, as is frequently the case, it is wise to employ an adjuvant, usually Freund's adjuvant. Great care should be taken, however, in preparing and injecting the oily emulsion. The great forces that must be used to emulsify and inject the adjuvant often cause syringe breakage or inadvertent leakage of precious material. The novice will do well to practice these procedures in advance. Blenders can be used to prepare emulsions, but a double-hubbed needle with two glass syringes is a common method of procedure. A stable emulsion should be formed. The material can be examined for stability microscopically, but it is probably sufficient to emulsify it until a small droplet retains its shape when placed on distilled water. Preparing such emulsions is a time-consuming, difficult operation requiring sturdy glassware and appliances. Injections into the animals, too, are best accomplished using glass Luerloc syringes and careful technique. A slip while forcefully making an injection into an animal's skin can result in the injection of Freund's adjuvant into the operator's skin or a spray of emulsion droplets into the eye. This can result in an intense local inflammatory

---

*Even this amount is excessive, and frequently the maximum response may be achieved with as little as 50–100μg (see Chapter 3).

reaction (particularly in the tuberculin-sensitive worker). Accidental injection of laboratory workers with antigens in Freund's adjuvant has resulted in severe but, fortunately, limited allergic illnesses including encephalitis.

Injections of Freund's adjuvant are often made into the skin of animals. The result is an intense inflammatory reaction, usually with ulceration. If appropriate titers of antibodies can be obtained from subcutaneous or intramuscular injection of the animal, these more humane immunization methods are desirable. Immunization into the footpad is often recommended, but this procedure is difficult to perform and is probably uncomfortable for the animal, particularly when caged on wire. If footpad immunization is attempted, the animals should be caged in straw. Readministration of Freund's adjuvant produces a heightened inflammatory response. Consideration should be given to decreasing or omitting the mycobacteria after the first injection.

The heterogeneity of antibody response mentioned previously requires rather frequent evaluations of sera for proper assessment. Two-week intervals may be appropriate during the early phases of immunization. In addition, the animals should be observed for a considerable period of time if appropriate serum has not been obtained, since continued immunization may eventually produce an effective antiserum. Immunization should always begin in a respectably sized group of animals, 6 to 12 rabbits for instance. There is always likely to be a small number of animals who fail to respond to the antigen entirely, and the desired response may be present only in a minority of animals. If a desired antiserum cannot be developed in one species of animal, it is sometimes effective to immunize other species.

Since immune responses are under genetic control, it has been suggested for some time that an appropriate way to deal with weakly immunogenic antigens is to breed animals for immune response. This idea, however, has never been used effectively for the development of sera for immunoassay.

MONOCLONAL ANTIBODIES FROM HYBRIDOMAS

Kohler and Milstein (3) opened up a whole new field of immunologic investigation by their demonstration that mouse antibody-forming cells could be fused with mouse myeloma cells, with subsequent isolation of hybrid clones of antibody-forming cells. In subsequent work, they and others have shown that these clones can be grown as stable cell lines secreting monospecific antibody, since the clone is derived from a single antibody-secreting cell. The availability of these hybrid clones and their monospecific antibody products has stimulated a huge number of investigative efforts. Modifications of the system have included the use of a myeloma that secretes only light chains and does not grow in the selective medium used for the tissue culture, so only the hybrid, fused cells grow. Antibody-forming cells from rats and mice and immunoglobulin-forming cells from human peripheral blood have all been successfully fused with myeloma cells with the aid of Sendai virus or, more recently, polyethylene glycol (4). After fusion, the cells are distributed in multiple-well tissue culture plates. Wells found to contain growing cells are then screened for antibody production. Those making desired antibodies are selected for cloning. Cloning has been done both by dilution in multiple wells or by disbursement in soft agar. After growth and selection of antibody-producing clones, hybrid cell lines can either be grown in tissue culture flasks or implanted in animals to grow as solid or ascites tumors. Monoclonal antibody concentrations on the order of 2 mg/ml can be obtained from in vitro cultures of cell lines. Amounts of monoclonal antibody as great as 40 mg/ml have been obtained from ascitic fluid or peripheral blood of animals bearing solid tumors.

The key to the use of this technique is a convenient, sensitive method for detection of the desired antibody, allowing the selection of cell clones for further culture. Fluorescence-activated cell sorters are one of several innovative approaches being used for this purpose. Cell cultures producing a desired antibody can be frozen with dimethyl sulfoxide and preserved. Continual checks on antibody production by the cultures and its quality are necessary, since there is a tendency for the antibody-secreting clone to mutate.

The availability of large amounts of monoclonal antibody and the associated genetic machinery for producing this antibody have led to some dramatic insights into the structure of the genes responsible for antibody synthesis. There has also been intensive use of this technology to develop specific antibodies to cell surface antigens where difficulties in preparing highly purified antigen have previously necessitated the use of typing antisera containing multiple specificities. The hybridoma technology also appears to offer solutions to a number of problems in preparing antisera for immunoassay, particularly where there is difficulty in preparing purified antigen for immunization. Enthusiastic investigation of this approach is clearly warranted. A possible problem looms in that monoclonal antibodies are likely to have a relatively low affinity despite their extraordinary specificity. It is well known that continued immunization results in increases in antibody affinity. This is thought to be due to the selective effects of antigen, selecting out clones of cells that bind antigen with high affinity, hence manufacture antibody with similar high affinity. Since this selective pressure is no longer effective in an antibody-forming cell clone, to develop high-affinity antibodies it will probably still be necessary to immunize animals until antibody with appropriately high affinity is manufactured and use antibody-forming cells from such animals for hybridoma production.

IMMUNOREGULATION

It has long been known that the dose and route of administration of a stimulating antigen are important in determining the amounts and characteristics of the antibody produced. Optimal quantities of antigen stimulate maximal antibody response. Smaller or much larger amounts of antigen may produce forms of tolerance, hence less antibody. The physical and chemical characteristics of the antigen also contribute to increased antibody formation, as well as exert an influence on the form of the immune response. Not the least of these factors is the importance of genetic constitution. Genetic predispositions to certain types of immune responses take several forms. There are characteristic immune responses in some species; rabbits and horses produce precipitins, whereas guinea pigs express cell-mediated immunity readily. Certain strains of inbred animals have been found to have increased or decreased immune responses to distinct antigens, and there is the familiar human example of variation in sensitivity to environmental antigens. Knowledge of the regulation of the immune responses responsible for these variations has increased strikingly in recent years, so that the mechanisms underlying these variations are now being clarified.

Much of the new information concerns the regulation by T cells of B-cell responses (5). In most instances, B cells produce antibody after stimulation with antigen only with the aid of helper T cells. Antigenic stimulation promotes the development of these helper T cells and other cells, suppressor T cells. The latter tend to inhibit the immune response by their action on T cells or T-cell products. The amount of antibody produced by a stimulated B-cell clone is the result of a balance between these two influences, this balance shifting gradually to suppression within weeks of antigen administration. Immunoregulation is tuned even finer by interaction between T cells. Suppressor T cells are induced from a presuppressor population by helper T cells. Cell replication is necessary for this transformation. Consequently, suppressor T-cell activity is usually inhibitable by antimitotic influences such as ionizing radiation. Excess antigen, too, may promote T-cell suppression by promoting T-cell mitogenesis. Both antigen-specific and nonspecific T-cell help and suppression have been described, and T-cell help and suppression may be immunoglobulin class-specific, too. Both helper and suppressive influences on B cells can be expressed through soluble factors derived from T cells.

In addition to T cells and B cells, a third cell is usually necessary to produce antibody in in vitro systems and presumably also in the animal. The nature of these accessory cells had been uncertain but, as discussed in the section on immunization, it now seems quite clear that they are derived from the monocyte–macrophage family. Monocytes can inhibit as well as promote immunoglobulin production and mitogenesis. In some patients with multiple myeloma, for instance, immunoglobulin production is suppressed by monocytes. A prostaglandin-secreting, glass-adherent, mononuclear suppressor cell inhibits mitogenesis in Hodgkin's disease and normal older people, possibly accounting for decreases in cell-mediated immunity in these groups.

Genetically governed variations in immune response appear to be largely regulated by immune response genes. These genes are located near the major histocompatibility complex, so that immune response genes are frequently linked with histocompatibility types. The effects of immune response genes appear to be manifest only with antigens dependent upon T-cell help (T-dependent antigens). These immune response genes give rise to Ia proteins, distinctive markers found on the surface of B cells and monocytes. Current hypotheses suggest that these proteins act as recognition units promoting cellular interactions. The locus of the cellular interaction has not yet been completely determined, since some studies have suggested that the important interactions are not confined to interactions of T and B cells but that macrophages or monocytes have the primary role in the expression of immune response gene function.

Antibody itself is a most important immunoregulatory factor. Removal of large amounts of antibody by plasmapheresis has the effect of greatly stimulating antibody production, indicating that the presence of antibody in the animal controls antibody synthesis. Jerne's network hypothesis provides a likely explanation for this most sensitive type of immunoregulatory activity. Briefly, the hypothesis states that each antibody has specific antigenicity as a result of its specific structural characteristics. This specific antigenicity is referred to as an *idiotype*. In making a specific antibody to the antigen, the immunized animal produces a new protein with idiotypic characteristics unique for the antibody, hence foreign and antigenic to the immunized animal. In consequence, antibodies to the idiotype are also manufactured. These anti-antibodies, in turn, have unique idiotypic determinants stimulating production of yet another antibody with yet another idiotype in this network of regulatory antibodies. The effects of the anti-idiotypic antibodies presumably are mediated through their effects on the membrane immunoglobulins of the clones of B cells making the antibodies of the network, since B cells express their unique antibody in their membrane immunoglobulin. The potentialities for exquisite control, both by facilitation and suppression of immune responses, through variations in the activities of the components of the network are easily understood.

Some confirmation of the theory now exists, since anti-idiotypic antibodies that influence both antibody synthesis and cell-mediated immunity have been detected (6).

Immunization sets in motion a fascinating series of cellular events. The immune response and its control have been briefly reviewed with emphasis on the phenomena of importance to immunoassay work.

REFERENCES

1. Cambier JC, Ligler, FS, Uher JW, et al: Blocking of primary in vitro antibody responses to thymus-independent and thymus-dependent antigens with antiserum specific for IgM and IgD. *Proc Natl Acad Sci USA* 75:432, 1978.
2. Weigle WO, High GJ, Nakamura RM: The role of mycobacteria and the effect of proteolytic degradation of thyroglobulin on the production of autoimmune thyroiditis, *J Exp Med* 130:243, 1969.
3. Kohler G, Milstein C: Continuous cultures of fused cells secreting antibody of predefined specificity, *Nature* 256:495, 1975.
4. Melchers F, Potter M, Warner N (eds): *Lymphocyte Hybridomas.* Berlin, Springer-Verlag, 1979.
5. Cantor H, Gershon RK: Immunological circuits: cellular composition, *Fed Proc* 38:55, 1979.
6. Sy M-S, Moorhead JW. Claman, HW: Regulation of cell mediated immunity by antibodies: possible role of anti-receptor antibodies in the regulation of contact sensitivity to DNFB in mice, *J Immunol* 123:2593, 1979.

READING LIST

Roitt IM: *Essential Immunology,* ed 3. Oxford, Blackwell Scientific Publications, 1977.
Weir DM: *Handbook of Experimental Immunology,* ed 3. (3 volumes). Edinburgh, Blackwell Scientific Publications, 1978.

CHAPTER 3
ANTIBODY PRODUCTION FOR IMMUNOASSAY

Paul Franchimont
Jean-Claude Hendrick
Aimée-Marguerite Reuter

Antibodies are one of the constituents of the immunologic reaction basic to immunoassays in general and to radioimmunoassays in particular. In their production, the aim should be to obtain an amount sufficient for many years and that can be used for the assay of hundreds of thousands of samples by as large a number of investigators as possible in order to achieve uniformity of results. Antisera for immunoassay should have two characteristics: high affinity and defined specificity.

Antibody affinity for the antigens used to raise them determines assay sensitivity (1). The higher the affinity, the better the sensitivity, and a high degree of sensitivity is essential for the measurement of antigens such as ACTH, ρ-endorphin, calcitonin, and vasopressin whose concentrations in biologic fluids are very low. Antibodies against these hormones must therefore be of high affinity. On the other hand, the measurement of antigens whose concentration in biologic fluids is greater, such as human placental lactogen (HPL) and human chorionic gonadotrophin (HCG), can be achieved with antibodies of lower affinity (2).

Antibodies must also be specific, that is, react only with the antigen to be measured. Such specificity implies that the antiserum contains no antibodies against antigenic contaminants in the immunogen. Further, they should be directed against a specific antigenic sequence in the immunogen that is not present in the structure of any other molecule. If the antibody is directed against an antigenic group that is common to different immunogens, cross-reaction with these substances is possible.*

In certain cases, antiserum specificity is incomplete. This is the case for steroids with similar structures, for example, testosterone and dihydrotestosterone, and for peptides that differ by only one amino acid, for example, methionine-enkephalin and leucine-enkephalin. This is also the case

---

*Depending in large part on the quality of the label for protein assays.

when one substance is a complete portion of another molecule that is frequently its precursor, for example, β-endorphin in relation to β-lipotrophin. Under these circumstances, methods for separating these related substances are necessary.

It is also useful to determine against which of the antigenic determinants the antibodies are directed. This knowledge allows one to interpret the results obtained with the assay method. Thus, depending on the sequence against which they are directed, the antibodies can be used to measure either only the native molecule or the native molecule as well as its metabolic fragments with a longer biologic half-life. This is the case with parathormone (PTH). Antibodies directed against the N-terminal portion of the intact molecule and/or the 1–33 fragment, which has a half-life of less than 3 minutes, may be compared with antibodies against the C-terminal portion that measure the intact hormone but also the 34–84 C-terminal fragment and its cleavage products, which have a half-life of about 3 hours (3).

ANTIBODY PRODUCTION

Antibodies may be produced either in vivo by active immunization of animals or in vitro using the hybridization technique and selecting the secretory clones.

ACTIVE IMMUNIZATION IN VIVO

It is difficult to formulate general rules for immunization, as there are problems particular to each antigen in obtaining specific antibodies in sufficient quantities. Furthermore, the production of a good antibody in an animal appears to be more a result of chance than of the use of particular immunization schedule. However, we shall attempt to describe certain factors that enhance and affect the animal's immunologic activity.

The Animals
A number of animals have been used for antibody production: rabbits, guinea pigs, goats, sheep, and horses. The choice has been influenced more by practical considerations, such as the availability of accommodations in the animal house and the amount of antiserum required, rather than by a scientific approach. Usually, species of animals are used that do not possess antigens identical to the immunogen. This is the situation for a number of polypeptide hormones (growth hormone, prolactin, gonadotrophins, calcitonin) that have immunologic species specificity.

The use of inbred animals may sometimes be helpful and at other times inhibitory. As immunologic responsiveness is determined genetically, probably by genes transmitted as Mendelian dominants, it is best to use random-bred animals unless a given strain is known to respond to a given antigen. The potential of an animal for producing antibodies against an immunogen is individual and unpredictable. Immunization should therefore be undertaken in several animals simultaneously. The choice of a good antibody producer should be made during the immunization schedule by regular assessments of the antibody titer and specificity. When one or more animals produce satisfactory antibodies, great care must be taken of them, repeated blood samples taken, and booster injections given.

Antigens and Immunogens

It is generally agreed that proteins and polypeptides of molecular weight greater than 10,000 are good immunogens and produce a good antibody response. On the other hand, small peptides of molecular weight equal to or less than 5,000 are weak immunogens that give rise to antibodies with difficulty. The immunogenicity of these small peptides is increased by their physical or chemical linkage to carriers: inert particles (charcoal), synthetic macromolecules (poly-L-lysine), naturally occurring proteins (egg albumin, thyroglobulin). These small peptides then behave as haptens (see Chapter 4).

It should, however, be pointed out that antisera of excellent quality have been obtained by using nonconjugated antigens with a molecular weight less than 5,000: ACTH (MW $\sim$ 4,500), glucagon (MW $\sim$ 3,500), calcitonin (MW $\sim$ 3,200), gastrin (MW $\sim$ 2,100), β-endorphin (MW $\sim$ 3,465), luteinizing hormone-releasing hormone (LH-RH) (MW 1,148), and vasopressin (MW 1,100).

A pure immunogen allows one to obtain an antiserum containing antibodies directed only against itself. However, the purity of the immunogen is not essential in obtaining an antiserum useful for radioimmunoassay. Radioimmunoassay specificity is determined above all by the purity of the tracer and not by the monospecificity of the antiserum (5).

Apart from the lower cost of immunization with semipurified preparations, it appears that the latter are often better immunogens than antigens in their pure state, as if the contaminants had an adjuvant role.

The amount of immunogen that must be injected varies from one antigen to another. The experiments of Odell et al. (2) have shown that antibody titer rises with the amount of immunogen used. On the other hand, the phenomenon of tolerance is rarely seen.

The Adjuvants

Soluble antigens such as peptide hormones are rapidly absorbed from the injection site, diluted in the circulation, and metabolized. Furthermore, such rapid absorption may lead to the expression of unfortunate biologic properties in the animal used for immunization when the antigen has such characteristics, as in the case of hormones such as insulin and PTH. Adjuvants ensure that the absorption of the antigen will be very slow over several days or weeks.

Freund (6) introduced emulsions of water in mineral oil and showed them to be efficient for antigens incorporated in the dispersed (water) phase. A single injection of the water-in-oil emulsion stimulates a long-lasting antibody response. A simple water-in-oil emulsion is called *incomplete Freund's adjuvant*. The adjuvant is complete when dried, and heat-killed *Mycobacterium tuberculosis* is added to the medium.

The use of adjuvants also has a marked effect on the immunologic reaction. They stimulate and facilitate antigen phagocytosis and macrophages and then pass their information on to the immunocompetent cells that produce antibodies (antigen uptake, antigen processing, and presentation of processed antigen). Further, they give rise to the formation of granulomata which become veritable furnaces of antibody formation. Last, the mycobacteria in the adjuvant have a major role in stimulating cell-mediated immunity. The main disadvantage of the use of adjuvants is the extensive granuloma and abcess formation at the inoculation site.

Injection using the intradermal and the subcutaneous routes (see following paragraph) also contributes to slow absorption, thus allowing the antigen access to lymph nodes.

An important aspect of the problem is antigen stability. A stable antigen is one that can be stored at 37°C for long periods without losing its antigenic character. Labile antigens are rapidly denatured at 37°C by chemical, physical, or enzymatic damage. Some of these materials may remain active long enough after incorporation in complete Freund's adjuvant to stimulate an adequate immune response. In these circumstances, it appears better to incorporate the freeze-dried antigen into an oil emulsifier mixture. This material is ground up with oil in a mortar and administered to rabbits by the subcutaneous route. Booster injections are given in saline intravenously.

Routes of Inoculation

Whereas the immune response is a systemic reaction, the route of injection of the antigen is of importance as it affects the degree of persistence of the antigen at the site of injection, its absorption from the resulting granuloma, and its speedy and easy access to histocytic structures such as the lymph nodes and the spleen.

Intradermal and subcutaneous injections allow rapid access of the antigen to the draining lymph nodes. At this level, absorption of antigen mixed with Freund's adjuvant is slower, permitting the use of small quantities of diluted antigens in small volumes, thus conserving antigens that are difficult to obtain. The use of complete Freund's adjuvant often leads to abcess formation and, when this drains, to loss of part of the injected immunogen. The subcutaneous route is usually used for booster injections, as it minimizes the risk of anaphylactic shock.

Intramuscular injection also allows rapid access of the antigen to the circulation and lymph nodes, but the persistence of the antigen is shorter than for the two routes of injection described above. It is recommended when complete Freund's adjuvant is used and when it is desirable to avoid abcess formation.

The intravenous route is rarely used. The antigen is then taken up by histiocytic cells of the spleen and the lungs. Sometimes this route is used for booster injections, but there is always a risk of anaphylactic shock.

In the mouse, intraperitoneal injections are usually given. The antigens are drained into the mesenteric nodes.

Some investigators have used intra-articular injections or direct injections into lymph nodes and into the footpad. None of these modalities leads to immunization superior to that achieved with intradermal and subcutaneous injections. In fact, they are technically more difficult to carry out and lead to great distress for the animal (see review by Herbert [7]).

Immunization Schedule

The time intervals between the first injection and boosters, and the amount of immunogen used, vary considerably from one report to another. However, all investigators agree on the following principles:

1. Primary responses: The first injection should be given by the intradermal, subcutaneous, or intramuscular route, the antigen having been emulsified in an adjuvant.

2. The immunologic response is relatively independent of the amount of antigen used for immunization once a threshold quantity has been reached. With the use of adjuvant, a satisfactory response can often be obtained with a primary dose of 100 μg or less of a polypeptide antigen of molecular weight greater than 15,000 and booster injections of half the primary dose.

3. Booster injections: When a depot-forming adjuvant has been employed, the best results from a booster dose are obtained if it is given after the primary response has had time to reach a plateau. In rabbits, antibodies appear 7–8 days after the primary injection of an immunogen emulsified in Freund's adjuvant and reach their maximum about 6 weeks later. There is thus no point in repeating injections weekly if Freund's adjuvant has been used. On the contrary, no booster doses should be given earlier than 4 weeks after the first injection and no more frequently than once each month thereafter. The antibody titer rises to a maximum 10 days after the booster injections, so that bleeding should be undertaken 7–10 days (8).

4. Highly specific antibodies are produced by short immunization programs, and the production of antibodies against trace quantities of unwanted antigens in the immunogen is minimized. A schedule of immunization that is too long can lead to the induction of nonspecific
   antibodies against contaminants in the antigen (9).

An immunization method was described by Vaitukaitis et al. (10) that
leads to the production of high-titer antibodies following the injection of
very small quantities of immunogen: 20–100 μg. This method is very useful when one has a very small quantity of material.

Equal volumes of complete Freund's adjuvant (1 ml) and of a saline solution of the immunogen (1 ml) are carefully emulsified. The fur is shaved
from the back and proximal portion of the limbs of rabbits, and the emulsion (2 ml) is injected intradermally at 35 to 50 sites. At a separate site, 0.5
ml of crude *Bordetella pertussis* vaccine is injected intradermally. A single
immunization with 20 μg of the α subunit of HCG and 50 μg of the
β subunit was sufficient to produce an antiserum with a maximum titer
80–90 days after immunization. In certain circumstances, a booster injection was necessary: 20 μg of immunogen emulsified in incomplete
Freund's adjuvant.

PRODUCTION OF MONOCLONAL ANTIBODIES

Kohler and Milstein (11) showed that it was possible to produce a single
antibody molecule in a cultured cell line obtained by hybridization of nonse-
cretory myeloma cells with lymphoid cells from a hyperimmunized individual.

The steps in this method consist of hyperimmunization of the animals,
fusion techniques and isolation of cultures, screening of the culture product, and selection of stable clones secreting the desired antibody in sufficient quantities (12).

There are already on the market several dozen monoclonal antibodies
such as anti-prostatic alkaline phosphatase, anti-carcinoembryonic antigen=
CEA, and anti-α-fetoprotein.

ANTIBODY ASSESSMENT

Antibodies should be characterized by their concentration, affinity, specificity, and the antigenic group against which they are directed. Let us ex-
amine these characteristics.

DEFINITION OF THE TITER

The presence of antibody in a biologic fluid and in an antiserum can be established by its reaction with labeled antigen. The amount of antibody present is often defined by the titration curve established when the same quantity of labeled antigen is incubated with progressively increasing dilutions of antiserum. The titer is usually defined as the final dilution of antiserum in the incubation medium that allows the binding of a sufficient quantity of labeled antigen in the absence of unlabeled antigen and ensures optimal sensitivity and precision. This level of binding varies from 30 to 60% depending on the assay. In all cases, there must be an excess of labeled antigen in relation to antibody. As a result, unlabeled antigen (to be quanti-

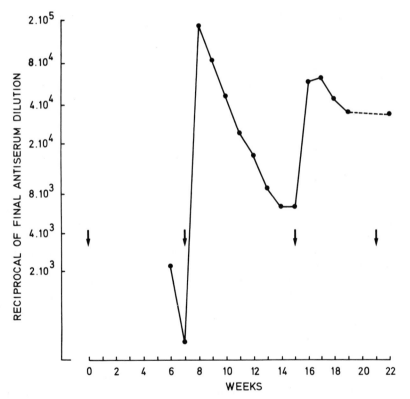

Figure 1. Immunization schedule with human prolactin. Abscissa: time after the first prolactin injection. Ordinate: the highest dilution of antiserum still able to bind 30% of labeled hormone. The arrows indicate the days of injections and boosters. The first multisite intradermal injection was made with 50 μg of human prolactin in complete Freund's adjuvant, and 0.5 ml of *Bordetella pertussis* vaccine was injected intramuscularly at the same time. Booster injections were made with the same amount of prolactin emulsified in incomplete Freund's adjuvant.

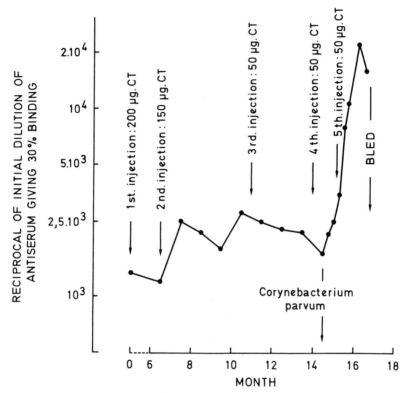

Figure 2. Development of anti-human calcitonin during immunization. Abscissa: months after the primary injection. Ordinate: the highest dilution of antiserum still able to bind 30% of labeled hormone. Antibody titer did not increase from the beginning of immunization to the fourteenth month despite the three booster injections. One week after the last booster, 4 mg of *Corynebacterium parvum* preparation (Merieux Institute, Lyon, France) was injected by the intramuscular route. This bacterial preparation is known to stimulate macrophage and B-lymphocyte functions. A final booster injection of 50 μg of calcitonin was given 1 month later (the fifteenth month). These last two treatments lead to a marked increase in the antibody titer of the antiserum.

fied) effectively competes with labeled antigen* for binding. Two examples illustrate the development of antibody titers obtained by the method of Vaitukaitis et al. (10), on the one hand, against human prolactin (Fig. 1) (13) and, on the other hand, against synthetic human calcitonin (Fig. 2) (14). Optimal binding of labeled antigen to antibody was established in both cases at 30%.

*Antigen-antibody interactions are described by the Mass Action equation. Therefore, even with labeled antigen in excess, free antibody is never zero. With high affinity antibodies under such conditions, however, free antibody concentrations become very small.

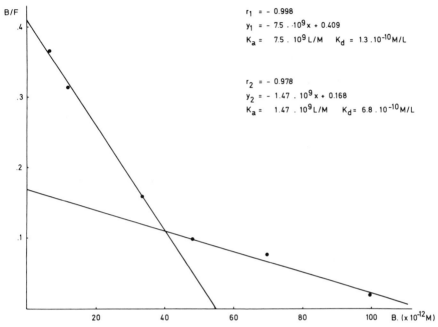

Figure 3. Affinity of antibody for β-endorphin is calculated using Scatchard analysis. There are two populations of antibodies with $K_d = 6.8 \times 10^{-10}$ mole/liter and 1.3×10^{-10} mole liter, respectively.

AFFINITY

A discussion of antibody affinity can be found in Chapter 8. We note, however, that a standard curve allows estimation of the equilibrium constant (K) by means of a Scatchard plot (15–17). The ratio of antibody bound to free antigen is plotted against the concentration of bound antigen expressed in moles per liter. A linear relationship is found if there is only a single order of combining sites (i.e., the antibody population is homogeneous with respect to its equilibrium constant). The affinity is then given by the slope of this line, and the binding capacity of antibody by its intercept on the abscissa. An example of this calculation of affinity and binding capacity of antibody is given in Figure 3 for an antiserum against human β-endorphin.

As sensitivity is a function of affinity (1), one can in practice determine whether an antiserum has sufficient sensitivity by using several dilutions. A simple preliminary procedure is to set up duplicate titration curves with and without the addition of a small, constant amount of unlabeled antigen. Antisera with high sensitivity are identified by a wide separation between the two curves (8).

ANTIBODY SPECIFICITY

In this paragraph, we discuss only the specific interference existing at the level of the antigen–antibody reaction, since nonspecific interference (pH, ionic concentrations, effects of serum proteins) is discussed in Chapter 8.

Two situations may occur: The antiserum may contain antibodies directed against contaminants or the antibody may be directed against antigenic groups shared by different molecules.

Antibodies Directed against Contaminants

In principle, antibodies directed against contaminants do not interfere in the radioimmunoassay if the tracer is reasonably pure. The purity of the labeled hormone is an absolute necessity to ensure the specificity of the immunologic reaction, since the technique is based on changes in radioactivity bound to antibody. The existence of significant quantities of labeled contaminants can mask changes in the binding of the labeled hormone itself to the antibody. Furthermore, if the antiserum contains nonspecific

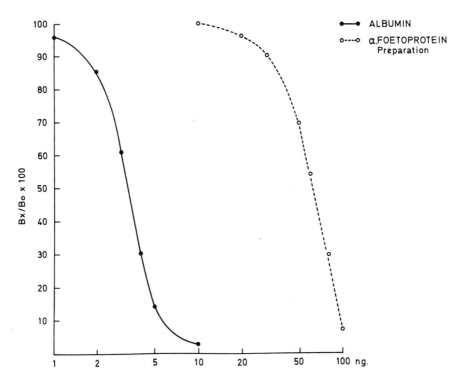

Figure 4. Inhibition curves of the labeled albumin–anti-albumin antibody reaction obtained with pure human albumin and with a preparation of α-fetoprotein. The immunoreactivity of the α-fetoprotein preparation is about 20 times less than that of the albumin preparation.

antibodies against these contaminants, the relationship between free radio-activity and radioactivity bound to γ-globulin can be altered in the absence of any effect of the hormone to be measured.

Thus, the contaminants against which the antibodies are directed must be established and neutralized. Such a situation is found in the assay of α-fetoprotein which is usually contaminated with albumin. Anti-σ-fetoprotein antisera contain antibodies against α-fetoprotein and against albumin, as shown by the binding of labeled albumin by the anti-α-fetoprotein antisera and the cross-reaction of α-fetoprotein in the radioimmunoassay of albumin (18). Under the latter circumstances, the inhibition curves for the reaction of labeled albumin with antialbumin produced by unlabeled albumin and α-fetoprotein are parallel, proving that there is identical affinity of the antibodies for the antigen present in both preparations. However, the immunoreactivity of the α-fetoprotein preparation is 20-fold less than that of lactalbumin. It can therefore be calculated that the α-fetoprotein preparation is contaminated by 5% albumin (Fig. 4). The antialbumin antibodies can be neutralized with albumin (20) or removed by affinity chromatography.

Cross-reactivity

In these circumstances, the antibodies are directed against an antigenic grouping common to different substances. This is the case for hormones and their precursors. Thus, antibodies against β-endorphin always react with its precursor β-lipotrophin, a molecule with 91 amino acids. β-endorphin is the 61–91 sequence of β-lipotrophin.

Likewise, the glycoprotein hormones [follicle stimulating hormone (FSH), luteinizing hormone, (LH), thyroid stimulating hormone (TSH), and human chorionic gonadotrophin (HCG)] have common antigenic groupings. Each of these glycoprotein hormones is made up of two subunits termed α and β (21). The α subunit is immunologically identical for all four hormones in the same animal species. In contrast, the β subunits that determine the biologic activity are hormone-specific and do not appear to be species-specific (22). There is, however, incomplete cross-reactivity between the LH and β subunits (19). The presence of the common α subunit makes it difficult to obtain antisera specific to any single one of the hormones. Thus, to prepare an antiserum directed specifically against one glycoprotein hormone or another, the following experimental methods may be used (20).

Selection of Antiserum.   As already mentioned, virtually all anti-HCG sera cross-react with LH. However, of 43 anti-HCG sera tested in our laboratory only 1 was found to be directed specifically against HCG. Thus, unlabeled LH, FSH, and TSH in doses up to 200 ng failed to decrease the percentage of HCG* bound to this antibody (Fig. 5).

*HCG indicates radioiodinated HCG (label).

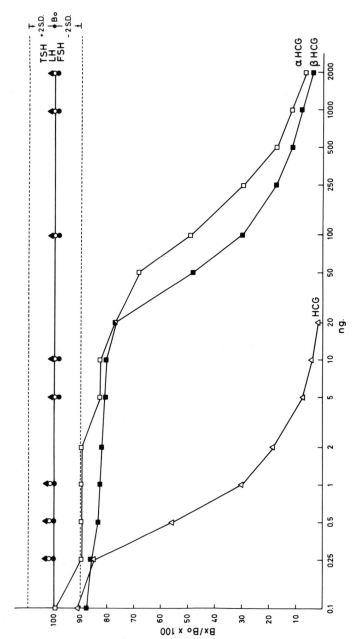

Figure 5. Absence of cross-reaction of FSH, LH, and TSH in HCG radioimmunoassay (labeled HCG and specific anti-native HCG serum). Weak cross-reaction of α and β subunits with native HCG immunoassays.

This particular antibody is not directed specifically against the HCG β subunit, and the immunoreactivity of the α and β subunits is 100 and 200 times less, respectively, than that of the native HCG molecule (Fig. 5). The reactivity of these preparations of α and β subunits could be due to contamination with native HCG. In this case, the antibodies are directed against an antigenic grouping peculiar to the tertiary structure of the HCG molecule, permitting the specific assay of HCG (19).

Neutralization. Antisera obtained after immunization with FSH, LH, and TSH usually contain two populations of antibodies. The first reacts nonspecifically with all the glycoprotein hormones and is undoubtedly directed against the antigenic groupings of the α subunit. This effect can be neutralized by incubation with HCG which contains the same σ subunit but differs in its β subunit (Figs. 6 and 7). The second population is directed specifically against the individual hormone.

Use of Anti-β-subunit Serum. An alternative to the method of neutralizing nonspecific antisera with cross-reactive hormone is the use of an anti-β-subunit serum, as the β subunit differentiates the four glycoprotein hormones from each other. For assay of the native hormone, the latter must be used as tracer and standard.

These antisera may, however, incompletely recognize the antigenic groups of the subunit when associated with α subunit in the native glycoprotein hormone. As a result, the amount of native hormone present in a biologic fluid may be underestimated.

Use of Heterologous Radioimmunoassay Systems. A heterologous radioimmunoassay system may be defined as one in which the antibodies are directed against the hormone of one animal species and the labeled antigen (tracer) is the same hormone but derived from another species (23). The reference preparation may be of the same origin as the tracer but can also be derived from a third animal species. Such heterologous systems have been used under various circumstances (see review of Franchimont et al., [20]). The study of glycoprotein subunits has shown that the immunologic behavior of the common α subunit of the glycoprotein hormones of one species of animal is completely different from that of another. Thus, in the radioimmunoassay system HCG α subunit–anti-HCG α subunit the α subunits of porcine TSH and LH show no interference, nor do native TSH, FSH, and LH from species other than humans (20). Likewise, Pierce et al. (24) showed by means of immunoelectrophoresis that the α subunit of human TSH did not react with the anti-porcine α-subunit serum. It thus seems that there is an absolute species specificity between the α subunit of the glycoproteins of humans and those of other animal species, though the α subunits of various ruminant species are very similar, if not identical (25). On the other hand, the β subunits of the same glycoprotein hormone of different animal species appear to have common antigenic determinants

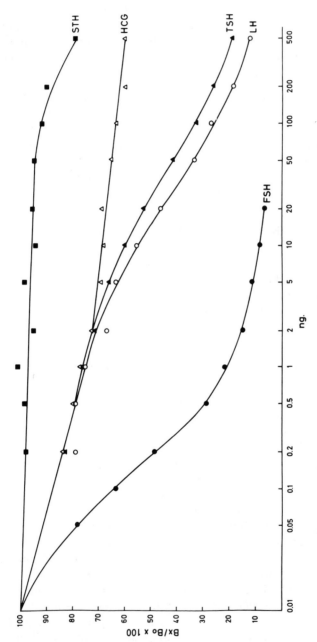

Figure 6. Inhibition curve obtained with labeled FSH and anti-FSH antiserum diluted 2.5×10^{-4} before neutralization. GH does not cross-react. HCG displays an incomplete cross-reaction, whereas TSH and LH completely cross-react with FSH but the slope of the inhibition curve for FSH is steeper than those of TSH and LH. $B_0 = 38\%$ of total radioactivity.

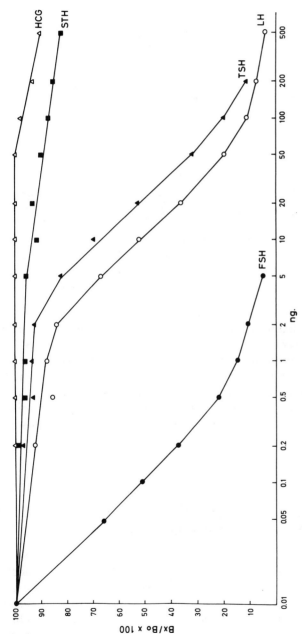

Figure 7. Inhibition curve obtained with labeled FSH and anti-FSH serum after neutralization with HCG. Antiserum dilution 1×10^{-4}. $B_0 = 39\%$ of total radioactivity. Growth hormone and HCG do not cross-react. LH and TSH completely cross-react, and inhibition curves for FSH, TSH, and LH are parallel. FSH is 100 and 200 times more immunoreactive than LH and TSH, respectively. Thus, the effect of these preparations appears to be due to their FSH contamination being 1 and 0.5%, respectively.

47

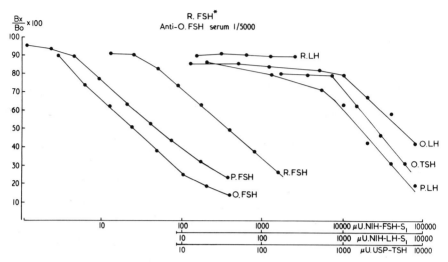

Figure 8. Example of heterologous radioimmunoassay for FSH: Inhibition of the binding of labeled rat FSH to antibody against ovine FSH with ovine (O), porcine (P), rat (R) FSH, LH, and TSH.

(22, 25). Thus, with heterologous systems, particularly when the materials come from human species and are very different [e.g., human TSH and anti-porcine TSH serum (26), human or rat FSH and anti-ovine FSH serum (27)], the immunologic reaction is concerned with the antigenic groupings of the β subunit. As this subunit is specific for each glycoprotein hormone, the reaction is thus highly specific for each of these hormones in different animal species. An example of a heterologous system is illustrated in Figure 8.

DETERMINATION OF THE ANTIGENIC SITE
AGAINST WHICH THE ANTIBODY IS DIRECTED

The determination of the antigenic grouping is important in the interpretation of the results given by radioimmunoassay methods. An antigenic grouping may appear or disappear during the hormone's passage through the kidney. Also, the immunoreactivity of the same hormone may change depending on whether it is present in urine or in blood. This is the case for the gonadotrophins. It appears that the pituitary FSH molecule has a num-

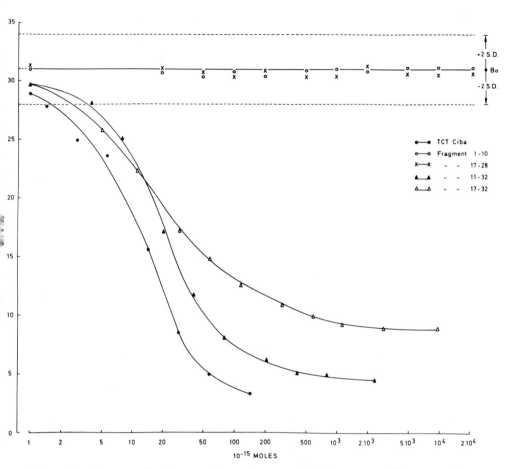

Figure 9. Cross-reaction between the various synthetic fragments of human calci-tonin (final dilution of antiserum 4.5×10^{-4}). Fragments 1–10 and 17–28 up to a concentration of 10^{-11} M showed no cross-reaction. On the other hand, fragments 11–32 completely inhibited the binding of labeled 1–32 CT. The molar ratio of immunoreactivity of fragment 11–32 as compared with the intact 1–32 hormone was 2.1 at 20% inhibition and 3.1 at 50% inhibition. Fragment 17–32 caused incom-plete displacement of labeled 1–32 antibody. The complete cross-reactivity of the 11–32 fragment, lack of immunoreactivity of the 17–28 fragment, and the incom-plete cross-reaction of the 17–32 fragment means that two types of antibodies exist: the first directed against the 11–16 fragment and the second directed against the 29–32 fragment.

ber of antigenic determinants, one or more of which may be lost during its conversion to urinary FSH (28). In addition, in the course of being metabolized, the tertiary structure of the molecule may become altered so that certain antigenic sites that were hidden on the pituitary molecule become exposed and are thus capable of inducing antibody formation. We have prepared anti-urinary FSH serum which contains antibody directed specifically against the antigenic determinants of urinary FSH and which is incapable of reacting with pituitary FSH (29). On the other hand, the antibodies may be directed against part of the molecule, leading to recognition of the native hormone and its metabolic fragments which may have a longer half-life than the intact hormone. This is the case for PTH. Intact PTH is rapidly eliminated from the circulation and cleaved enzymatically in the cells of kidney and bone into fragments 1–33 and 34–84. The 1–33 fragment may not reenter the circulation and has a very short half-life, on the order of 5 minutes. In contrast, the clearance of the C-terminal fragment is much slower, and it thus has a much longer half-life (30), on the order of 3 hours.

Thus anti-C-terminal antisera (34–84) and anti-N-terminal antisera (1–34) provide different results and have different uses. In view of the respective half-lives of the two fragments, PTH levels are much lower when measured using an anti-N-terminal antiserum than when using an anti-C-terminal antiserum which mainly assays fragments of PTH in the circulation.

Furthermore, knowledge of the molecular sites against which the populations of antibodies are directed is useful. Immunochemical studies of this kind have been pursued particularly for peptide hormones of lower molecular weight, fragments of which have been synthesized: PTH, calcitonin, β-lipotrophin, ACTH, bradykinin, vasopressin, LH-RH, etc.

The simplest and most reliable method is to set up standard curves with a variety of synthetic unlabeled fragments. In general, fragments containing a group identical to the antigenic determinant in the intact hormone give complete inhibition of the reaction between labeled intact hormone and antibody when there is a single population of antibody. The inhibition of

Figure 10. Immunoreactivity of anticalcitonin antiserum pretreated with the fragment 17–32. Under these conditions, the binding of labeled CT to the antibody fell considerably. Before neutralization 31% of labeled CT was bound to antibody at 4.5 $\times 10^{-4}$, whereas after neutralization the same amount of labeled CT showed 23% binding to antiserum diluted 1.5 $\times 10^{-4}$. Labeled 1–32 CT was really not further displaced from the antibody by the 17–32 fragment but was completely displaced by the 11–32 fragment. The steric configuration of the native 1–32 hormone nevertheless affected the immunoreactivity for antibiotics directed against the 11–16 fragment, as the slopes of the inhibition curves were different for 1–32 and the 11–32 fragments, the first being steeper than the second.

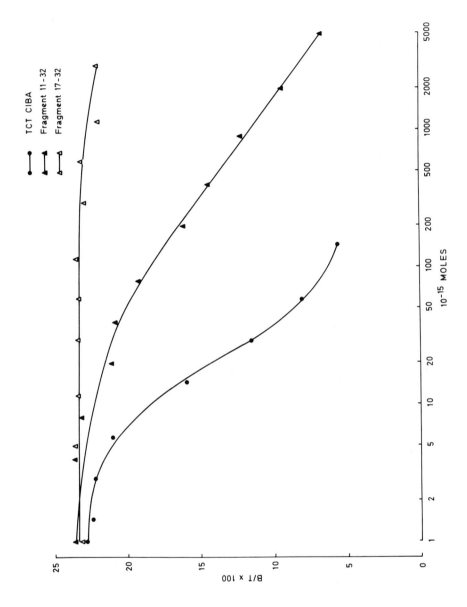

TCT CIBA
Fragment 11-32
Fragment 17-32

10⁻¹⁵ MOLES

B/T x 100

51

binding is parallel when the affinity of the antibody for the fragment is similar to that for the native hormone. The inhibition curves are nonparallel when the affinity differs. When there are two or more populations of antibody, the cross-reaction will be complete if the fragment contains all the antigenic determinants that generated the antibody populations. If the fragment contains only some of these antigenic determinants, the cross-reaction will be incomplete; that is, the fragment will not be capable of inhibiting completely the binding of labeled intact hormone to the antibody. This discussion of antigenic determinants is illustrated in the case of calcitonin in Figures 9 and 10.

REFERENCES

1. Berson SA, Yalow RS: Measurement of hormones—Radioimmunoassay, in Berson SA, Yalow RS (eds): *Methods in Investigative and Diagnostic Endocrinology.* New York, American Elsevier, 1973, p 84.

2. Odell WD, Abraham GA, Skawsky WR, et al: Production of antisera for radioimmunoassays, in Odell WD, Daughaday WH (eds): *Principles of Competitive Protein-Binding Assays.* Philadelphia, J.B. Lippincott, 1971, p 57.

3. Segre GV, Niall HD, Habener JF, et al: Metabolism of parathyroid hormone: Physiologic and clinical significance, in Proceedings of the 3rd Memorial Symposium on Parathyroid Hormone, Calcitonin and Vitamin D: Clinical Considerations. *Amer J Med* 32, 1974.

4. Green I, Paul WE, Benacerraf B: Genetic control of immunological responsiveness in guinea-pigs to 2,4-dinitrophenyl conjugates of poly-*l*-arginine, protamine and poly-*l*-ornithinic. *Proc Natl Acad Sci* 64:1095, 1969.

5. Yalow RS, Berson SA: Problems of validation of radioimmunoassays, in Odell WD, Daughaday WH (eds): *Principles of Competitive Protein-Binding Assays.* Philadelphia, J.B. Lippincott, 1971, p 374.

6. Freund J: The effect of paraffin oil and mycobacteria on antibody formation and sensitization. *Am J Clin Pathol* 21:645, 1951.

7. Herbert WJ: Mineral-oil adjuvants and the immunization of laboratory animals, in Weir E (ed): *Handbook of Experimental Immunology.* London, Blackwell Scientific Publications, 1978, pp A3.1–A3.15.

8. Hurn BAL, Landon J: Antisera for radioimmunoassay, in Kirkham KE, Hunter WM (eds): *Radioimmunoassay Methods.* Edinburgh, Churchill Livingstone, 1971.

9. Odell WD, Abraham G, Raud HR, et al: Influence of immunization procedures on the titer, affinity and specificity of antisera to glycopolypeptides. Proceedings of the Karolinska Symposia on Research Methods in Reproductive Endocrinology, in Diczfaluzy E (ed): *Immunoassay of Gonadotrophins. Acta Endocr* (Suppl. 142) 54, 1969.

10. Vaitukaitis J, Robbins JB, Nieschlag E, et al: A method for producing specific antisera with small doses of immunogen. *J Clin Endocr* 33:988, 1971.

11. Kohler G, Milstein C: Continuous culture of fused cells secreting antibody of pre-defined specificity. *Nature* 256:495, 1975.

12. Melchers F, Potter M, Warner N: Lymphocyte hybridomas, in *Proceedings of the Workshop on Functional Properties of Tumours of T and B Lymphocytes, Bethesda*. Berlin, Heidelberg, Springer Verlag, 1978, p 246.

13. Reuter AM, Kennes F, Gevaert Y, et al: Homologous radioimmunoassay for human prolactin. *Int J Nucl Med Biol* 3:21, 1976.

14. Reuter A, Vrindts-Gevaert Y, Pirlot D, et al: Radioimmunoassay of human calcitonin and its clinical applications, 1980 (in press).

15. Scatchard G: The attraction of proteins for small molecules and ions. *Ann NY Acad Sci* 51:660, 1949.

16. Yalow RS, Berson SA: Immunoassay of endogenous plasma insulin in man. *J Clin Invest* 39:1157, 1960.

17. Ekins RP, Newman GB, and O'Riordan JLH: Theoretical aspects of saturation and radioimmunoassay, in Hayes RL et al (eds): *Radioisotopes in Medicine: "in vitro" Studies*. Oak Ridge, Tenn, USAEC, 1968, p 59.

18. Franchimont P, Zangerle PF, Debruche ML, et al: Dosage radioimmunologique de l'alpha foeto protéine dans les différentes conditions normales et pathologiques. *Ann Biol Clin (Paris)* 33:139, 1975.

19. Franchimont P: A study of the cross reaction between human chorionic and pituitary luteinizing hormones (HCG and HLH). *Eur J Clin Invest* 1:65, 1970.

20. Franchimont P, Hendrick JC, Reuter AM, et al: Radioimmunoassays of glycoprotein hormones, in: *Radioimmunoassay and Related Procedures in Medicine*. Vol. 1. Vienna, International Atomic Energy Agency, 1974, p 195.

21. De La Llosa P, Courte C, Jutisz M: On the mechanism of reversible inactivation of LH by urea. *Biochem Biophys Res Commun* 26:411, 1967.

22. Pierce JG, Liao TH, Cornell JS, et al: Thyrotropin and its subunits, in Margoulies M, Greenwood FC, (eds): *Protein and Polypeptide Hormones*. Amsterdam, Excerpta Medica Foundation, ICS 241, 1971, p 91.

23. Midgley AR: Heterologous and homologous radioimmunoassays: Species specificity considerations, in Odell WD, Daughaday WH (eds): *Principles of Competitive Protein-Binding assays*. Philadelphia, J.B. Lippincott, 1971, p 419.

24. Pierce JG, Bahl OP, Cornwell JS, et al: Biologically active hormones prepared by recombination of the α chain, of human chorionic gonadotropins and the hormone specific chain of bovine thyrotropin or of bovine luteinizing hormone. *J Biol Chem* 246:2321, 1971.

25. Ketelslegers JM, Hennen G, Franchimont P: Immunological behavior of LH subunits from different species, in Margoulies M, Greenwood FC (eds): *Protein and Polypeptide Hormones*. Amsterdam, Excerpta Medica, 241:148, 1971.

26. Ketelslegers JM, Franchimont P: TSH radioimmunoassay, in Marois M (ed): *Frontiers of Hormone Research*. Basel, S. Karger, 1971, p 22.

27. Hendrick JC, Legros JJ, Franchimont P: Le dosage radioimmunologique de la FSH de rat et étude radioimmunologique de la réaction croisée entre la FSH de rat, de mouton et de porc. *Ann Endocrinol (Paris)* 32:241, 1971.

28. Faiman C, Ryan RJ: Radioimmunoassay for human follicle-stimulating hormone. *J Clin Endocrinol Metab* 27:444, 1967.

29. Franchimont P, Donini P: Immunologic behavior of follicle-stimulating hormone extracted from postmenopausal urine and the pituitary. *J Clin Endocrinol Metab* 31:18, 1970.

30. Papapoulos SE, Hendy GN, Tomlinson S, et al: Clearance of exogenous parathyroid hormone in normal and uremic man. *Clin Endocr* 7:211, 1977.

CHAPTER 4

CONJUGATION TECHNIQUES – CHEMISTRY

Pyara K. Grover

The specific binding proteins used in radioimmunoassay are antibodies elicited by active immunization with the substance to be measured in bioliogic fluids. This substance may be any hapten, but for this presentation it could be a peptide, steroid, or another compound, such as a drug. Substances with a molecular weight of less than 1000 are essentially nonantigenic (1). To produce antibodies against these substances they must be covalently coupled to large molecules which we will call proteins; most commonly used is serum albumin (bovine or human), although thyroglobulin, ovalbumin, fibrinogen, and synthetic polypeptides have also been used. During the past decade an enormous amount of work has been published on the preparation of hapten–protein conjugates for producing primary antibodies for all kinds of compounds vis-à-vis development of their immunoassays (2,3). In this chapter an attempt will be made to present sufficient information on the chemistry involved in making a hapten–protein conjugate, with special reference to peptides, steroids, and drugs.

There are a few important factors that should be taken into consideration when covalently coupling a hapten to a carrier protein:

1. The conditions for the reaction should be such that no molecular rearrangement of the hapten takes place and it maintains its basic chemical structure.
2. The reagent used for coupling should not be strong enough to denature the protein.
3. A suitable reactive group should be present on the hapten, which could under suitable conditions form a covalent bond with the carrier protein. If a suitable reactive group is lacking, it is desirable to introduce chemically a group that can be easily coupled to the carrier protein.

Hapten derivatives with free amino groups can be coupled with the carboxyl group of protein by using a water-soluble carbodiimide (4). Alternatively, hapten with amino groups can be conveniently conjugated to amino groups of proteins by using a bifunctional reagent such as gluteraldehyde

(5), or with the use of toluene 2,4-diisocyanate (6). Bisdiazotized benzidine has been used to prepare a conjugate for thyrotropin-releasing hormone (TRH) (7). If the amino group of the hapten forms part of an aromatic ring, it can be converted to the diazonium compounds by nitrous acid which at mildly alkaline pH reacts with the tyrosine, histidine, or tryptophan residues of the protein carrier (8). Hapten or hapten derivatives with a free carboxyl group can be conjugated to the amino groups of carrier proteins by the water-soluble carbodiimide (2) or by the mixed anhydride method (9). Water-soluble carbodiimide has also been used to make active esters of carboxyl groups on a hapten, which in turn can be covalently coupled under very mild conditions. A hapten carrying a free hydroxyl group cannot be conjugated as such to a carrier protein and so must be functionalized either as a hemisuccinate by treatment with succinic anhydride or as a carboxymethyl derivative (10) by treatment with chloroacetic acid for covalent linkage to a carrier protein by using carbodiimide or the mixed anhydride method. The hydroxyl group on the hapten can also be made to react with phosgene to yield a very reactive chlorocarbonate derivative (9) which reacts directly with the amino groups of proteins under alkaline conditions. A bifunctional reagent such as sebacoyl dichloride (11) has also been used to convert an acid to acid chloride which under mild alkaline conditions reacts with amino groups of protein. Phenols react readily with diazotized p-aminobenzoic acid, and the resulting derivative containing the carboxyl group (12) can be coupled to the amino group of a protein by either the carbodiimide or the mixed anhydride method. A chemical substance that carries vicinal hydroxyl groups can be converted to the corresponding dialdehyde by the use of sodium metaperiodate which reacts with the amino groups of protein carriers under alkaline conditions (13).

Haptens carrying a ketone group in the form of an aldehyde or a ketone can be converted to oximes which can be reduced to the corresponding amine and coupled to the carboxyl group on the protein by methods mentioned earlier, or alternatively they can be converted to the O-(carboxymethyl)oxime (2) and the carboxyl group coupled with the free amino groups of proteins by the mixed anhydride or carbodiimide method.

In chemical substances such as steroids (testosterone) both functional groups, ketones and hydroxyl groups, are present and by choosing the proper reagent it is possible to make conjugates to the carrier proteins at a given position at will (14).

Recently it also has been possible to functionalize steroids at different parts of the molecule with specific stereochemistry which, when conjugated to carrier protein, has resulted in very specific antibodies (15).

For making conjugate of catecholamines (16) or lysergic acid (17) the Mannich reaction has been used. By this method an aromatic compound carrying a phenolic hydroxyl function or any reactive position is covalently linked to the protein by a methylene bridge.

The methods mentioned above will be illustrated with figures by giving examples for each category of compounds under consideration—peptides, steroids, and other compounds such as drugs. Efforts will be made to cite only those examples in each category where a novel procedure either for preparing a suitably substituted hapten or for preparing a conjugate has been used.

The most commonly used reagent for conjugation reaction is water-soluble carbodiimide—the reactive group being a free carboxyl group on the hapten or in the form of a hemisuccinate or carboxymethyl or carboxymethyloxime. It will be of interest to understand the mechanism of this reaction (Fig. 1). The pK of the acid (I) is very important for the participation of the acidic group to form an active ester with carbodiimide. From the reaction sequence (Fig. 1) the attack of the acid group takes place on the electron-deficient carbon atom of the carbodiimide only in the ionized form to give II. It is not possible to isolate II in pure form, as it is not stable. To keep the acidic function in the ionized form it is important to keep the pH of the reaction mixture higher than the pK of the acid. This is one reason why this reaction does not work very well with acids having a pK of 7 or higher. There are side reactions involving anionic species in the solution at higher pH that also react with the electron-deficient carbon atom in carbodiimide. The active ester (II) can give rise to different products— some desirable and some undesirable. It can react with the amino groups of the protein to give the desired conjugate (V) and urea (VI), or it can react with another molecule or carboxyl acid to give an anhydride (III) which in turn can react with the amino group of protein giving the desired product (V). Alternatively the active ester I can undergo intramolecular rearrangement, giving the undesired product, acylurea (IV). This undesired side product seems to be solvent-dependent.

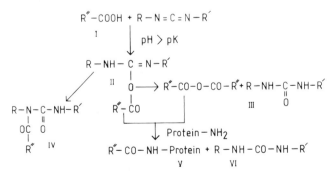

Figure 1. Carbodiimide reaction.

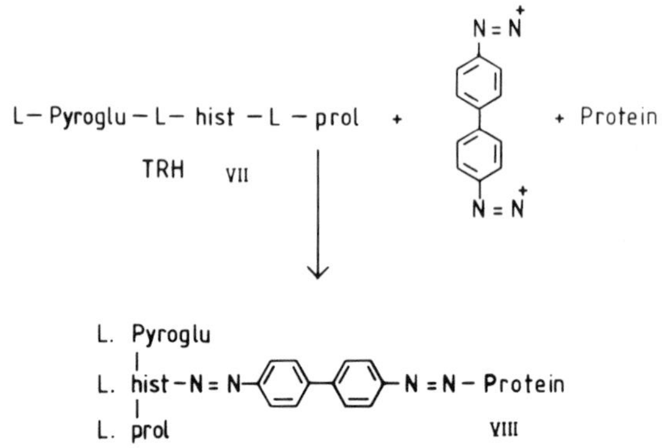

$$L-Pyroglu-L-hist-L-prol \quad + \quad + \quad Protein$$

TRH   VII

L. Pyroglu
|
L. hist−N=N−⟨◯⟩−⟨◯⟩−N=N−Protein
|
L. prol   VIII

Figure 2. Thyrotropin-releasing hormone protein (VIII).

PEPTIDES

In this group two peptides, TRH and bradykinin, have been chosen.

THYROTROPIN RELEASING HORMONE PROTEIN

Treatment of TRH (VII) with bisdiazotized benzidine and protein gives a conjugate (VIII) (7) in which one diazotized group in benzidine is linked to histidine of TRH, and the other diazotized group with the protein (Fig. 2). In this reaction one may by chance end up with a single product which would be difficult to repeat. Usually this kind of reaction can produce several side products which also produce antibodies when animals are immunized with a mixture of conjugates.

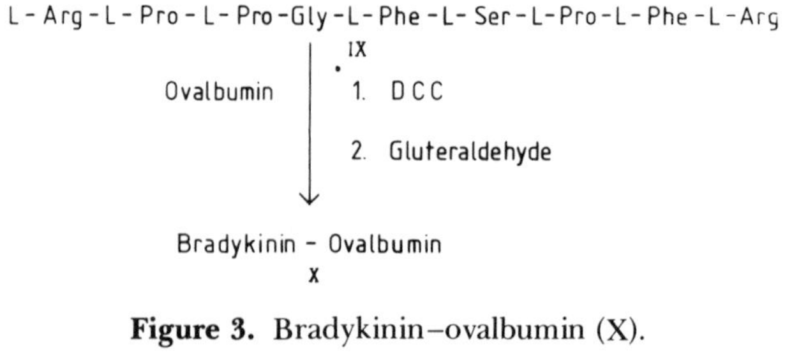

L - Arg - L - Pro - L - Pro - Gly - L - Phe - L - Ser - L - Pro - L - Phe - L - Arg
                                                        IX

Ovalbumin   1. DCC

                 2. Gluteraldehyde

Bradykinin - Ovalbumin
                 X

Figure 3. Bradykinin–ovalbumin (X).

BRADYKININ–OVALBUMIN

Bradykinin (IX) has been successfully conjugated to ovalbumin in two steps (18): (1) treatment with water-soluble carbodiimide, and (2) treatment with gluteraldehyde of the resulting product to yield the bradykinin–ovalbumin conjugate (X) (Fig. 3).

STEROIDS

Steroids are a class of compounds having a rigid coplanar tetracyclic structure. They are amenable to chemical modification to introduce different functional groups at different carbon atoms in the molecule without any alteration in the basic structure for conjugation. In several cases the group introduced by chemical modification acquires a specific stereochemistry. A good correlation between the stereochemistry of the group conjugated and the specificity of the antibodies with little or no cross-reaction with compounds of closely related structure has been made (15). This is illustrated by the following examples from different groups of steroids.

17β-SUCCINYL ESTRADIOL–BOVINE SERUM ALBUMIN

Under normal conditions it is rather difficult to esterify the 17β-hydroxyl group in preference to the 3-hydroxyl group, as the hydroxyl group at C-3 is more reactive, being phenolic in nature. However, estradiol (XI) when treated with succinic anhydride in pyridine at reflux temperature gives the 3,17β-disuccinyl derivative (XII) which under mild alkaline conditions (sodium bicarbonate–methanol) gives 17β-monossuccinate (XIII), which is a good crystalline compound and can be purified to chemical purity by crystallization (2). When conjugated with bovine serum albumin (BSA) and carbodiimide, it gives the required conjugate (XIV) (Fig. 4).

ESTRADIOL-6-CARBOXYMETHYLOXIME–BOVINE SERUM ALBUMIN

The introduction of a keto group at the C-6 position imparts coplanarity to the molecule and gives specific antibodies with very little cross-reaction

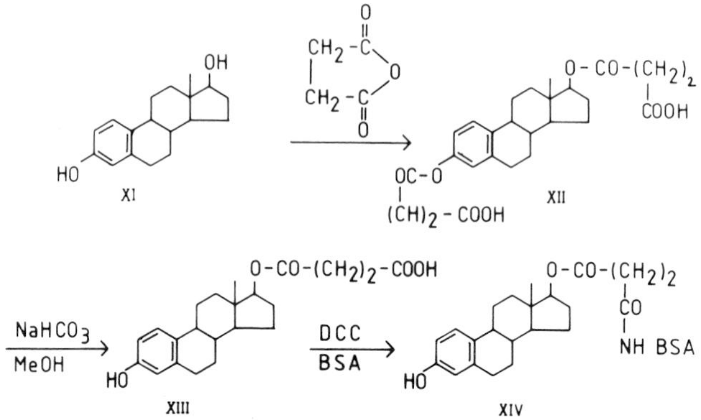

Figure 4. 17β-Succinylestradiol–BSA (XIV).

with compounds with similar structures. Estradiol diacetate (XV), on treatment with chromium trioxide in acetic acid, gives the 6-keto derivative (XVI). Hydrolysis with alkali gives XVII which can be converted to estradiol-6-carboxymethyloxime by treatment with carboxymethoxylamine hydrochloride in good yields, and further treatment with BSA or thyroglobulin (15) and carbodiimide gives the conjugate (XIX) (Fig. 5).

17β-SUCCINYL TESTOSTERONE–BOVINE SERUM ALBUMIN AND TESTOSTERONE-3-CARBOXYMETHLYOXIME–BOVINE SERUM ALBUMIN

Testosterone XX has both functional groups—a keto group at the C-3 position and a secondary hydroxyl group at the C-17 position. So treatment with succinic anhydride in pyridine at reflux temperature gives the 17β-succinate (XXII), and treatment of XX with carboxymethoxylamine hydrochloride gives the 3-oxime (XXI) (14). When treated with carbodiimide and BSA both derivatives give the required conjugates, XXIV and XXIII, respectively (Fig. 6).

1α-THIOCARBOXYMEHTYL-5α-DIHYDROTESTOSTERONE–BOVINE SERUM ALBUMIN

Introduction of the thiocarboxymethyl group at the 1-position, which takes an axial conformation, has been known to give fairly specific antibodies to

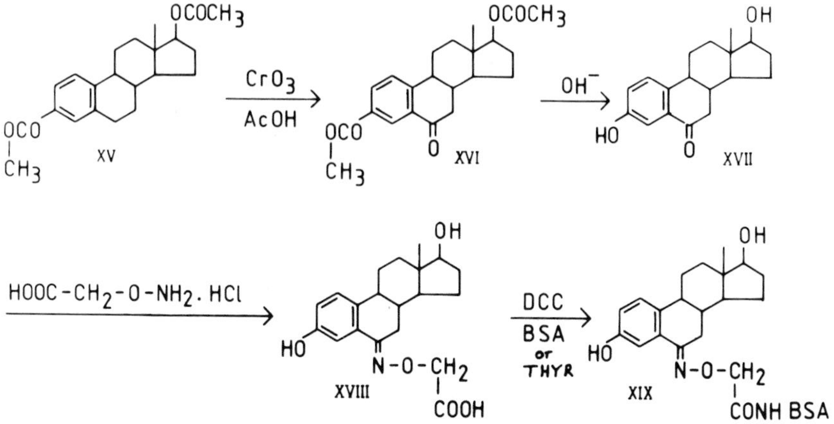

Figure 5. Estradiol-6-carboxymethyloxime–BSA (XIX).

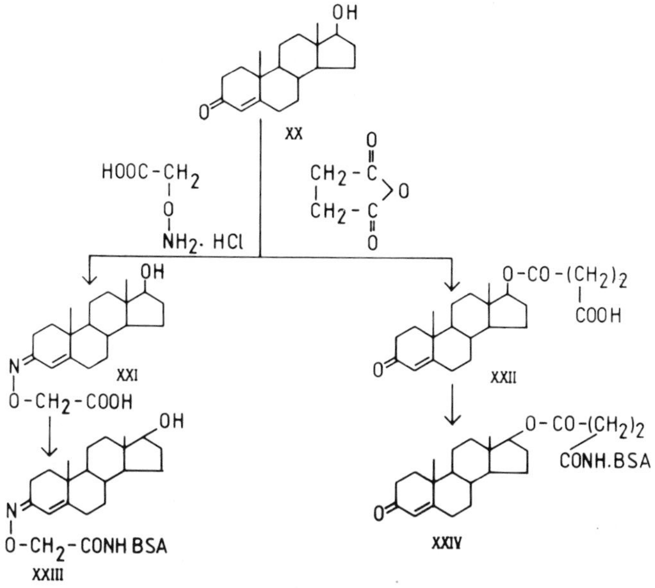

Figure 6. 17β-Succinyltestosterone–BSA (XXIV) and testosterone-3-carboxy-methyloxime–BSA (XXIII).

61

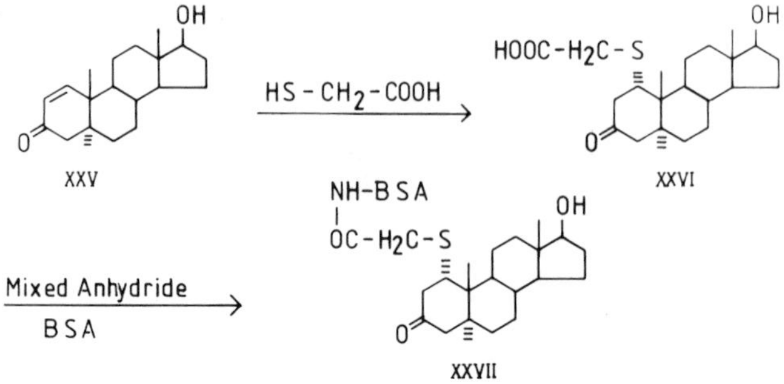

Figure 7. 1α-Thiocarboxymethyl-5α-dihydrotestosterone–BSA (XXVII).

dihydrotestosterone with very little cross-reaction with testosterone (19). The compound (XXVI) is easily obtained by the addition of thiocarbolic acid to 17λ-hydroxy-5α-androst-1-ene-3-one (XXV) which is conjugated to BSA with carbodiimide giving XXVII (Fig. 7).

6α-THIOCARBOXYMETHYLTESTOSTERONE–BOVINE SERUM ALBUMIN

Substitution at C-6 in a steroid molecule attains an equatorial conformation, and antibodies made from a conjugate at this position also are fairly specific. When treated with N-bromosucciniimide, testosterone (XX) gives the 6β-bromo derivative (XXVIII) which by SN_2 displacement with thiocarbolic acid yields XXIX (20). On conjugation with carbodiimide and BSA this compound gives the conjugate (XXX) (Fig. 8).

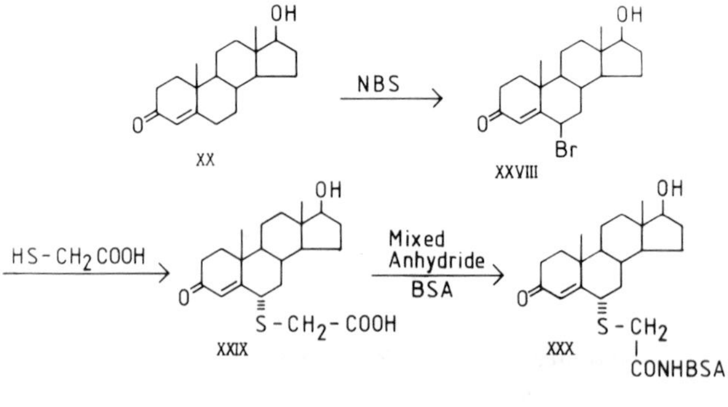

Figure 8. 6α-Thiocarboxymethyltestorterone–BSA (XXX).

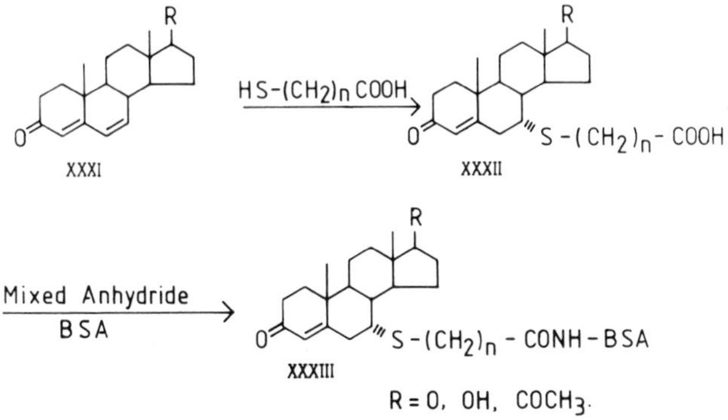

Figure 9. 7σ-Thiocarboxyalkyl steroid–BSA (XXXIII).

7α-THIOCARBOXYALKYL STEROID–BOVINE SERUM ALBUMIN

The 7α-substituent in a steroid takes an axial conformation and is shown to give nonspecific antibodies. This is a general reaction and is applicable to androstendione, testosterone, and progesterone. As a typical example, where R is hydroxyl; 6-dehydrotestosterone (XXXI) on addition with thiomethyl carbolic (in this case one can vary the length of the alkyl chain) gives the 7α-thiocarboxy derivative (XXXII) (21) which was conjugated to BSA by the mixed anhydride method, giving XXXIII (Fig. 9).

DRUGS

Unlike steroids where the derivative to be conjugated can be purified and characterized, in most cases involving drugs all the steps are carried out without purification and characterization. The following examples show some variance from the normal reactions cited so far.

HALOPERIDOL–BOVINE SERUM ALBUMIN

In this case BSA was first converted to the hydrazide (XXXIV) by treatment with hydrazine hydrate which was subsequently made to react with the keto group of haloperidol (XXXV), giving the conjugate (XXXVI) (22) (Fig. 10). No attempt was made to purify either the hydrazide or the conjugate.

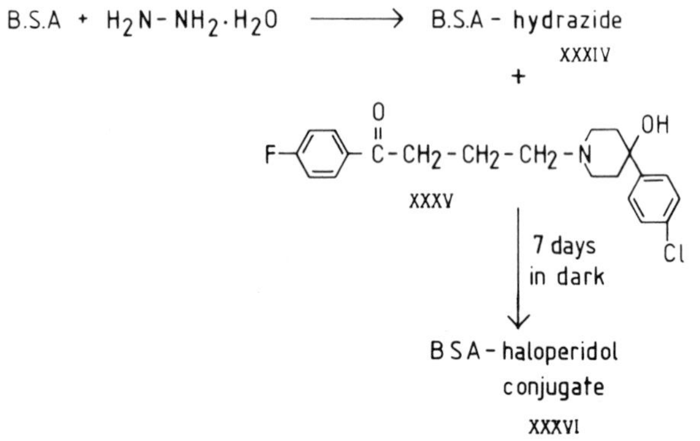

Figure 10. Haloperidol–BSA (XXXVI).

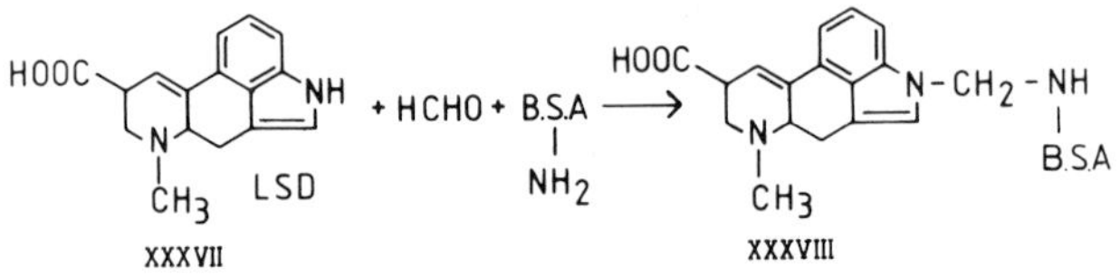

Figure 11. Lysergic acid–BSA (XXXVIII).

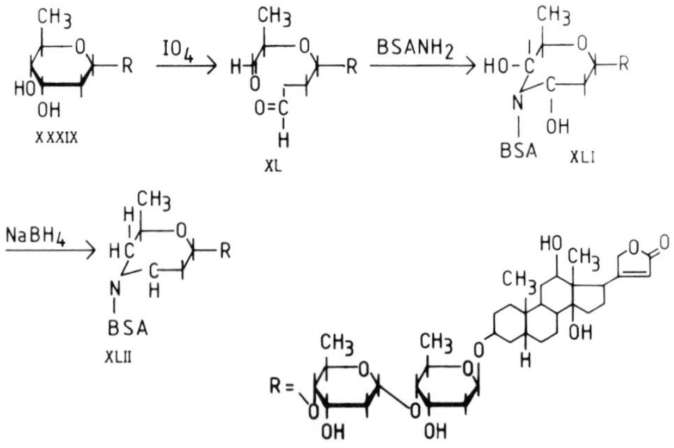

Figure 12. Degoxin–BSA (XLII).

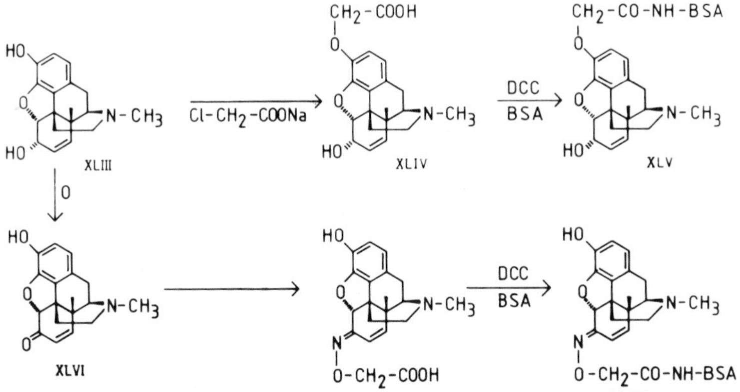

Figure 13. Morphine–BSA (XLV and XLVIII).

LYSERGIC ACID–BOVINE SERUM ALBUMIN

By Mannich addition of BSA and formaldehyde to lysergic acid (XXXVII), the conjugate (XXXVIII) (Fig. 11) was obtained in which BSA was linked to indole nitrogen in lysergic acid by a methylene bridge (17).

DEGOXIN–BOVINE SERUM ALBUMIN

Degoxin (XXXIX), when treated with sodium metaperiodate, gives a dialdehyde by fission at the carbon atoms in terminal glycoside moiety carrying vicinal hydroxyl groups (XL), which when treated with BSA gives the aldimine (XLI), and this is stablized on reduction with sodium borohydride (13), yielding the right conjugate (XLII) (Fig. 12).

MORPHINE–BOVINE SERUM ALBUMIN

Like testosterone, morphine has two positions at which chemical manipulation conjugation can be achieved, namely, positions 3 and 6. Morphine (XLIII), when treated with sodium salt of chloroacetic acid, gives the 3-carboxymethyl ether (XLIV) (23), which can give the conjugate with BSA (XLV). Alternatively, morphine, when treated with a suitable oxidizing agent, gives morphone (XLVI), which gives 6-carboxymethyloxime (XLVII), of morphone (24). This on treatment with BSA and carbodiimide gives a conjugate (XLVIII) (Fig. 13).

REFERENCES

1. Gilliland PF, Prout TE: Immunologic studies of Octapeptides. II. Production and detection of antibodies to oxytocin. *Metabolism* 14:918, 1965.

2. Abraham GE, Grover PK: Covalent linkage of hormonal haptens to protein carriers for use in radioimmunoassay, in Odell WD. Daughaday WH (eds): *Principles of Competitive Protein-Binding Assays.* Philadelphia, JB Lippincott, 1971, pp 134, 140.

3. Butler VP: The immunological assay of drugs. *Pharmacol Rev* 29:103, 1978.

4. Goodfriend TL, Levine L, Fasman GD: Antibodies to bradykinin and angiotensin: A use of carbodiimide in immunology. *Science* 144:1344, 1964.

5. Riceberg LJ, Van Vunakis H, Lavine L: Radioimmunoassays of 3,4-5-trimethoxyphenylethylamine (muscaline) and 2,5-dimethoxy-4-methylphenylisopropylamine (DOM). *Anal Biochem* 60:551, 1974.

6. Liehite V, Sehon A: Protein-protein conjugation. In Williams CA, Chase MW (eds): Methods in Immunology and Immunochemistry Vol. 1. New York, Academic Press, 1967, p 150.

7. Bassiri S, Uttiger RD: The preparation and specificity of antibody to thyrotropin releasing hormone. *Endocrinol* 90:722, 1972.

8. Parker CW: Nature of immunological responses and antigen–antibody interaction, in Odell WD, Daughaday WH (eds): *Principles of Competitive Protein-Binding Assays.* Philadelphia, JB Lippincott, 1971, p 25.

9. Erlanger BF, Borek F, Beiser SM, et al: Steroid protein conjugates. I. Preparation and characterisation of conjugates of bovine serum albumin with testosterone and cortisone. *J Biol Chem* 228:713, 1957.

10. Spector S, Parker CW: Morphine: radioimmunoassay. *Science* 168:1347, 1970.

11. Beiser SM, Butler VP Jr, Erlanger BF: Hapten protein conjugates: Methodology and applications. In Miescher PA, Muller-Eberhard HJ (eds). Textbook of Immunopathology, 2nd edition, Vol. I. New York, Grune and Stratton, 1976, p 15.

12. Gross SJ, Campbell DH, Weetall HH: Production of antisera to steroids coupled to protein directly through the phenolic-A ring. *Immunochemistry* 5:55, 1968.

13. Butter, VP Jr, Chen JP: Digoxin-specific antibodies. *Proc Nat Acad Sci USA* 57:71, 1967.

14. Odell W, Swerdloff RS, Bain J, et al: The effect of sexual maturation in testicular sensitivity to LH stimulation to testosterone secretion in the intact rat. *Endocrinology* 95:1380, 1974.

15. Grover PK, Odell WD: Specificity of antisera to sex steroids. *J Steroid Biochem* 8:121, 1976.

16. Miwa A, Yoshida M, Tamura Z: Preparation of specific antibodies to catecholamines and L-3,4-dihydroxyphenylalanine: II. The site of attachment of catechol moity in the conjugates. *Chem Pharm Bull (Tokyo)* 26:2903, 1978.

17. Ratcliff WA, Fletcher SM, Moffat AC, et al: Radioimmunoassay of lysergic acid diethylamide (LSD) in serum and urine by using antisera of different specificities. *Clin Chem* 23:169, 1977.

18. Odya CE, Goodfriend TL: Bradykinin, in Abraham GE (ed): *Handbook of Radioimmunoassays.* New York, Marcel Dekker, 1977, p 499.

19. Bauminger S, Kohen F, Lindner HR, et al: Antiserum to 5-dihydrotestosterone: Production, characterization and use in radioimmunoassays. *Steroids* 24:477, 1974.

20. Lindner HR, Perel E, Friedlander A, et al: Specificity of antibodies to ovarian hormones in relation to the site of attachment of the steroid hapten to the peptide carrier. *Steroids* 22:357, 1972.

21. Weinstein A, Lindner HR, Friedlander A, et al: Antigenic complexes of steroid hormones formed by coupling to protein through position 7: Preparation from Δ^4-3-oxosteroids and characterization of antibodies to testosterone and androstenedione. *Steroids* 20:789, 1972.

22. Clark BR, Tower BB, Rubin RT: Radioimmunoassay of haloperidol in human serum. *Life Sci* 20:319, 1977.

23. Spector S, Berkowitz B, Flynn EJ, et al: Antibodies to morphine, barbiturates and serotonin. *Pharmaco Rev* 25:281, 1973.

24. Koida M, Takahashi M, Muraoka S, et al: Antibodies to BSA conjugates of morphine derivatives: Strict dependency of the immunological specificity on the hapten structure. *Jpn J Pharmacol* 24:165, 1974.

CHAPTER 5
RADIOLABELING TECHNIQUES

William D. Odell

The optimized radioimmunoassay or radioreceptor assay requires as one reagent a highly purified radioisotopic analyte. For steroid assays, tritium-labeled steroids are used and are available from commercial sources in varying degrees of purity. Although steroid assays are discussed separately, it is essential to emphasize that it is prudent to assess the purity of tritiated steroids before use in assays, for example, to be certain that purchased tritiated estradiol is only estradiol. Purity may be assessed in a high-discrimination separation system, such as thin-layer or LH-20 chromatography [see Abraham and Grover (1) and Murphy (2)]. Similarly, assessment of the purity of radioiodinated materials is desirable for commercially purchased thyronines, and purification may be required. The latter is discussed in a separate chapter.

This chapter concerns itself with the preparation of highly purified radioiodinated proteins and peptides. (Table 1 lists the methods commonly available.)

In the early publication of Berson and Yalow (3) describing the kinetics of the interaction of radioiodinated insulin and antiserum against insulin, Scatchard analysis failed to reveal a linear plot. This was interpreted as indicating that more than a single population of antibody-binding sites or more than one antigenic site existed on insulin. During the past 15 years, we have similarly analyzed a number of radioimmunoassays and obtained similar nonlinear Scatchard plots. However, as the quality of the radioiodinated label has improved, Scatchard analysis using antisera from a number of optimized immunoassays has subsequently yielded linear Scatchard plots. We believe that, in the earlier immunoassays, the radioiodination procedure produced a spectrum of iodinated products with varying affinities for the antiserum, whereas more recent procedures usually result in more homogeneous preparations. Furthermore, we believe that, in most optimized radioimmunoassays using very highly diluted antisera, often only a single population of antibodies is involved. Thus, linear Scatchard plots are typically or commonly obtained using highly diluted antisera reacting with a high-quality labeled hormone.

In addition, it is commonly true that a radiolabeled preparation adequate for immunoassay use may be inadequate for radioreceptor assays.

Table 1. Methods of Radioiodination

Chloramine-T
Lactoperoxidase
Bolton–Hunter
TCDPG

This can occur because the tyrosine or histidine iodinated is involved in receptor binding and/or the protein is "damaged" (e.g., oxidized) by the iodination process, destroying receptor binding although maintaining the ability to react with the antiserum.

These examples underscore the importance of preparing and using the highest-quality label possible. In addition to accuracy in analysis of antigen–antibody or receptor–hormone kinetics, the optimization of all radioimmunoassays depends on the production of a high-quality radiolabel. We observed, for example, a 10-fold improvement in the sensitivity of the parathormone radioimmunoassay when a low-specific-activity, average-quality label was replaced by a monoiodinated, highly purified radioiodinated parathormone and the assay reoptimized (i.e., the antisera retitered and the separation method modified).

The iodination procedure using chloramine-T as an oxidizing agent originally described by Hunter and Greenwood (4) and Greenwood et al. (5) greatly simplified the preparation of radioiodinated proteins. This procedure was later modified, and a second procedure (lactoperoxidase) was introduced (6,7) and in turn modified (8) in attempts to minimize damage to the peptide. A number of publications indicate that enzymatic oxidation (lactoperoxidase) produces a higher-quality radiolabel than chloramine. We believe most investigators use excess chloramine-T, thereby producing a damaged product. In fact, it has been our experience with most peptide hormones that there is little reason to prefer one oxidation method over another, *as long as each is optimized for use with the particular protein.* It is necessary to assess carefully the organification of iodine versus the amount of time and exposure to chloramine-T. When chloramine-T was limited (amount and time of exposure), we obtained identical preparations of several peptides with both optimized lactoperoxidase and chloramine-T. As a result, our preference is to use chloramine-T rather than enzymatic iodination for both radioimmunoassays and radioreceptor assays because it yields more easily reproducible results with higher rates of iodine incorporation.

Over the past 15 years, we have evolved three general procedures for preparing the following three kinds of radioiodinated proteins: (1) small peptides, that is, below MW 6000, (2) glycoproteins [e.g., thyroid-stimulating hormone (TSH), luteinizing hormone (LH), (FSH), and human chorionic gonadotropin (HCG)], and (3) larger proteins not containing carbohydrate [e.g., prolactin and growth hormone (GH)].

ISOTOPES, STABILITY, AND LABEL MASS

As a generality in a competitive protein binding assay system, it is desirable to use a quantity of radiolabel equal to or smaller than the quantity of nonlabeled analyte the assay is capable of quantifying. In this way, the sensitivity of the assay is not impaired by the radiolabel itself. We have, on several occasions, visited laboratories to troubleshoot receptor assays and found that the mass of the radiolabel was so large that, in effect, it was not too different from the largest dose of hormone the assay could quantify. That is, the bound/free ratio with radiolabel alone in the assay tube was extremely small. After improving label quality and decreasing label mass by 10 to 100-fold, the assay performed satisfactorily. While it is important to keep the amount of label small, from a practical standpoint it is important to have an adequate counting rate. The counting rate should be *at least* 10 times the background produced by the counter. Much greater counting rates are often desirable and, if the assay is not affected adversely, may greatly decrease counting times. Typically, counting rates of between 3000 and 20,000 cpm are used for radioimmunoassays.

A number of radioisotopes are available. For selected purposes, proteins labeled with ^3H (half-life 12.3 years) or ^{14}C (half-life 5.730 years) have been prepared. However, in the molar concentrations required for assays, counting rates and specific activities of labeled proteins have been so low as to preclude their use. Sulfur-35 might be used and is available in a high-quality, carrier-free state but has not yet been exploited for radioimmunoassay.

Generally, radioisotopic iodine has been the compound of choice because of the ease of obtaining reagents and the simplicity of procedures. ^{131}I was used earlier (half-life 8 days), because high counting rates resulted from the short half-life when radioiodinated proteins were prepared. In the mid-1960s, ^{125}I (half-life 60 days) of high isotopic abundance became available. The longer half-life was of practical significance, since it prolonged the shelf life of radioiodinated proteins and theoretically decreased the counting rate as a result of the longer half-life. However, the increased isotopic abundance in available materials plus increased counting efficiency (perhaps twice as high as ^{131}I) resulted in excellent counting rates. In addition, the increased safety of handling this isotope as compared to ^{131}I has made ^{125}I the reagent of general choice.

THE IODINATION PROCEDURE

[125]I is received as a solution of $Na^{125}I$, usually at a high pH. The first step in any of the iodination methods is to lower the pH to 7, where iodination occurs optimally. Once this is accomplished, the ^{125}I is oxidized, producing free iodine (I_2) which then reacts with water to produce the iodinium species. This in turn reacts with tyrosine in the protein, exchanging an iodine for a hydrogen. Diiodination can also occur, particularly in the presence of increased quantities of iodine.

THE CHLORAMINE-T METHOD

As stated previously, the first descriptions of the chloramine-T method represented an important advance in iodination procedures. If one prepares dose–response curves for the amount of chloramine-T versus iodination efficiency, the studies used what, retrospectively, is a great excess of chloramine-T. When iodinating 1–2 μg of protein hormone (10^{-9}–10^{-10} mole) iodination efficiency begins to decrease when less than 2.5–3 μg (10^{-8} mole) is used.

A detailed sample protocol is as follows:

Chloramine-T Iodination

1. Add the following reagents in the order given to a reaction vial: Microcaps are preferred to quantify the reagents, and small plastic vials (Brinkman) are recommended for use as the reaction vial.
    a. 20 μl of 0.05 M phosphate, 0.15 M NaCl buffer, pH 7.4, containing 1–2 μg of the protein to be radioiodinated
    b. 50 μl of 0.5 M phosphate buffer, pH 7.0
    c. 1 MCi of carrier-free, high-specific activity $Na^{125}I$ (generally about 2.5 μl)
    d. 5 μl, containing 2.5 μg chloramine-T, of 0.15 M NaCl, 05 M phosphate, pH 7.4; this mixture is prepared immediately before use, using preweighed reagents (e.g., 5 mg in 10 ml); mix by finger-flicking for 15–40 seconds (depending on the particular protein being iodinated).

2. Stop the reaction by adding 300 μl of bovine serum albumin (BSA) (10 g/liter) or 10 μl sodium metabisulfite (5 μg).

3. Rapidly transfer the contents of the reaction vial to the selected column for purification; this procedure will be discussed later.

The details of protein storage for iodination will subsequently be discussed. The 50 μl of 0.5 M phosphate buffer is added to bring the pH of the radioisotopic iodine down to neutral, because it is shipped in NaOH. Reagents 1a and b are mixed in the reaction vial by finger-flicking. Next, the ^{125}I is added, great care being exercised not to contaminate the syringe with the protein being iodinated. Since 10 or more proteins are commonly labeled with a single batch of ^{125}I, contamination can adversely affect many studies. We recommend placing the droplet of ^{125}I solution, using a Hamilton syringe, on the side of the iodination vial, not in contact with the other reagents. The reaction vial is then finger-flicked to mix the ^{125}I and the reagents in steps 1a and b. Next, the chloramine-T is added and the reaction vial continuously finger-flicked for the desired reaction time. This time is short (10–15 seconds) for labile proteins and long (45–60 seconds) for hardy proteins that are difficult to iodinate. The chloramine-T solution is prepared fresh during iodination. We recommend weighing out the chloramine-T just a few minutes before iodinating (5 mg) and quantifying the buffer in a separate tube (10 ml) when the chloramine-T is desired. The tube of 5 ml of buffer is added to the 5 mg. The contents are mixed, and 5 μl of this fresh solution is used for the iodination process (step 1d).

LACTOPEROXIDASE METHOD USING HYDROGEN PEROXIDE

The lactoperoxidase method using hydrogen peroxide (5) was originally described for the labeling of immunoglobulins by Marchalonis (6) and was later applied to radioiodination of protein hormones by Thorell and Johansson (7) and Miyachi et al. (8). The procedure involves the oxidation of iodide by the enzyme lactoperoxidase. Hydrogen peroxide is used as a substrate. We have emphasized that the optimal iodination procedure must be determined for each homone, no matter which oxidation method is used (chloramine-T or lactoperoxidase). Miyachi et al. (8) gives examples of rather marked differences in requirements, even among biochemically related glycoproteins (FSH, LH, and HCG) and different preparations of the same hormone (human FSH, LER > 80 versus LER 1366). The lactoperoxidase–hydrogen peroxide method is schematically shown as follows:

The Lactoperoxidase–Hydrogen Peroxide Method*

Add all reagents to the reaction vial (10 × 75 mm glass tube) at room temperature in the following order.

1. 2–5 μg of the protein to be labeled in 5 μl of 0.01 M phosphate, 0.15 M NaCl, pH 7.4, buffer
2. 50 μg of lactoperoxidase in 10 μl of 0.1 M sodium acetate, pH 5.6
3. 1 MCi carrier-free Na^{125}I
4. 25 μl of 0.4 M sodium acetate buffer, pH 5.6.

The reaction is initiated and maintained by the addition of 100–200 μg of hydrogen peroxide at 10-minute intervals, usually for a total of three times. For hydrogen-sensitive proteins (such as HCG), smaller amounts of hydrogen peroxide are permissible.

The Lactoperoxidase–Glucose Oxidase Method

Add all reagents at room temperature except the glucose-oxidase, which is kept at 4°C until addition.

1. 15 μl 0.01 M phosphate buffer–0.15 M NaCl, pH 7.5
2. 2–5 δg of the protein to be iodinated
3. 1 MCi of ^{125}I
4. 50 μg of lactoperoxidase in 10 μl of 0.1 M sodium acetate, pH 5.6
5. 5 μl of glucose oxidase
6. 25 μl of 0.1% glucose.

Mix the reaction vial by finger-flicking continually for 1.5 minutes. Then add 0.5 ml of 0.01 M phosphate buffer, pH 7.5, and transfer to a separation–purification column (to be discussed later).

THE BOLTON-HUNTER REAGENT

The Bolton–Hunter reagent (9) is the N-hydroxysuccinimide ester of iodinated p-hydroxypenylpropionic acid. This compound acylates terminal amino groups with the ^{125}I-labeled p-hydroxyphenylpropionic acid residue. The compound was originally described by Rudinger and Ruegg (10). Bolton and Hunter (9) described the preparation of TSH, growth hormone,

*For these enzymatic methods, sodium azide, a common antibacterial added to buffers, is avoided since enzyme activity can be impaired.

and LH with excellent immunoreactivity. The reagent is commercially available and may be expensive. It is advertised as being a more mild labeling procedure, and in our hands is quite satisfactory for proteins over MW 10,000 (although it does not appear to be superior to previous optimized methods). In addition, for small peptides such as vasopressin and GnRH analogues, the large iodinated reagent may interfere with antibody or receptor binding.

1,3,4,6-TETRACHLORO-3α,6α-DIPHENYLGLYCOLURIL METHOD

The 1,3,4,6-tetrachloro-3α,6α-diphenyglycoluril (TCDPG) method (11) is based on the interesting principle of iodinating at the aqueous interface of this sparingly soluble material. Like chloramine-T, TCDPG is a chloramide. However, whereas chloramine-T is quite soluble in water, TCDPG is poorly soluble. It forms a solid-phase-like material that can be used for iodination. Fraker and Speck (11) first described this method, comparing chloramine-T and TCDPG for iodination of immunoglobulins, two types of living cells (sheep erythrocytes and mouse tumor cells), and chicken lysozyme. In contrast to investigators describing other methods, Fraker and Speck carefully determined dose–response relations of chloramine-T and TCDPG versus iodine incorporation. With smaller amounts of TCDPG, greater amounts of iodine were incorporated into the proteins. Unfortunately, sodium metabisulfite was used to stop the chloramine-T reaction, and the iodination reaction with chloramine-T was carried out in pH 8.2 buffer, which may not have been adequate to buffer commercial Na^{125}I (as discussed previously). No enzymatic activity could be shown for the chloramine-T–sodium metabisulfite–lysozyme, whereas considerable activity remained after TCDPG iodination. In addition, the cells iodinated using TCDPG retained viability.

Since the article by Fraker and Speck appeared, McGregor et al. (12,13) have used this method for TSH and recommend it highly. The latter group made no direct comparisons with the optimized chloramine-T method but did prepare very highly receptor-active TSH with ease. At the time of manuscript preparation, this author has had no direct experience with the TCDPG chloramide method, but from the theoretical standpoint it appears to be an excellent technique and may prove to be the preferred one if the reagents become easily available.

In practice, the method appears quite simple once the TCDPG is prepared. It is dissolved in methylene glycol, and a 20-μl aliquot is evaporated to dryness, layering the bottom of the reaction vial. Buffer, carrier-free ^{125}I, and the protein to be iodinated are added rapidly, and the reaction permitted to occur. For rabbit IgG, Fraker and Speck reacted at 0–2°C for 5 minutes. The reaction is stopped by aspirating or decanting reagents and rapidly transferring them to the selected purification column.

STORAGE OF PROTEINS AND PEPTIDES FOR RADIOIODINATION

Proteins or peptides to be radioiodinated must be available in highly purified form; any protein present in the storage tubes will be radioiodinated along with the protein desired. However, the storage of highly purified proteins in a solution free of other proteins presents problems, especially if the highly purified proteins are stored in dilute solutions. Adsorption to glass occurs, resulting in loss of protein. Spontaneous lyophilizaion occurs in storage in freezers, and many proteins slowly change structure in these dilute protein-free solutions. No practical storage plan is perfect. For very labile proteins such as human prolactin, it is probably best to freshly weigh dry protein and place it in solution immediately preceding iodination. Alternatively, small aliquots of solutions might be stored for thawing and use in 6–8 weeks only. For rugged proteins such as growth hormone, frozen solutions can be used over several years.

The pH of the storage solution should be selected for optimal stability, but it is important to be certain that the buffers employed for iodination are capable of returning the pH to neutrality for the iodination procedure. A common technique used for a wide range of protein hormones is to pipet 50–200 μl volumes of a 100 to 400-μl/ml concentration into small tubes. These are "snap-frozen" in dry ice–alcohol and kept in a suitable freezer. For iodination, one vial is thawed, the aliquot removed and used, and the tube refrozen (snap-frozen). A more desirable alternative method is to pipet just the amount needed for iodination (1–2 μg of protein) into small plastic vials containing attached tops. These are then stored frozen; one is thawed and used for iodination, the process occurring directly in the storage vial.

Table 2. Purification of Radioiodinated Proteins

Glycoproteins—concanavalin A
Peptides (under MW 4000)—ion exchange
Proteins—gel filtration

PURIFICATION OF RADIOIODINED PROTEINS AND PEPTIDES

Regardless of which method is used to prepare the radioiodinated peptides or proteins, it is essential to purify them following preparation. The optimal method not only separates nonreacted ^{125}I from iodinated protein but also separates partially or fully denatured proteins, fragmented proteins, and di- or noniodinated proteins from the reagent desired—a monoiodinated peptide. Any high-resolution purification method may be satisfactory. From the theoretical standpoint, one could purify the reagent by reacting it with antibody or receptor, discarding what failed to react and then disassociating the reacted label. Thus, solid-phase-conjugated immunoabsorbent or receptor columns fulfill this purpose. However, for almost all purposes, we recommend simpler purification methods, as mentioned in Table 2, and have routinely used three general kinds, depending on the protein hormone.

PURIFICATION OF RADIOIODINATED GLYCOPROTEIN HORMONES

For purification of the glycoprotein hormones, TSH, LH, FSH, and HCG, we prefer use of the plant lectin concanavalin A (Con A) (14). We employ this method routinely for these hormones from several species of animals. Small Con A columns (8.5 × 50 mm) are prepared at room temperature and washed with 1–2 ml of 10 g/liter BSA in phosphate-buffered saline (PBS). The iodination mixture is placed on top of the column. Free iodine, iodinated albumin (albumin is used to stop the reaction mixture during iodination), and damaged glycoproteins are eluted with 60–100 ml of PBS. After this, the buffer is changed to PBS with 0.2 M methyl-α-D-glucopyranoside which elutes the glycoproteins from the column. Three-milliliter fractions are collected in tubes containing 50 μl 5% BSA. Immunoreactivity is determined for 5-μl (or smaller) aliquots from each tube by incubating with excess antiserum at room temperature for 12 hours. In this manner, radiolabeled glycoproteins of known immunoreactivity are available for assay use within 1 day. Figure 1 illustrates this method.

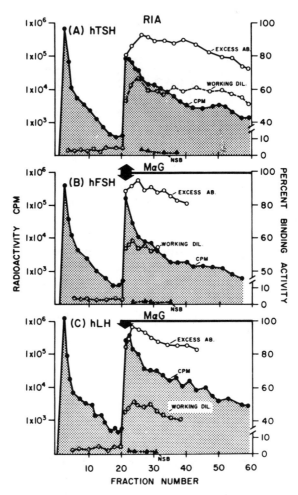

Figure 1. Elution patterns of (*a*) radioiodinated human thyrotropin (hTSH), (*b*) human follicle stimulating hormone (FSH), and (*c*) human luteinizing hormone (hLH) on concanavalin A–Sepharose. [Reproduced with permission from Patritti-Laborde et al., 1979 (14).]

PURIFICATION OF SMALL PEPTIDES

For peptides with molecular weights under about 5000, we prefer ion-exchange column chromatography (CM-Sephadex, SP-Sephadex, or OAE-Sephadex, Pharmacia, Inc.) (15). When cation exchange was chosen, chromatography was done 1 pH unit below the estimated pK$_a$ of the peptide to be purified. When anion exchange was chosen, chromatography was done at a pH 1 unit above the pK_a. Alternatively, one may empirically determine the pH at which binding of the radioiodinated peptide is maximal by batch addition of small amounts of ion exchanger to aliquots of radioiodinated peptide in tubes containing dilute buffers at varying pH values. After centrifugation, the supernatant is decanted, and the fraction of radiolabel binding to the exchanger calculated.

For cation exchange, we use 0.9 ∓ 12 cm columns packed by gravity and eluted in two steps. In the first elution step, low-ionic-strength buffer is used, and unreacted iodine that did not adsorb to the column is eluted. In the second step, a buffer at the same pH, but of higher molarity, is used to elute the peptide gradually in 300–400 ml of elution volume. A flow rate of 40–50 ml/h is recommended. When anion exchange is used, untreated iodide is retained on the column. Thus, only the second or elution step is required. When developing such a procedure for new peptides, we use as initial evaluation a shallow elution gradient to determine the approximate range of molarities. From such data, a molarity just below the molarity that elutes the peptide is selected and used as the second-step molarity for rou-

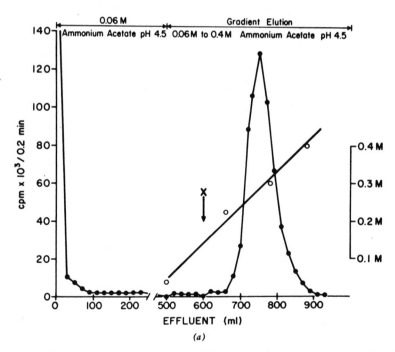

Figure 2. (a) Linear gradient elution of ^{125}I-labeled gonadotropin-releasing hormone (a 10-amino-acid peptide) on CM-Sephadex-C-25. O, Osmolarity, determined by freezing point depression; •, counts per minute; X, approximate molarity chosen for delayed elution.

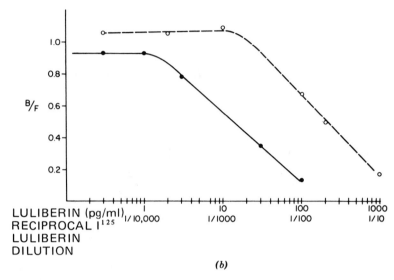

(b) Separation of iodinated (•) and uniodinated (○) gonadotropin-releasing hormone by cation-exchange chromatography. (Luliberin is another name for gonadotropin-releasing hormone.)

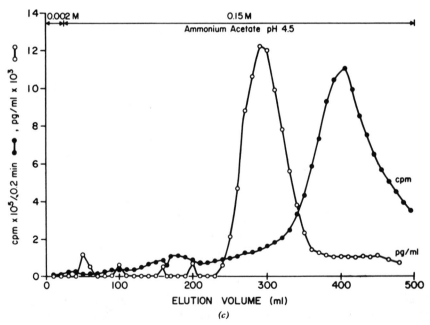

(c) Autodisplacement of ^{125}I-labeled gonadotropin-releasing hormone used to determine specific activity. •, Dilution of ^{125}I-labeled hormone ○, unlabeled hormone.

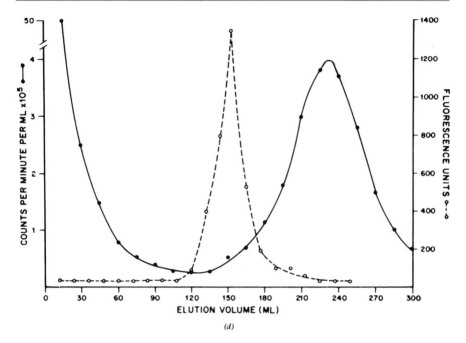

(d) Separation of ^{125}I-labeled corticotropin (ACTH) on carboxymethylcellulose. ●, cpm; ○, picograms of unlabeled corticotropin. [Reproduced with permission from Heber et al., 1978 (15).]

tine use. Such a molarity delays elution and is optimal for better separation of radioiodinated from noniodinated peptide. Figure 2 illustrates these principles.

PURIFICATION OF NONCARBOHYDRATE CONTAINING PROTEINS

Proteins over MW ~ 5000 that do not contain carbohydrate may usually be purified by Sephadex column chromatography or gel electrophoresis. The former is usually the most simple, and we prefer adding the iodination mixture to 0.8 × 50 cm columns and eluting ½-ml fractions in tubes containing 20 μl of 5% BSA. Damaged iodinated proteins appear with the first peak of radioactivity. The highest immunoreactivity is generally on the trailing edge of the assymmetric peak.

Free iodide (unreacted) elutes with the salt peaks. Optimally used, Sephadex column chromatography can result in the preparation of proteins with 80–95% immunoreactivity, which is adequate for routine immunoassay.

STORAGE OF RADIOIODINATED PROTEINS AND PEPTIDES

The shelf life of purified radioiodinated proteins varies from protein to protein. Some are quite stable and, once prepared, may be stored in solution at 4°C for 4–6 weeks with little loss of immunoreactivity. This is true for optimally prepared ^{125}I-labeled TSH, LH, HCG, and GH where initial immunoreactivity should be about 95%. For labile proteins (such as calcitonin, parathormone, and ACTH), we prefer to iodinate and use the label within 2–3 days of preparation. In our hands immunoreactivity falls considerably after a week. Other proteins easily remain adequate for use for 2–3 weeks (e.g., prolactin, FSH). We recommend that maximal immunoreactivity be determined weekly for each iodinated protein before setting up assays that week. After 2–4 months of "in-house" experience, guidelines for routine assay use can be developed. It is highly recommended, however, that radioiodinated peptides or proteins with maximal immunoreactivity (with excess antibody) of over 85% be used for assay purposes. Assessing maximal receptor activity is considerably more difficult and is not dealt with in this chapter.

REFERENCES

1. Abraham GE, Grover PK: Covalent linkage of hormonal haptens to protein carriers for use in radioimmunoassay, in Odell WD, Daughaday W (eds): *Principles of Competitive Protein-Binding Assays.* Philadelphia, JB Lippincott, 1971, p 134.

2. Murphy BEP: Hormone assay using binding proteins in blood, in Odell WD, Daughaday W (eds): *Principles of Competitive Protein-Binding Assays.* Philadelphia, JB Lippincott, 1971, p 108.

3. Berson SA, Yalow RS: Preparation and purification of human insulin-I^{131}; binding to human insulin-binding antibodies. *J Clin Invest* 40:1803, 1961.

4. Hunter WM, Greenwood FC: Preparation of iodine-131 labeled human growth hormone of high specific activity. *Nature* 194:495, 1962.

5. Greenwood FC, Hunter WM, Glover JS: The preparation of ^{131}I-labelled human growth hormone of high specific radioactivity. *Biochem J* 89:114, 1963.

6. Marchalonis JJ: An enzymic method for the trace iodination of immunoglobulins and other proteins. *Biochem J* 113:299, 1969.

7. Thorell JI, Johansson BG: Enzymatic iodination of polypeptides with I^{125} to high specific activity. *Biochem Biophys Act* 251:363, 1971.

 8. Miyachi Y, Vaitukaitis JL, Nieschlag E, Lipsett MB: Enzymatic radioiodination of gonado-tropins. *J Clin Endocrinol Metab* 34:23, 1972.

 9. Bolton AE, Hunter WM: The labelling of proteins to high specific radioactivities by con-jugation to a ^{125}I-containing acylating agent. *Biochem J* 133:529, 1973.

10. Rudinger J, Ruegg U: Preparation of N-succinimidyl 3-(4-hydroxyphenyl) propionate. *Biochem J* 133:538, 1973.

11. Fraker PJ, Speck JC Jr: Protein and cell membrane iodinations with a sparingly soluble chloroamide,1,3,4,6-tetrachloro-3α,6α-diphenylglycoluril. *Biochem Biophys Res Comm* 80:849, 1978.

12. McGregor AM, Petersen MM, McLachlan SM, et al: Carbimazole and the autoimmune response in Graves' disease. *N Engl J Med* 303:302, 1980.

13. McGregor AM, Petersen MM, Robb S, et al: Changes in thyroid autoantibodies during therapy for Graves' disease. Read before the Sixth International Congress of Endocrinol-ogy, Melbourne, February 1980.

14. Patritti-Laborde N, Yoshimoto Y, Wolfsen A, Odell WD: Improved method of purifying some radiolabeled glycopeptide hormones. *Clin Chem* 25:163, 1979.

15. Heber D, Odell WD, Schedewie H, Wolfsen AR: Improved iodination of peptides for radioimmunoassay and membrane radioreceptor assay. *Clin Chem* 24:796, 1978.

CHAPTER 6
REFERENCE MATERIALS AND STANDARDIZATION

Derek R. Bangham

STANDARDIZATION: AIMS, ASPECTS, AND REQUIREMENTS

The primary aim of standardization in assays is to make assay results reliably accurate and reproducible so that results obtained with different reagents, in different laboratories, and at different times can be validly compared. Achieving standardization involves understanding the purposes for which assays are carried out, the nature of and differences among various kinds of assays—bioassays and limited and excess binding reagent in vitro assays—hence the principles and assumptions that underlie the validity of the results. Standardization involves the proper preparation and matching of the component reagents, characterization of the whole assay system (reagents and procedure), and control of quality. Standardization requires that certain biometric principles be followed in each assay and that suitable reference materials be used as calibration yardsticks and for assessment of the specificity of the assays. This in turn involves evaluation of the reliability characteristics (precision, bias, sensitivity, validity, reproducibility, and ruggedness) of the assay system and the sustained monitoring of assay performance and requires a common and correct way of reporting the results. At present, standardization also badly needs a common exact terminology; many terms used in assay methodology require exact, agreed upon definitions so that they can be used more accurately by the scientific, clinical, and manufacturing communities.

Many of the precepts and problems of assays and biologic standardization have been known since the early days of classic pharmacology. But the immense diversity and scope of application of recently developed in vitro binding assay procedures requires that further thought be given to the principles underlying all kinds of assays (1).

This chapter is concerned mainly with reference materials and their role in standardization, and a brief reminder of the well-known precepts of standardization will explain the problems in complying with theory, hence their advantages and limitations, and the scientific implications of their use.

85

ASSAYS: PURPOSES, COMPONENTS, TYPES, AND VALIDITY

PURPOSES

Assays are carried out for one of two purposes: either to estimate the amount (concentration) of a substance (analyte) in a test specimen or to compare two dissimilar substances in a particular test system, for example, when the specificity of an assay system is tested with other substances (such as those structurally related to the analyte) that might influence the assay.

The great majority of immunoassays in research and clinical practice are carried out for the former purpose, to quantify the amount of an analyte. Certain of them are carried out to determine the relative change in analyte concentration in response to a stimulus. Others, such as tests for chorionic gonadotrophin (pregnancy tests) and for hepatitis antigen, are designed to give a yes or a no answer. Although in these tests quantification is simple, they too require standardization with reference materials so that their specificity and detection limit (the minimum amount of analyte they can detect with a stated confidence) can be measured.

Thus for their quantification (by calibration) and for assessment of their specificity, virtually all in vivo and in vitro protein binding assays rely on comparisons with measured quantities of reference materials.

COMPONENTS OF ASSAY SYSTEMS: THE BINDING REACTION—THE NEED FOR COMPARISON OF LIKE WITH LIKE

Essentially all assay systems have the same main components: the analyte in the specimen and the standard; the binding protein (e.g., an antibody or cell receptor); and a mechanism for generating, amplifying, and measuring the response signal.

BIOASSAYS AND IMMUNOASSAYS

It is often stated that bioassays are fundamentally different from immunoassays—and other protein binding (e.g., receptor) assays—but no general agreement has been reached on the nature of the distinction between

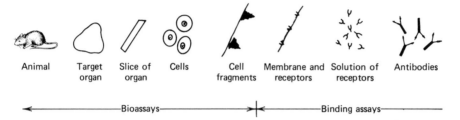

Figure 1. Transition from classic in vivo biological assays to typical in vitro immunoassays.

them (2). There appears to be a continuous transition (Fig. 1) involving whole animals at one end and successively target organs (slices, dissociated cells, fragmented cells, membranes with a minimal amount of cytoplasm attached, membranes with receptors but no cytoplasm, solutions of solubilized receptors) and solutions of antibodies at the other end.

Perhaps the most fundamental way in which binding assays differ is based on whether the amount of the binding protein in the assay system is limited or in excess (1). Analyzed in this way most typical hormone bioassays are excess binding reagent assays, and it is the biologic response initiated by the binding of the analyte to the receptor that is the amplifier and that provides the signal parameter measured. In this respect, these assays are different from radioimmunoassays (limited binding agent, analyte tracer measured) and immunoradiometric assays (excess binding reagent, labeled binding agent measured) (Table 1). In practice the distinction is that of different types of specificity (and not necessarily different degrees of

Table 1. Comparison of Protein-Binding, Receptor and Biological Assays

	Radioimmuno-assay	Immuno-radiometric assay	Receptor assay	Bioassay
Example of typical hormone assay				
Type of assay	Limited binding reagent	Excess binding reagent	Limited or excess binding reagent	Excess binding reagent
Component measured as response parameter	Labeled analyte	Labeled binding reagent	Labeled analyte or labeled receptor	Response of biologic matrix (cells or enzyme system) activated by analyte

specificity). Although a suggestion has been made for distinguishing two types of assays, those depending on structure and those depending on function, in fact the structure of an agonist is as relevant in a bioassay as it is in an immunoassay; there is essentially a difference in specificity and the way in which the signal is generated.

The ability to describe the specificity of an assay has far-reaching implications. A reference material shown to be suitable for one type of assay may not be suitable for another of different specificity, and calibration of a standard by one procedure may be quite inappropriate for use in other types of assays of other specificities.

THE BINDING REACTION: COMPARISON OF LIKE WITH LIKE—PARALLELISM

Virtually all in vivo bioassays and in vitro immunoassays involve the binding of analyte to a binding protein with a high order of affinity and specificity for the analyte. This strong binding forms the basic reaction of an assay. The strength of the binding depends on the closeness of fit of the binding sites on the binding protein and the complementary site(s) on the analyte or standard. Any difference between the molecular structure or conformation of the analyte in the specimen and that in the standard may give different binding characteristics, and hence dissimilar or unreproducible assay results.

It is thus one of the basic assumptions underlying the validity of an assay to determine the concentration of an analyte, that the analyte in the test specimen be compared in the assay with a standard of the identical substance. Only when complete identity occurs, and specimen and standard are free of interfering substances, can parallelism be expected in any assay system in which they are compared. Whenever this does not occur—as happens in almost all bioassays and immunoassays—it is necessary to show that the analyte in the specimen and the standard at least behave identically in the particular system(s) in which they are compared (i.e., in each individual assay). This is one reason why, in classic biologic standardization, parallelism is required to be demonstrated in each assay as part evidence of the validity of the estimate of relative potency.

It is a weakness of many routine clinical assay services that specimens are assayed at one dose level only, since specimens containing abnormal forms of the analyte (such as those produced by tumors), which would give non-parallelism and an invalid erroneous estimate, go unrecognized.

Thus the work of setting up an assay system involves demonstration that the standard used and the specificity of the system are such that parallelism will reliably be obtained with forms of the analyte that the assay system (kit) is intended to measure. While parallelism is essential for the validity of such assays, it is not by itself proof of validity of an assay or of the identity of an analyte in two preparations.

The problems of compliance with the axiom that like should be compared with like are manifold and have been discussed in detail (3–5). These problems arise mainly from two interrelated causes. One of them is that the specificity (the extent to which the result of an assay is not influenced by cross-reacting substances or other factors) in many assay systems is inadequate, inappropriate, or unknown. The other relates to the difficulty of exactly matching the molecular form(s) of the analyte in the test specimen with a suitable reference material (standard).

HETEROGENEITY OF ANALYTES: METABOLIC, INTRINSIC, ARTIFACTUAL: SYNTHETIC PEPTIDES

There are various types of heterogeneity of common analytes (Table 2). Many analytes that are commonly assayed—notably peptide hormones—occur in biologic fluids together with their precursors and metabolic forms; since each form may be partly similar to the analyte and able to cross-react in the assay system, they can influence the result. The family of peptides derived from the parent molecule proadrenocorticotrophin is a particularly well-analyzed example (6). Specimens of sera may contain different proportions of such structurally related forms, which in systems with even only slightly different binding characteristics can give rise to markedly dissimilar results. Many analytes (glycoprotein hormones, immunoglobulins, heparins) are themselves "intrinsically" heterogeneous and occur as groups of similar molecules, all with largely similar biologic activity. For certain of them, for example, human pituitary luteinizing hormone, individual groups have been isolated and their biologic characteristics analyzed (7). Natural polymorphism also occurs as genetic variants of viruses, certain hormones, and enzymes, and in the various and sometimes bizarre forms of proteins and peptide hormones produced by tumors. When preparations of synthetic peptides are assayed, it is essential to consider them po-

Table 2. Common Types of Heterogeneity of Analytes

Genetic:	isohormones, isoenzymes
Metabolic:	precursor and metabolic forms
Intrinsic:	glycoprotein hormones, immunoglobulins
Tumor:	normal and abnormal forms
Artefact:	degradation in biologic specimens, during extraction and purification and in preparation of synthetic peptides

tentially heterogeneous too, as explained below. Artifactual changes in the analyte can also occur in the handling and storage of specimens. Of course there are many immunoassay systems that can discriminate between individual metabolic forms even when they are only slightly different from each other; but evidence of such specificity requires particularly thorough tests.

When the particular molecular form(s) of the analyte that an assay has been designed for has been identified, the next problem is the preparation of a suitable reference material.

REFERENCE MATERIALS: DISTINCTION BETWEEN PURE CHEMICALS AND BIOLOGICALS

Reference material is a nonspecific term for a standard for calibration, a reference preparation, or a reference reagent; a standard or a reference preparation is an identified preparation of material of attested suitability, containing a specific analyte and intended for quantification or for assessment of the quality of an assay system.

An important distinction should be made between a so-called pure chemical, a substance such as a steroid or a drug whose exact structure can be determined completely by chemical and physical means alone, and substances such as proteins of complex molecular structure and usually of biologic origin, whose structure cannot be so determined. By tradition these substances are called *biologicals*. In this connection it should be said that preparations of synthetic peptides, particularly those of more than 10 residues, should not be assumed to be pure. The most rigorous testing is required to establish the identity and purity of peptides made by in vitro synthesis or by recombinant DNA procedures. To make such products pure requires that scrupulous purification procedures be used during and after synthesis; as evidence of the purity of such a product, information should be obtained from such tests as amino acid sequencing, end-group analysis, electrophoresis on various media, isoelectrophoresis, isotachophoresis, high-performance liquid chromatography using various separation systems, separation of molecules of different size and, where possible, bioassay against a measured quantity of the natural substance. Even such testing may fail to detect racemic isomers and certain other peptide impurities; and for certain purposes therefore it is advisable to regard a preparation of a synthetic peptide as a "biological".

As a standard for a simple chemical (such as a steroid or thyroxine), any pure sample of it is likely to be suitable, providing it complies with appropriate exact specifications of identity and purity.

In contrast, for biologicals it is necessary to have available suitable reference preparations. Moreover, so as to be able to compare validly the results of assays in which they are used, it is essential that each reference preparation of the substance be related to another by its calibration directly (or indirectly via another calibrated preparation), by one or more well-defined and attested assay procedures, against a single one of recognized international status.

PREPARATION AND CHARACTERIZATION OF REFERENCE MATERIALS

It is for this purpose that a service of international biologic standards and reference preparations has been provided since 1925. This service, set up by the League of Nations (used first, for example, for determination of the potency of insulin preparations), is now administered under the aegis of the Expert Committee on Biological Standardization (ECBS) of the World Health Organization (WHO).

Essential attributes of a reference material are that each sample of it must be identical to another and that the preparation must have measured suitable stability. The setting up of an international standard (8) entails the careful selection and testing of candidate materials, their ampuling under certain fastidious conditions to avoid damage to the analyte and to ensure its long-term stability; and assessment of the stability and suitability to serve as standards in various widely used bioassay and protein binding assay procedures in an international collaborative study. The report of each such study contains the collected data of chemical and physical analyses, the assay designs and methods of use, and the statistical assessment and interpretation of the results. The large scale of such studies, in which results of several hundred assays from 10 to 30 expert laboratories may be accumulated, often provides new information, seldom otherwise obtained, about the materials and the validity and precision of various assay procedures. The reports of such studies are therefore usually published in scientific journals (e.g., reference 9, and references in the Appendix). Such information constitutes the evidence on which a particular batch of ampuled material is considered suitable to be designated an international standard or an international reference preparation on the authorization of the ECBS and with the agreement of the participants in the collaborative study. Detailed guidance on how to prepare, ampul and characterize international, national, and laboratory standards has been published by WHO (10).

Table 3. Causes of Instability

Instability is loss, or chemical or configuration alteration commonly due to:

enzymes, e.g., peptidases, during extraction from biologic materials or present in other reagents, e.g., carrier proteins

oxidation, deamidation, alkylation

configurational change, dimerization, β-aspartyl shift

adsorption onto surfaces or on other molecules, e.g., denatured proteins

STABILITY: CAUSES OF INSTABILITY, MEASUREMENT OF STABILITY OF MATERIAL IN DRY FORM AND IN SOLUTION

It is axiomatic that a reference material have measured and adequate stability. The stability of a substance may be defined as its lack of alteration under defined conditions.

Common causes of instability of reference materials are listed in Table 3. Steps taken in the ampuling of biologic reference materials include avoidance of contamination with enzymes such as peptidases from biologic tissues or from microorganisms by making the preparation "clean" if not sterile, prevention of adsorption onto surfaces by adding a carrier substance, avoidance of oxidation by containing the preparation in an atmosphere of inert gas such as pure dry nitrogen, in neutral glass ampuls sealed by fusion of the glass, and limiting of moisture by desiccation so that the water content is below about 1–2%; ampuls are then stored in the dark at −20°C.

Instability is the result of a chemical change, and such changes can be accelerated by keeping the material at elevated temperatures. The rate of change of the material can be estimated with precision by accelerated thermal degradation studies (11) in which samples of the standard kept at various high temperatures (20, 37, and 56°C) for periods of time are assayed against samples kept at a low temperature such as −20°C. The large proportion of activity lost at the higher temperature can be estimated with greater precision than can the much smaller proporation lost at the lower temperature. In this way, using the Arrhenius equation, the log rate constant of change can be plotted against the reciprocal of the absolute temperature at which each sample was stored. If the plot is linear, it will then be possible to calculate the rate of loss at other temperatures. Results of accelerated degradation studies with international standards of a wide variety of biologic substances have given, in all instances, plots that were linear and thus shown that a first-order reaction was involved in the dry form in which the materials were ampuled.

Most international standards change by less (usually much less) than 1% per year at the temperature at which they are stored ($-20°$). Thus they are stable enough to last virtually unchanged for about 10–20 years, if need be, and to withstand transit in the mail for several days even under tropical conditions.

On the other hand, the stability of substances in solution is influenced by other conditions, and simple first-order change is less likely. Practical steps that can be taken to ensure the stability of proteins in solution (10, p. 140) include making a relatively concentrated solution of the protein; in addition, a suitable buffer with a relatively high eutectic freezing point and one that does not change pH at low temperatures should be used, thus potassium phosphate buffers are better in this respect than buffers made with sodium phosphate. The addition of a suitable carrier (e.g., 0.5% protein) helps to prevent the loss of certain peptides by adsorption onto glass and plastic surfaces, but the protein must be free of peptidase activity (12). A suitable bacteriostat such as azide is almost always advisable, as standards are clean but not necessarily sterile. To conserve stock solutions of standards it is advisable to subdivide them in small quantities into several small containers which, after they have been tightly closed, are rapidly frozen to a low temperature, for example in liquid nitrogen or solid CO_2, and then stored at a temperature below the eutectic freezing point of the constituents, that is, usually below $-40°C$. A fresh container can then be used every 1 or 2 weeks, or when necessary. Experience has shown that incorrect storage of standards is one of the most frequent causes of assay problems such as bias drift.

EXPRESSION OF ASSAY RESULTS: UNITS, MASS, NOMINAL CONTENT

Standardization requires a common way of expressing assay results. For substances considered pure chemicals, estimates of analyte concentration are usually stated as mass concentration (grams per liter) or substance concentration (molar per liter). Where it is desirable to relate the concentrations of analyte metabolites, it may be more convenient to state the results as substance concentration.

For biologic substances (q.v.) assayed in terms of biologic standards, the use of units defined by an identified and suitably calibrated reference material is recommended (5). International units of biologic activity have long been used satisfactorily for many substances such as insulin, human chorionic gonadotropin, and thyrotropin.

Similarly, for example, results of immunoassays for thyrotrophin are reported in units defined by the IRP of human thyrotropin for immunoassay.

The use of units in this way should be retained until there is general sustained agreement on the complete characterization of the substance by chemical means.

The statement of results in terms of mass of heterogeneous analyte or impure reference materials can cause endless confusion when it is necessary to relate potencies of more than two or three reference materials; it can be logically invalid to equate the mass of one heterogeneous analyte with the mass of a different unknown mixture unless the specificity of the method of comparison is completely defined.

Further confusion often arises from misunderstandings of statements of the mass content of a substance in a reference material. *Standard* or *reference material* always refers to the whole material, which may contain other unknown materials (as in the case of an impure extract) or added carrier substances, buffer salts, and water in addition to the substance itself. The proportion of the substance present may be extremely small, and it is often impossible to determine or calculate with accuracy the actual mass of pure substance present in an ampul of such material. Thus, whereas the unitage of an ampul of a standard is accurate by definition, the content of pure substance is stated as an approximate "nominal" amount.

Until assays are entirely analyte-specific, and while hetergoeneous mixtures are assayed, it is strongly recommended (8) that the result of each assay be stated as an estimate (with confidence limits) of mass and amount of substance (moles) or units per volume of the test specimen, together with a statement of the assay method and the standard used, the definition of the unit, the concentration of the standard, and the assay method used to assign this concentration.

ASSIGNMENT OF A UNITAGE: CONTINUITY OF THE UNIT

The unitage of WHO reference materials may be assigned on various grounds (3,10). It may be based on a unit already in widespread use, for example, a national standard or research standard, it may be made equivalent to the estimated mass or molar content, or it may be an empirical number, especially for a material of unknown purity. The ECBS of WHO has recommended that a first standard for a substance (e.g., a hormone) intended for immunoassays should have its unitage assigned on the basis of estimates of its units of biologic activity.

When an international reference material is replaced, the continuity of the unit is made by extensive assay of the replacement against the existing standard by a variety of well-established assay procedures, so as to determine whether there are consistent disparities between them. Where the standard and replacement are of similarly pure preparation, estimates generally agree well and continuity of the unitage is straightforward. On the other hand, when the materials are impure or mixtures are of slightly dissimilar molecular forms or of differing quality, then discrepancies in estimates by different assay procedures may be significant (5, p. 21). In this case a particular unitage must be decided upon by the ECBS. Such a decision may lead to a discontinuity of units for certain assays, and this must be made widely understood by publication of the report of the collaborative study of the ECBS.

It follows that such discontinuities will be less frequent and widespread if international and other standards are made to last a long time (normally 10–15 years) and to be used as widely as possible; the provision of international working standards based on a stock of master ampuls of the same bulk material has been strongly advocated (10, p. 129). It also follows that each manufacturer's new replacement standard should be calibrated by assays directly against the primary (international) one by the assay procedure(s) with which it will be used.

AVAILABILITY OF REFERENCE MATERIALS

Preparations used as standards come from various sources, including research workers, manufacturers, national organizations such as the American National Pituitary Agency, the National Institute for Biological Standards and Control (NIBSC), and WHO. The extent to which they have been ampuled, characterized, and shown to be suitable for their purpose varies considerably. The information about its preparation and characterization is an essential attribute of a standard and should be made available; a memorandum on international reference materials is routinely provided with ampuls.

The service of WHO reference materials is the result of international collaborative work on a very extensive scale. It is fully documented in successive reports of the ECBS and in unpublished documents of this committee, in publications in the scientific literature, and in information provided by the custodian laboratory. A list of such preparations made available by WHO and NIBSC is given in the Appendix.

There is also of course an immense range of substances for which official international reference materials have not yet been, or will not be, provided. There are great advantages in providing reference materials in the early stages of research on a biological, particularly when new methods of assay are being developed. There are indeed other pragmatic grounds for the organized provision of working reference materials even though they may not all be strictly defined as biologicals (Table 4).

Table 4.

Reference preparations are particularly useful for substances that are:

Unable to be completely characterized by chemical and physical means alone (e.g., WHO biologic standards and reference preparations)

Of unknown composition or complex and ill-defined (e.g., erythropoietin)

Heterogeneous (e.g., glycoprotein hormones)

Difficult to isolate in pure form (e.g., synthetic peptides)

Scarce or costly (e.g., gastrins, parathyroid hormone)

Unstable or easily altered during isolation (e.g., secretin, human growth hormone)

Difficult or costly to be assayed or characterized (e.g., prolactin, thyrotrophin)

ESTABLISHMENT OF INTERNATIONAL STANDARDS: SCIENTIFIC AND LEGAL IMPLICATIONS

New international standards and reference preparations, consisting where possible of the most highly purified preparations, are established each year by the ECBS of WHO. Each is recorded in successive reports of this committee. The formal establishment of an international standard has both scientific and legal implications. One feature of a biologic reference material is that it forms part of the scientific definition of the substance. A hormone such as thyrotrophin is identified by its activity in stimulating thyroid cells to produce thyroxine, and it is the standard used to quantify the activity in suitable bioassay procedures. What the scientific community calls erythropoietin is the entity that has the highest biological activity when bioassayed against the International Reference Preparation (IRP) of erythropoietin (13).

The editorial policies of scientific journals propagate this by insisting, rightly, that reported estimates of biological substances should relate to international reference materials where appropriate. But it should not be forgotten that it is a basic assumption that the ampuled reference material is the "right" material, even when it is backed by all the evidence from an international collaborative study.

The establishment of WHO reference materials also has legal implications insofar as member nations of WHO undertake to use them—and the international units they define. These units are used in official WHO and national manufacturing requirements (14) and specifications. Manufacturers who sell their products and assay kits in different countries normally calibrate their working standards against the WHO reference materials, and any country or individual purchasing a kit can expect it to be so calibrated.

GENERAL MEASURES TO IMPROVE STANDARDIZATION

Considerable improvements may be expected to follow publications on various aspects of standardization formulated jointly by WHO, the Expert Panel on Immunoassay of the International Federation of Clinical Chemists, the International Society for Endocrinology, and the International Atomic Energy Agency. These include papers on the nature and types of assays, a proposed classification of in vitro protein binding assay systems, requirements for the manufacture of assay kits and reagents (annex 10, 31st Report, WHO ECBS, 1980), recommendations on the control of quality of assay performance, guidance on the preparation and characterization of international, national, and laboratory standards (10), including advice on the storage of protein solutions at low temperatures (p. 140), and proposals for terminology and definitions in assay methodology.

Improvements are already coming from the introduction into several countries of organized systems for affecting external quality control by monitoring the performance of assays in individual laboratories and from other steps for reducing interlaboratory bias and within-laboratory imprecision.

ACKNOWLEDGMENT

I am grateful to Fiona Forrester for help in preparation of the manuscript.

REFERENCES

1. Ekins RP: General principles of hormone assay, in Loraine JA, Bell ET (eds): in *Hormone Assays and Their Clinical Application,* ed 4, 1976.
2. Bangham DR: Biological standards in clinical endocrinology: Some soluble and insoluble problems, in Wilson DW, Gaskell SJ, Kemp KW (eds): *Quality Control in Clinical Endocrinology.* Cardiff, Wales, Alpha Omega Publ. Ltd, 1982, pp 43–49.
3. Bangham DR, Cotes PM: Reference standards for radioimmunoassay, in Kirkham KE, Hunter WM (eds): *Radioimmunoassay Methods.* Edinburgh, London, Churchill Livingstone, 1971, pp 345–368.

4. Bangham DR, Cotes PM: Standardization and standards. *Br Med Bull* 30:12, 1974.

5. WHO Expert Committee on Biological Standardization, 26th report. *WHO Tech Rep Ser No 565,* 1975, p 21.

6. Eipper BA, Mains ER: Structure and biosynthesis of proadrenocorticotropin/endorphin and related peptides. *Endocrinol Rev* 1(1):1, 1980.

7. Robertson DM, Froysa B, Diczfalusy E: Biological and immunological characterization of human LH. IV: Biological and immunological profile of 2 IRPs after electrofocusing. *Mol Cell Endocrinol* 11:91, 1978.

8. Bangham DR: Standardization in peptide hormone immunoassays: Principle and practice. *Clin Chem* 22(7):957, 1976.

9. Storring PL, Gaines-Das RE, Bangham DR: International reference preparation of human chorionic gonadotrophin for immunoassay: Potency estimates in various bioassay and protein binding assay systems; and IRPs of the α and β subunits of human chorionic gonadotropin for immunoassay. *J Endocrinol* 84:295, 1980.

10. WHO Expert Committee on Biological Standardization, 29th report, Annex 4: Guidelines for the preparation and establishment of reference materials and reference reagents for biological substances. *WHO Tech Rep Ser No 626,* 1978.

11. Jerne NK, Perry WLM: The stability of biological standards. *Bull WHO* 14:167, 1956.

12. Caygill CPJ: Detection of peptidase activity in albumin preparations. *Clin Chim Acta* 78:507, 1977.

13. Cotes PM, Annable L, Mussett MV: The second international reference preparation of erythropoietin, human, urinary, for bioassay. *Bull WHO* 47:99, 1972.

14. WHO Expert Committee on Biological Standardization, 31st report, Annex 10: Requirements for immunoassay kits and reagents. *WHO Tech Rep Ser* No. 658, 1981.

APPENDIX

Standard	Ampoul Code No.	Defined Activity	Approximate Composition of Ampoul Contents	Other Information
Angiotensin I (Asp-Isoleu^5)	71/328	9 μg/ampul, nominal	9 μg synthetic angiotensin I, 2 mg mannitol	*Clin Sci Mol Med* 48:135S, 1975
Angiotensin II (Asp-Ileu^5)	70/302	24 μg/ampul, nominal	24 μg synthetic angiotensin II, 2 mg mannitol	*Clin Sci Mol Med* 48:135S, 1975
1st IS for Arginine Vasopressin	77/501	8.2 IU/ampul	20 μg synthetic arginine vasopressin, 5 mg human albumin, citric acid	WHO unpublished working document WHO/BS/78.1231
1st IRP of Calcitonin, human, for bioassay	70/324	1.0 U/ampul	10 μg synthetic calcitonin of sequence found in tumors, 5 mg mannitol	*Acta Endocrinol.* 1980, 93:37
1st IRP of Calcitonin, porcine, for bioassay	70/306	1.0 IU/ampul	10 μg purified extract, 5 mg mannitol	T$_3$ and T$_4$ trace amounts WHO/BS/74.1077
1st IRP of Calcitonin, salmon, for bioassay	72/158	80 IU/ampul	20 μg synthetic salmon calcitonin II, 2 mg mannitol	WHO unpublished working document WHO/BS/74.1077
1st IRP of Chorionic gonadotropin for immunoassay	75/537	650 IU/ampul	70 μg chorionic gonadotropin, 5 mg human albumin	*Bull WHO* 1976, 54:463–470 *J Endocrinol* 1980, 84:295–310.
1st IRP of α subunit of chorionic gonadotropin	75/569	70 IU/ampul	70 μg chorionic gonadotropin α subunit, 5 mg human albumin	*Bull WHO* 1976, 460–470 *J Endocrinol* 1980, 84:294–310.

APPENDIX (Continued)

Standard	Ampoul Code No.	Defined Activity	Approximate Composition of Ampoul Contents	Other Information
1st IRP of β subunit of chorionic gonadotropin	75/551	70 IU/ampul	70 μg chorionic gonadotropin β subunit, 5 mg human albumin	Bull WHO 1976, 54:463–470 J. Endocrinol 1980,84:295–310
2nd IS for chorionic gonadotropin for bioassay	61/6	5300 IU/ampul	2 mg chorionic gonadotropin, 5 mg lactose	Bull WHO 1964, 31:111–125
Corticotropin, human	74/555		11.6 μg corticotrophin, 5 mg human albumin, 2.5 mg mannitol	Bioassay versus 3rd IS: s.c. adrenal ascorbate depletion assay, 3.19 IU/ampul
3rd IS for corticotrophin (ACTH), porcine, for bioassay, international working standard	59/16 Various	5.0 IU/ampul 5.0 IU/ampul	50 μg pituitary extract, 5 mg lactose	Bull WHO 1962, 27:395 J Endocrinol 1980, 85:533–539 Vasopressin <25 MU/ampul by rat blood pressure assay in terms of IS
1st IS for desmopressin	78/573	27 IU/ampul	27 μg purified desmopressin, 5 mg human albumin, citric acid	WHO unpublished working document WHO/BS/80.1226
2nd IRP of erythropoietin, human, urinary, for bioassay	67/343	10 IU/ampul	2 mg urinary extract containing erythropoietin, 3 mg sodium chloride	Bull WHO 1972, 47:99–122

Preparation	Code No.	Unitage	Contents	Reference
2nd IRP of FSH/LH, human, pituitary for bioassay	78/549	FSH:10 IU/ampul LH:25 IU/ampul	0.5 mg FSH/LH, 1.25 mg lactose	*J Clin Endocrinol Metab* 1973, 36:647–660
IS FSH/LH, human, urinary, for bioassay	70/45	FSH:54 IU/ampul LH:46 IU/ampul	1 mg human postmenopausal urine extract, 5 mg lactose	*Acta Endocrinol* 1976, 83:700–710
Gastrin, human	68/439	12 U/ampul	12.6 μg synthetic gastrin, as hexamonium salt, 5 mg lactose, phosphate buffer	
Gastrin II, porcine	66/138	10 U/ampul	10 μg gastrin II, 5 mg sucrose, phosphate buffer	
1st IRP of glucagon, porcine, for bioassay	69/194	1.49 IU/ampul	1.5 mg glucagon, 5 mg lactose, 0.24 mg sodium chloride	*Acta Endocrinol* 1974, 77:705–714 *J Biol Stand* 1975, 3:263–265
1st IS for glucagon, porcine, for immunoassay	69/194	1.49 IU/ampul	1.5 mg glucagon, 5 mg lactose, 0.24 mg sodium chloride	*Acta Endocrinol* 1974, 77:705–714 *J Biol Stand* 1975,3:263–265
1st IRP for Gonadorelin for bioassay	77/596	31 IU/ampul	31 nmol synthetic gonadorelin, 2.5 mg lactose, 0.5 mg human albumin	Ovine/porcine sequence WHO unpublished working document WHO/BS/78.1219
1st IRP of growth hormone, human, for immunoassay	66/217	0.35 IU/ampul	175 μg growth hormone, 5 mg sucrose, phosphate buffer	Prolactin activity: pigeon, 1 IU/ampul; rabbit, 7 IU/amp; decidual response (mice) 1 IU/amp

APPENDIX (Continued)

Standard	Ampoul Code No.	Defined Activity	Approximate Composition of Ampoul Contents	Other Information
Insulin C-peptide for immunoassay	76/561	2.5 nm/ampul approx.	10 μg synthetic human insulin, C-peptide analogue, 50 μg human albumin, .05 nmole phosphate buffer	Synthetic (64-formyl-lysine) human proinsulin 31–65. *Diabetologia* 1980, 18:197–204
1st IRP of insulin, human, for immunoassay	66/304	3.0 IU/ampul	130 μg insulin, 5 mg sucrose	WHO unpublished working document WHO/BS/74.1084
4th IS for insulin, bovine and porcine, for bioassay	58/6	24.0 IU/mg	100–125 mg crystals, 42% porcine insulin, 58% bovine insulin	*Bull WHO* 1959,20:1209 *Diabetologia* 1975, 11:581–584
1st IRP of LH, human pituitary, for immunoassay	68/40	77 IU/ampul	11.6 μg LH, 5 mg lactose, 1 mg human albumin, 1 mg sodium chloride	*Acta Endocrinol* 1978,88:250–259
1st IS for lysine vasopressin	77/512	7.7 IU/ampul	30 μg synthetic lysine-vasopressin acetate, 5 mg human albumin, citric acid	WHO unpublished working document WHO/BS/78.1227
4th IS for oxytocin	76/575	12.5 IU/ampul	24 μg synthetic oxytocin acetate, 5 mg human albumin, citric acid	WHO unpublished working document WHO/BS/78.1230
Parathyroid hormone, human, for immunoassay	75/549	0.025 U/ampul	250 ng extract of human adenomata, 250 μg human albumin, 1.25 mg lactose	Estimated to contain ~25 ng parathyroid hormone *J Endocrinol* 1980, 86:291–304

Preparation	Code	Potency	Contents	Reference
1st IRP of parathyroid hormone, human, for immunoassay	79/500	0.100 IU/amp	100 ng purified extract of human adenomata, 250 μg human albumin, 1.25 mg lactose	—
1st IRP of parathyroid hormone, bovine, for bioassay	67/342	200 IU/amp	0.6 mg gland extract, 5 mg lactose	WHO unpublished working document WHO/BS/74.1078
1st IRP of parathyroid hormone, bovine, for immunoassay	71/324	2.0 IU/amp	1 μg purified extract, 200 μg human albumin, 1 mg lactose	WHO unpublished working document WHO/BS/74.1078
IRP of placental lactogen, human, for immunoassay	73/545	0.000850 IU/amp	850 μg placental lactogen, 5 mg mannitol	Br J Obstet Gynaecol 1978, 85:451–459
2nd IS for prolactin, ovine, for bioassay	57/8	22 IU/mg	10 mg extract	Bull WHO 1963, 29:721
1st IRP of renin, human, for bioassay	68/356	0.1 IU/amp	0.27 mg renal extract, 5 mg lactose, phosphate buffer	Clin Sci Mol Med 1975, 48:135S
2nd IS for serum gonadotrophin, equine, for bioassay	62/1	1600 IU/amp	0.8 mg extract, 5 mg lactose	Bull WHO 1966, 35:761
1st IRP of tetracosactrin, for bioassay	80/590	490 IU/amp	490 μg tetracosactrin, 20 mg mannitol	—
1st IRP of TSH, human, for immunoassay	68/38	150 IU/amp	46.2 μg TSH extract, 5 mg lactose, 1 mg human albumin	Acta Endocrinol 1978, 88:291–297
1st IS for thyrotrophin, bovine, for bioassay	53/11	74 mU/mg	1 part pituitary extract, 19 parts lactose	Bull WHO 1955, 13:917

SUGGESTED READING

Bangham DR, Mussett MV: The fourth international standard for insulin. *Bull WHO* 20:1209, 1959.

Bangham DR, Mussett MV, Stack-Dunne MP: The third international standard for corticotrophin. *Bull WHO* 27:395, 1962.

Bangham DR, Mussett MV, Stack-Dunne MP: The second international standard for prolactin. *Bull WHO* 29:721, 1963.

Bangham DR, Grab B: The second international standard for human chorionic gonadotrophin. *Bull WHO* 31:111, 1964.

Bangham DR, Woodward PM: The second international standard for serum gonadotrophin. *Bull WHO* 35:761, 1966.

Bangham DR, Berryman I, Burger H, et al: An international collaborative study of 69/104, a reference preparation of human pituitary FSH and LH. *J Clin Endocrinol Metab* 36:647, 1973.

Bangham DR, Salokangas AA, Annable L, et al: The first international standard for glucagon. *Acta Endocrinol* 77:705, 1974.

Bangham DR, Robertson I, Robertson JIS, et al: An international collaborative study of renin assay: Establishment of the international reference preparation of human renin. *Clin Sci Mol Med* 48:135S, 1975.

Canfield RE, Ross GT: A new reference preparation of human chorionic gonadotrophin and its subunits. *Bull WHO* 54:436, 1976.

Caygill CPJ, Gaines-Das RE, Bangham DR: Use of a common standard for comparison of insulin C-peptide measurements by different laboratories. *Diabetologia* 18:197, 1980.

Cotes PM, Annable L, Mussett MV: The second international reference preparation of erythropoietin, human, urinary, for bioassay. *Bull WHO* 47:99, 1972.

Cotes PM, Gaines-Das RE: An international collaborative study of the assay of human placental lactogen: Establishment of WHO international reference preparation of human placental lactogen. *Br J Obstet Gynaecol* 85:451, 1978.

Cotes PM, Gaines-Das RE, Kirkwood RBL, et al: The stability of standards for radioimmunoassay of human TSH: Research Standard A and the international reference preparation initially 68/38. *Acta Endocrinol* 88:291, 1978.

Gaines-Das RE, Cotes PM: International reference preparation of human prolactin for immunoassay: Definition of the international unit, report of a collaborative study and comparison of estimates of human prolactin made in various laboratories. *J Endocrinol* 80:157, 1979.

Mussett MV, Perry WLM: The international standard for thyrotrophin. *Bull WHO* 13:917, 1955.

Storring PL, Greaves PL, Mussett MV, et al: Stability of the fourth international standard for insulin. *Diabetologia* 11:581, 1975.

Storring PL, Dixon H, Bangham DR: The first international standard for human urinary FSH and human urinary LH (ICSH) for bioassay. *Acta Endocrinol* 83:700, 1976.

Storring PL, Bangham Dr, Cotes PM, et al: The international reference preparation of human pituitary luteinising hormone for immunoassay. *Acta Endocrinol* 88:250, 1978.

Storring PL, Gaines-Das GE, Bangham DR: International reference preparation of human chorionic gonadotrophin for immunoassay: Potency estimates in various bioassay and protein binding assay systems; and international reference preparations of the α and β subunits of human chorionic gonadotrophin for immunoassay. *J Endocrinol* 84:295, 1980.

Storring PL, Gaines-Das RE, Tiplady RJ, et al: Stability of the third international standard for corticotrophin: Accelerated degradation study using different bioassays and isoelectric focusing. *J Endocrinol* 85:533, 1980.

Zanelli JM, Gaines-Das RE: International collaborative study of research standard A for human parathyroid hormone, for immunoassay. *J Endocrinol* 86:291, 1980.

CHAPTER 7

SEPARATION OF BOUND FROM FREE HORMONE

William D. Odell

Although many investigators study the interactions of the antiserum and analyte or receptor and hormone in great detail, few characterize as carefully the method of separating bound and free analyte. It is extremely important to recognize that the separation method is a major source of error in competitive protein binding assays (probably the largest single source of major error). The separation method must be characterized in detail for specificity and precision and be well enough understood to permit troubleshooting when assays "go bad." Errors in the separation step directly result in errors in measurement of the substance the assay is designed to quantify.

The ideal method for separating bound and free analyte would be simple, rugged,* precise, and inexpensive. The ideal method would never misclassify, that is, indicate some bound analyte as free, or vice versa, and would not be affected by variations in sample constituency (e.g., osmolality, protein content, pH). In practice, the ideal method does not exist. A large number of separation methods have been described, but each has its own limitations and problems. Table 1 lists the major categories of separation methods. Note that all these methods depend on a substantial size difference in free analyte and antibody-bound analyte (e.g., free insulin and bound insulin). Fortunately, most hormones are small proteins, or even smaller thyronines or steroids. However, competitive protein binding assays are also used to quantify large substances (e.g., viruses). For the separation of bound and free analyte with a high molecular weight (> 300,000), solid phase-conjugated antibodies may be used. More commonly, assay techniques based on different principles are used, for example, "sandwich" assays as discussed in Chapter 13.

Rugged indicates simply that the technique performs well, is not easily subject to errors, and is capable of being done in most laboratories on the first try. Modest errors do not greatly affect the result.

Table 1. Methods of Separating
Bound from Free Analyte

Chromatoelectrophoresis
Gel filtration
Immunoprecipitation
Chemical separation
Adsorbent techniques
Solid phase
Polymerized antibodies

CHROMATOELECTROPHORESIS

Chromatoelectrophoresis is seldom used anymore. However, it is of interest because it was the first separation method employed by Berson and Yalow for the insulin in radioimmunoassay, and understanding its principles makes easier the understanding of other methods. It is an empirical method and depends upon the fact that some radioiodinated peptides or proteins (or other analytes) have greater avidity for the cellulose of paper than does the antibody-bound analyte. This is not always true and varies with the type of paper (possibly even lots or batches of paper), pH, and protein content of the solution. Figure 1 illustrates this method from an early publication of Yalow and Berson (1). This method as used by these investigators appears to be principally a chromatography method, since strips of paper were placed in an electrophoresis unit open to the air, permitting evaporation. Radioiodinated insulin (free) remained at the origin, and radioiodinated insulin bound to antibody (bound) moved near the solvent front. By quantifying the radioiodine in two peaks, an estimate of bound and free insulin was obtained. However, when only radioiodinated insulin was run in this system, not all of it remained at the origin; a small (and variable) percentage moved or migrated in the same manner as an antibody-bound hormone and was defined by Yalow and Berson (2) as "damaged" hormone. It is important to realize that damaged hormone by this criteria may or may not be unable to bind to antibody or receptor and, furthermore, that the hormone remaining at the origin (defined as "undamaged" in this system) may or may not bind to antibody or receptor; if it does, it may not bind with a single affinity or avidity. The definition of damaged or undamaged applies to this separation method and applies using a constant batch or lot of a particular paper under defined conditions. If, for example, the protein content of the solution containing the radioiodinated analyte is increased, part or all of the radioiodinated analyte may move from the origin. This author has seen several laboratory groups

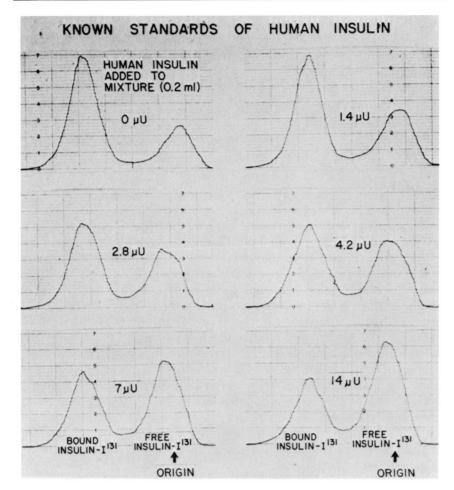

Figure 1. Radiochromatoelectrophoretograms of antiserum–insulin mixtures. Mixtures contained the same concentrations of guinea pig antibeef insulin serum and beef ^{131}I-labeled insulin but varying concentrations of human insulin as indicated. [Reproduced with permission from Yalow et al., 1960 (2).]

attempt to assess rigorously a variety of radioiodinated proteins using paper chromatoelectrophoresis and defining, without further evaluation, all radioiodinated analyte that adhered at the origin of a paper strip as high-quality or undamaged hormone. Assessment by antibody binding or receptor binding may reveal a very different answer.

Before leaving the discussion of this system, it might be noted that Berson and Yalow found some radioiodinated proteins so adherent to the paper used that, even when bound to antibody, they still remained at the origin. In the example of the growth hormone radioimmunoassay, they applied plasma or serum as a source of additional protein, determining empirically how much was required for the assay, under the conditions used, to permit bound growth hormone to migrate while free hormone remained at the origin.

As indicated in the first part of this discussion, this method is seldom used anymore because it is time-consuming and impractical for handling a large number of samples.

GEL FILTRATION

Separation of bound from free analyte using cross-linked dextrans (Sephadex) columns has also been used (3). This method, although simple, is slow and not applicable to large numbers of samples. It has been extensively used in developmental studies, particularly for steroids. Theoretically, the method is sound. "Mini"-Sephadex columns are generally used. If the immunoassays are being used to quantify analyte in buffer (as opposed to serum or plasma samples), it is important to saturate nonspecific surface binding sites on glass and Sephadex. This is usually done by passage through an albumin sample [e.g., 2% bovine serum albumin, (BSA)] before addition of the assay sample. We will not discuss this method further, since column preparation and collection of many effluents is time-consuming and much simpler methods are available.

IMMUNOPRECIPITATION

Immunoprecipitation is commonly called the double-antibody method and was originally described in an abstract by Feinberg (4) in 1956 and in a full-length paper by Skom and Talmage (5) in 1958. Subsequently, it was adapted for use in radioimmunoassays by Utiger et al. (6) for growth hormone, and for insulin by Morgan and Lazarow (7). The method involves precipitation of the antibody–analyte complex (bound) by a second antiserum, an anti-γ-globulin. For example, if the first antibody or antianalyte is a rabbit antiserum produced against human growth hormone, the second antiserum might be sheep or goat anti-rabbit γ-globulin. After incubation of the assay tubes containing radioiodinated analyte and the first antibody, the second antibody is added and the mixture incubated for additional time. Following this, tubes are centrifuged (commonly at 500g for 10 minutes), the supernatant is decanted or aspirated, and precipitates [containing the antigen–antibody complexes (bound)] assessed for radioactivity.

This method is very simple in practice, and large numbers of tubes can be handled in a short time using automatic pipetting devices. However, a number of problems can arise. It is of interest, historically, that this method could not be used on serum samples. Utiger (6) and Morgan et al. (8) found that serum or plasma interfered with the second-antibody precipitation step (i.e., it worked only with buffer). Morgan et al. (8) reported that this inhibitory activity was heat-labile and could be prevented by EDTA; they concluded that it was caused by a component of complement. Soeldner and Slone (9) reported that heparanized plasma had considerably less effect than serum and that the decrease in inhibitory activity was related to the amount of heparin added. However, other investigators failed to show striking differences with plasma and serum. Soeldner and Slone used a guinea pig anti-insulin as the first antibody and a rabbit anti-guinea pig γ-globulin as the second antibody. At present, it is most common to add EDTA routinely to all assays involving plasma or serum when employing the double-antibody separation system (generally 100 μl 0.5 M EDTA, pH 7.5, is added to each 900 μl of assay mixture—total volume of assay 1 ml).

Other factors also influence this separation system. Each batch of second antibody must be tested in detail for the amount required. This amount varies with the concentration of γ-globulin present in the assay tubes. Since most immunoassays use the first antiserum in very high dilutions (e.g., final dilution 1×10^6), the desired γ-globulin concentration is achieved by adding carrier γ-globulin in the form of normal (non-immunized) serum. For a rabbit immunoassay for human growth hormone, therefore, normal rabbit serum (NRS) is added.* Various publications suggest that wide ranges of NRS are used, varying from 0.1% to as high as 2% (e.g., contrast references 11 and 12). Whatever percentage of normal animal serum is selected, investigators should be aware that the time required to produce the separation of bound and free analyte is considerably longer for smaller amounts of carrier γ-globulin (e.g., NRS) than for larger amounts. For example, for assays employing 0.1 or 0.2% NRS, a common protocol is to incubate assay reagents for 48 hours at 4°C and then to add the second antibody and continue the incubation for 72 hours more. In contrast, using 1 or 2% NRS, a common protocol is to incubate assay reagents for 4 days at 4°C, and then to add the second antibody and incubate only 12–24 hours longer. Thus, variations in carrier χ-globulin determine different time requirements for the second-antibody incubation.

A second variable determining the time required to reach the separation of bound and free analyte using the double-antibody technique is temperature. A third variable is the amount of serum or plasma in the assay tube. Figures 2ab and 3 illustrates these points. Table 2 lists the variables to be

---

*Anti-γ-globulin antisera are usually highly specific. Thus, goat or sheep anti-rabbit γ-globulin does not react against the human γ-globulin present in human serum samples to be assayed. High species specificity exists.

assessed in detail when setting up a radioimmunoassay procedure using the double-antibody separation method. Figure 3 shows three titration curves for a single batch of sheep anti-rabbit γ-globulin using 0.2% NRS but incubated for three time periods at three temperatures. Note that, at 37°C, the amount of sheep anti-rabbit γ-globulin must be accurately pipetted at 50 µl. Any errors in this pipetting produce change in the amount of hormone interpreted as bound. However, at 4°C, once 75 γl or more of sheep anti-rabbit γ-globulin has been added, variations in the amount have little impact on the assay. If one chose to add 125 µl, the separation method could tolerate considerable variation in volume (pipetting error) as long as the temperature remained near 4°C. These details become particularly important when assays are shortened to reduce turnaround time. It therefore becomes essential to determine these details for the exact conditions under which the assay is to be performed and then not to deviate from these conditions unless one is prepared to reassess the separation step in detail.

Damaged* radiolabeled hormone is assessed two ways in the double-anti-

*Damaged hormone is hormone that shows no immunoreactivity.

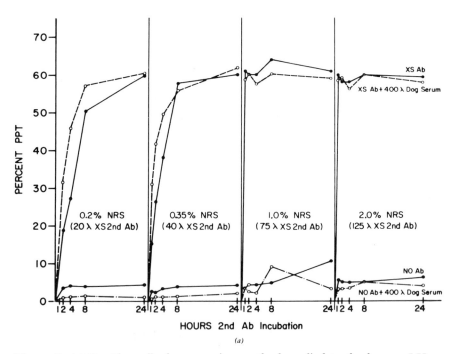

Figure 2. (a) Double-antibody separation method applied to the human LH radioimmunoassay. Influence of varying amounts of carrier α-globulin (normal rabbit serum, NRS) on the time characteristics incubated at 37°C.

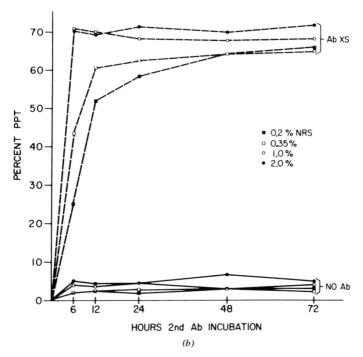

(b) Double-antibody separation method applied to the human LH assay. Influence of varying amounts of carrier γ-globulin (normal rabbit serum, NRS) on the time characteristics in the absence of serum. [Reproduced with permission from Odell et al., 1974 (10).]

body technique: (1) by incubation of radiolabeled hormone with excess first antibody to assess total immunoreactivity, and (2) by incubation of label in the absence of first antibody but using the separation method.† The latter also defines the blank of the system, which varies with the amount of carrier rabbit serum used. It is usually 2–3% of the total radioactivity when 0.2% NRS is used, and 6–7% when 2% NRS is used. Optimally, the total

†The precipitate can be washed, free trapped counts.

Table 2. Parameters Effecting Double-Antibody Separation of Bound and Free Analyte

Characteristics of the second antiserum (e.g., affinity titer)
Incubation temperature
Incubation time
Amount carrier γ-globulin
Quantity of analyte serum
pH of assay

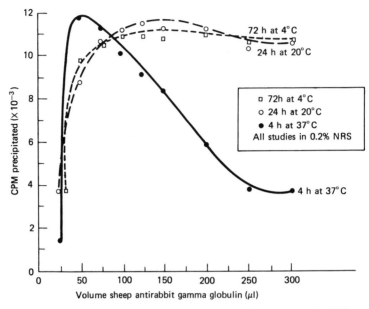

Figure 3. Dose–response curves for second antibody (sheep anti-rabbit α-globulin) precipitation of anti-HCG ^{125}I-labeled HCG immune complexes performed under three environmental conditions. Note that, at 4° and 20°C, there is a plateau of counts precipitated whereas at 37°, no plateau is seen. (γ-globulin diluted 1:5 before adding the volumes stated). (Data from M. Evans and W. Odell.)

immunoreactivity (in combination with excess first antibody) of a high-quality radioiodinated hormone is over 85%. These two tests do not indicate that a homogeneous label is present, nor do they assess possible variable effects on the label produced by different serum, plasma, or other analyte-containing samples.

CHEMICAL SEPARATION METHOD

As indicated previously, a considerable difference in molecular size usually exists between free analyte and bound analyte. In these instances, the bound analyte complex (usually larger) may be effectively separated from free analyte by chemical precipitation. Table 3 lists some of the reagents that have been employed. Obviously, a large number of chemicals can be selected, depending on the solubility characteristics of the analyte. The first use of this approach for immunoassays was by Grodsky and Forsham (13), who used sodium sulfite precipitation to separate bound and free insulin (the concentration was 17% in the assay tube). Odell et al. (14) used the

Table 3. Examples of Chemical
Separation Reagents

Ethanol–alcohol (TSH,LH)
Polyethylene glycol (many hormones)
Sodium sulfite (insulin)
Ammonium sulfate (steroids, cAMP)
Trichloracetic acid (growth hormone)

known solubility of the glycoprotein thyroid-stimulating hormone (TSH) in 55% ethanol–5% sodium chloride to devise a chemical separation method for the TSH radioimmunoassay. Perhaps the best chemical separation technique employs polyethylene glycol (PEG) (Carbowax) (15). This material may be prepared in solutions of varied concentration. The correct volume and concentration are rapidly pipetted into each assay tube, and tubes are then centrifuged. The method is particularly good for steroids and thyronines and is also quite satisfactory for some protein hormone and receptor assays.

To assess the adequacy of any chemical reagent as a separation method, it is wise to prepare a series of assay tubes containing the radiolabeled ana-

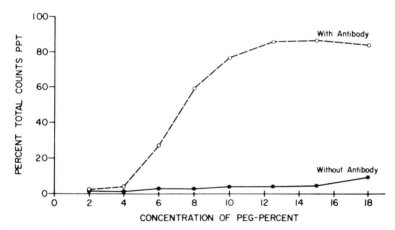

Figure 4. The testosterone radioimmunoassay. Assessment of PEG as separation method. Note that PEG is an excellent method of separation for this assay using this antiserum. No curves are shown, since for most steroid RIAs serum or plasma is first extracted using organic solvents; the solvent is then evaporated, and the steroid redissolved in buffer. Thus, assessment of this separation method was made only in buffer. However, for steroid RIAs performed on serum or plasma directly, such data are required before selecting a separation method. Note that PEG offers a very "precise" method, since an amount can be selected that is in the plateau region (i.e., 14%) of both curves; pipetting error, unless very great, would not affect assay results. [Reproduced with permission from Odell et al., 1974. (10).]

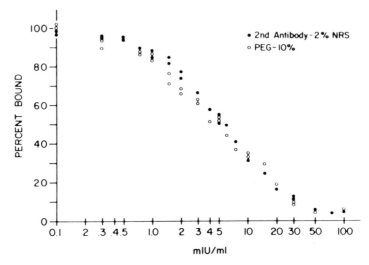

Figure 5. Comparison of dose–response curves for a human LH radioimmunoassay using two separation techniques in which each separation technique was independently selected as being satisfactory. In this study, all RIA tubes were prepared in duplicate and the two separation methods were then used. The second antibody was incubated at 4°C for 24 hours; the PEG was added and the tubes then centrifuged 10–15 minutes later. [Reproduced with permission from Odell et al., 1974 (10).]

lyte without antibody or receptor (zero percentage-bound tubes) and a second series of tubes containing excess antibody or receptor (100% bound or maximal bound tubes). After incubation to permit radiolabeled analyte to reach equilibrium with the antibody or receptor, the chemical separation reagent is added in varying amounts to pairs of tubes (0% series and 100% series). Figure 4 illustrates such a study with the testosterone radioimmunoassay. The PEG separation method was first applied by Desbuquois and Aurbach (15), who emphasized the importance of carefully assessing the effects of varying concentrations. Figure 5 shows dose–response curves for the human luteinizing hormone (LH) radioimmunoassay separated by both double-antibody technique and PEG. Each technique was optimized before use by the procedures described. Figure 6 illustrates a prostate cytosol androgen receptor assay using PEG as a separation method. Note that, in this assay, increasing amounts of PEG precipitated increasing amounts of receptor-bound dihydrotestosterone (DHT). When excess unlabeled DHT was added to define specific binding, increasing quantities of PEG also precipitated increased labeled DHT which was nonspecifically bound (i.e., not displaceable with excess cold); the dose–response relations differ. When only labeled DHT was present (without receptor), only a small change in precipitated DHT was produced by increasing concentrations of PEG. Analysis of these data indicates that PEG is not a good method for use

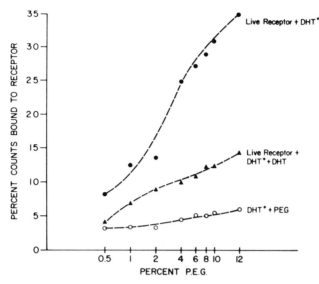

Figure 6. Rat prostate cytosol receptor assay for dihydrotestosterone (DHT); dose–response curves for varying amounts of polyethylene glycol. DHT* indicates [³H]DHT; DHT* + indicates [³H] + DHT plus excess unlabeled DHT. We have found that small amounts of protein affect the PEG precipitation curves. For example, all these curves are shifted to the right if the 2% γ-globulin (0.2% final concentration in tube) is omitted. [Reproduced with permission from Odell et al., 1974 (10).]

in the androgen–receptor assay. Unfortunately, charcoal, employed in an absorption method commonly used, is little better; no optimal method is known.

ADSORBENT TECHNIQUES

This technique depends upon the differential surface binding of small free hormone (analyte) and larger antibody-bound analyte. Because charge–charge interactions are involved, the concentration of electrolytes and proteins greatly affects this separation technique. Table 4 lists some of the adsorbent materials that have been used in competitive protein binding assays.

It was originally suggested by Gottlieb et al. (16) that one could coat charcoal with dextran (Sephadex) and create a molecular sieve that would permit adsorption of small molecules and prevent adsorption of larger molecules. Binoux and Odell (17) studied this phenomenon in detail and demonstrated that charcoal coated with several types of dextran adsorbed

Table 4. Examples of Adsorbents Used
to Separate Bound and Free Analyte

Charcoal
Talc
Silica
Resins
Florisil
Bentonite
Cellulose
Fuller's earth
Polystyrene resin
Staphylococcal protein A

both bound and free hormone, but that marked differences in the amounts of charcoal required existed. By detailed analyses of the dose–response relations between the amount of charcoal and the amount of free and bound analyte adsorbed, an amount of charcoal could be selected for some assays that permitted good separation. Changing the protein concentration shifted such dose–response curves considerably. Some of these data are illustrated in Figures 7a and b and 8. In Figure 7a, the adsorption of free analyte only is shown. Dextran coating of the charcoal shifted the dose–

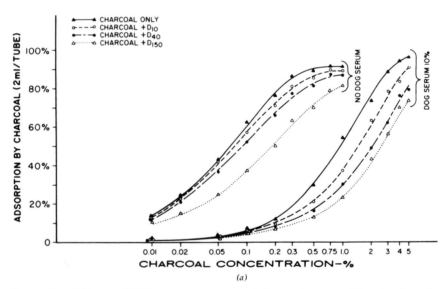

Figure 7. (a) Human TSH assay: assessment of charcoal as a possible adsorbent for free hTSH. Note that the addition of 10% dog serum results in marked rightward shifting of all dose–response curves. Note also that dextran coating with three different dextrans does not prevent hTSH (MW $\sim$ 28,000) adsorption, but merely shifts the curve slightly to the right.

response curves slightly to the right, presumably by decreasing the number of adsorbent surfaces. However, the addition of 10% dog serum (selected as a source of serum devoid of human TSH)* greatly shifted the curves to the right. In Figure 7b, the adsorption of bound analyte only is shown. Again, dextran coating did not prevent adsorption but produced a shift in the dose–response curves. In this instance, the addition of 10% dog serum produced a dramatic further shift. Although it is not shown, the addition of more dog serum (e.g., 20, 30, 40%) produced stepwise rightward shifting of all these curves. That is, if the protein content of an assay sample varied, a dose–response curve might be observed related to the volume of serum assayed, and not the hormonal content. The unwary would interpret factitious values as hormone values.

*Dog TSH shows no reaction in this human TSH assay.

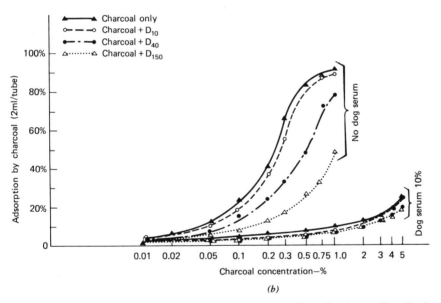

(b)

(b) Human TSH assay: assessment of charcoal as a possible adsorbent of antibody-bound TSH. This study was performed simultaneously with that shown in Figure a. Highly purified ^{125}I-labeled human TSH was prepared that was over 90% immunoreactive as tested by double antibody. This was incubated with excess anti-human TSH in the presence of varying amounts of charcoal. Note, as in Figure a, dextran coating does not prevent antibody-bound human TSH from being bound and that the addition of 10% serum causes a rightward shift of all dose–response curves. The magnitude of rightward shifting for any single dextran–charcoal preparation is related to the amount of serum added. In fact, a serum- dose–response curve can be shown to exist which could be interpreted by the unwary as representing a human TSH dose-response curve. [Reproduced with permission from Binoux and Odell, 1973 (17).]

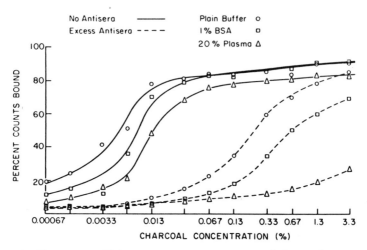

Figure 8. Glucagon radioimmunoassay: assessment of charcoal as a separation technique. Solid lines indicate dose–response curves for ^{125}I-labeled glucagon only; dashed lines indicate curves for ^{125}I-labeled glucagon in the presence of excess anti-glucagon. Note the marked differences in the dose–response curves depending on whether phosphate–saline buffer was used alone, whether 1% bovine serum albumin was used (1% BSA), or whether plasma was added (plasma to be assayed). [Reproduced with kind permission from doctoral thesis by C. Frame, 1973. From Odell et al., 1974 (10).]

Figure 8 shows charcoal binding of bound and free analyte in a glucagon radioimmunoassay. From these data, an amount of charcoal could be selected (e.g., approximately 0.04%) that might be satisfactory for radioimmunoassay use. However, if a different value, such as 0.13%, were selected and varying volumes of plasma assayed, large protein effects would be observed.

These comments on charcoal separation may be extended to any adsorbent separation technique. We recommend that the following steps be taken before using adsorbent methods to separate bound and free analyte:

1. For assays to be performed on neat serum or plasma, prepare a series of assay tubes containing free analyte and varying amounts of analyte-free serum or plasma. Since many assays are species-specific, serum or plasma from a different species might be used as a source of analyte-free serum. Alternatively, serum or plasma from an animal or human in which endogenous hormone is suppressed might be used.

2. Prepare a second series of tubes containing only bound analyte (use excess first antiserum or excess receptor and incubate for sufficient time to reach equilibrium). For assays to be applied to neat serum or plasma, tubes should also be prepared containing varying amounts of serum (or plasma) plus bound analyte. For assays performed on extracts (such as

most steroid immunoassays), tubes containing only buffer plus bound hormone need be studied.

3. Add varying amounts of the adsorbent to be used over a wide dose range. Separate adsorbent-bound from nonadsorbent-bound material and analyze data for selection of the optimal amount of adsorbent to be used for assay purposes.

For performing a routine assay, prepare a large batch of the adsorbent, assess in detail as discussed, and do not modify the conditions of the assay after the amount of adsorbent has been selected. When a new batch of adsorbent is prepared, reassess as before.

Different groups of investigators have recommended the addition of adsorbent in different ways. It may be added as a dry powder with a small spoon directly to the assay tube. Alternatively, it may be suspended in buffer, placed on a magnetic stirrer, and pipetted as a suspension. The latter is probably the simplest technique.

1. There is a dose–response curve for the amount of adsorbent versus the amount of both free and bound adsorbed material.
2. The dose–response curve for the binding of bound hormone is usually shifted to the right of that for free hormone.
3. The addition of serum causes a rightward shift in both bound and free curves and is related to the amount of serum added.
4. Dextran coating does not prevent the binding of bound hormone to charcoal.
5. Usually, or frequently, a dose of adsorbent may be selected that binds most of the free and little of the bound hormone.
6. For some assays, no dose of adsorbent can be found that binds all the free and none of the bound hormone.

Optimally, the use of an adsorbent as a separation method would permit the addition of an amount of adsorbent on the upper dose–response curve. Variation in the addition of adsorbent would then not lead to variation in answers in the assay.

SOLID-PHASE METHODS

While Catt et al. (18,19) extensively used a solid-phase separation method, they did not use covalently bound antibodies. Instead, antibodies were passively adsorbed onto the surface of the solid phase. With this technique, as discussed earlier, large protein effects occur and proper use demands the employment of constant amounts of protein in all the tubes, as well as knowledge of the principles discussed in the preceding paragraph. The passive adsorption of antibodies onto a solid phase (plastic tubes) has been used extensively by Abraham (20) for steroid radioimmunoassays. For steroid assays, since extracts of serum containing little protein are assayed, problems are considerably fewer (20). Although it is important to review these adsorption solid-phase methods, they are best classified under the heading of adsorption methods and are based on similar principles.

For our purposes, a solid-phase method involves covalent binding of the antibody (or other binding protein) to a solid matrix, such as dextran or Sepharose.

Wide et al. (21,22) described a procedure for covalently binding antibodies to Sephadex. This solid-phase method uses considerably more antiserum than the double-antibody or adsorption techniques but, once the Sephadex–antibody reagent has been made, it is stated to be quite stable at room temperature. Once the appropriate titer is known, whenever an assay is to be performed, the solid-phase conjugate suspension is simply pipetted into each tube. After appropriate incubation, low-speed centrifugation easily separates bound from free analyte. Other solid materials for binding, such as Sepharose, may be used with equal success. One disadvantage of such covalently bound solid-phase conjugation techniques appears to be the requirement for more antiserum than that used with other separation techniques. Approximately 1000-fold increases in quantities of antisera are required, compared to other separation methods.

We have used covalent linking to Sepharose and have noted that small, variable amounts of antibody may appear in solution and not be covalently bound. This occurs in spite of extensive washing at alternating pH values and at high osmolalities. Each assay can be assessed for the appearance of soluble antibodies by preparing two to four assay tubes containing only solid-phase antisera and buffer. After incubation of the entire assay, centrifuge to remove solid-phase antibodies, add radioiodinated hormone to the supernatant, incubate to reach equilibrium, and separate any soluble antibody-bound hormone by the double-antibody or the chemical separation technique. It is apparent that no antibody should be present in such a supernatant from a centrifuged solid-phase antibody reagent.

POLYMERIZED ANTIBODIES

Another method of separating bound and free hormone consists of polymerizing antibodies to form macromolecular aggregates, as described by

Avremeas and Ternynck (23). The polymerized antisera produce a gel that is suspended in buffer; titer is then determined, and specificity and affinity assessed as described under antiserum production. As for the solid-phase conjugates, once prepared, these polymerized antisera are stated to be stable for months, and separation is easily accomplished by low-speed centrifugation.

REFERENCES

1. Yalow RS, Berson SA: Immunological specificity of human insulin: Application to immunoassay of insulin. *J Clin Invest* 40:2190, 1961.

2. Yalow RS, Berson SA: Immunoassay of endogenous plasma insulin in man. *J Clin Invest* 39:1157, 1960.

3. Genuth S, Frohman LA, Lebovitz HE: A radioimmunological assay method for insulin using insulin-^{125}I and gel filtration. *J Clin Endocrinol Metab* 25:1943, 1965.

4. Feinberg R: Detection of non-precipitating antibodies coexisting with precipitating antibodies using I[131] labeled antigen abstracted. *Fed Proc* 13:493, 1954.

5. Skom JH, Talmage DW: Nonprecipitating insulin antibodies. *J Clin Invest* 37:783, 1958.

6. Utiger RD, Parker ML, Daughaday WH: Studies on human growth homone. I.A. radioimmunoassay for growth hormone. *J Clin Invest* 41:254, 1962.

7. Morgan CR, Lazarow A: Immunoassay of insulin: Two antibody system. *Diabetes* 12:115, 1963.

8. Morgan CR, Sorenson RL, Lazarow A: Studies of an inhibitor of the two antibody immunoassay system. *Diabetes* 13:1, 1964.

9. Soeldner JS, Slone D: Critical variables in the radioimmunoassay of serum insulin using the double antibody technic. *Diabetes* 14:771, 1965.

10. Odell WD, Silver C, Grover PK: Competitive protein binding assays: Methods of separation of bound from free, in: Cameron EHD, Hillier SG, Griffiths K (eds): *Steroid Immunoassay*, Proceedings of the Fifth Tenovus Workshop, Cardiff, Wales, 1974. England, Alpha Omega Publishing Ltd, 1975, p 207.

11. Midgley AR Jr: Radioimmunoassay: A method for human chorionic gonadotropin and human luteinizing hormone. *Endocrinology* 79:10, 1966.

12. Odell WD, Ross GT, Rayford PL: Radioimmunoassay for luteinizing hormone in human plasma or serum: Physiological studies. *J Clin Invest* 46:248, 1967.

13. Grodsky GM, Forsham PH: An immunochemical assay of total extractable insulin in man. *J Clin Invest* 39:1070, 1960.

14. Odell WD, Wilber JF, Paul WE: Radioimmunoassay of thyrotropin in human serum. *J Clin Endocrinol Metab* 25:1179, 1965.

15. Desbuquois B, Aurbach GD: Use of polyethylene glycol to separate free and antibody-bound peptide hormones in radioimmunoassays. *J Clin Endocrinol Metab* 33:732, 1971.

16. Gottlieb C, Lau KS, Wasserman LR, et al: Rapid charcoal assay for intrinsic factor (IF), gastric juice unsaturated B_{12} binding capacity, antibody to IF, and serum unsaturated B_{12} binding capacity. *Blood* 25:875, 1965.

17. Binoux MA, Odell WD: Use of dextran coated charcoal to separate antibody-bound from free hormone: A critique. *J Clin Endocrinol Metab* 36:303, 1973.

18. Catt KJ, Tregear GW: Solid-phase radioimmunoassay in antibody-coated tubes. *Science* 158:1570, 1967.

19. Catt KJ, Niall HD, Tregear GW, et al: Disc solid-phase radioimmunoassay of human luteinizing hormone. *J Clin Endocrinol Metab* 28:121, 1968.

20. Abraham GE: Solid-phase radioimmunoassay of estradiol-17β. *J Clin Endocrinol Metab* 29:866, 1969.

21. Wide L, Porath J: Radioimmunoassay of proteins with the use of Sephadex-coupled antibodies. *Biochim Biophys Acta* 130:257, 1966.

22. Wide L, Axen R, Porath J: Radioimmunosorbent assay for proteins. Chemical couplings of antibodies to insoluble dextran. *Immunochemistry* 4:381, 1967.

23. Avrameas S, Ternynck T: Biologically active water-insoluble protein polymers. *J Biol Chem* 242:1651, 1967.

24. Donini S, Donini P: Radioimmunoassay employing polymerized antisera, in Diczfalusy E (ed): *Karolinska Symposta on Research Methods In Reproductive Endocrinology, Immunoassay of Gonadotrophins*. Supp 142, *Acta Encodrinol,* 1969, p 257.

CHAPTER 8
MATHEMATICAL ANALYSIS OF COMPETITIVE PROTEIN BINDING ASSAYS

L. Arthur Campfield

The basic mathematical model we initially consider is the case of the competitive protein binding assay in which homogeneous populations of hormone (antigen or ligand) and antibody (binding protein or receptor) react to form hormone–antibody complexes. A portion of the antigen (hormone), in the reaction volume, is assumed to be labeled. This reaction can be represented as follows:

$$H^* + R \underset{k_{-1}}{\overset{k_1}{\rightleftharpoons}} H^*R \tag{1}$$

$$H + R \underset{k_{-2}}{\overset{k_2}{\rightleftharpoons}} HR \tag{2}$$

where H* is labeled free hormone (antigen or ligand), H is unlabeled free hormone, R is the antibody (binding protein or receptor) binding site, H*R is the labeled hormone–antibody complex, HR is unlabeled hormone–antibody complex, k_1, k_2 are association rate constants, and k_{-1}, k_{-2} are dissociation rate constants.

These reactions emphasize the fundamental concept on which the competitive protein binding assay is based: the competition of labeled and unlabeled hormone for a fixed number of antibody binding sites. Thus, as the total concentration of unlabeled hormone in the reaction mixture increases, less labeled hormone–antibody complex is formed.

ASSUMPTIONS

The following assumptions will be made to develop the basic mathematical model of the competitive protein binding assay:

1. The hormone is a homogeneous chemical species.

125

2. The antibody is a homogeneous chemical species.

3. One molecule of hormone binds to one molecule of antibody.

4. The hormone and antibody reaction is governed by first-order mass action (a bimolecular reaction). Thus, no cooperative effects are considered.

5. Labeled and unlabeled hormone have identical physical-chemical properties (except for the presence of the label) and participate in the reaction identically.

6. The reaction proceeds to complete equilibrium.

7. Hormone bound to antibody can be separated from free hormone perfectly without disturbing the equilibrium.

8. The ratio of bound hormone to free hormone can be measured perfectly.

The first three assumptions restrict the chemical complexity of the reaction mixture to two homogeneous components that react independently. Assumptions 4 to 6 define the kinetics of the reaction. Assumptions 7 and 8 idealize the separation and estimation procedures inherent in the method. The effects of relaxation of some of these limiting assumptions will be described in a separate section below.

The following differential equations can be written to describe the dynamics of the hormone–antibody reaction based on the assumptions given above. The rate of change of the labeled free hormone, H*, is:

$$\frac{d[H^*]}{dt} = k_{-1}[H^*R] - k_1[H^*][R] \tag{3}$$

where $[H^*]$ is the molar concentration of labeled free hormone (moles/liter), $d[H^*]/dt$ is the rate of change of the molar concentration of labeled free hormone (moles/liter $\cdot$ t), k_{-1} is the dissociation constant ($1/t$), k_1 is the association constant (liters/mole $\cdot$ t), $[H^*R]$ is the concentration of H*R complex (moles/liter). The rate of change of the unlabeled free hormone, H, is similarly given by:

$$\frac{d[H]}{dt} = k_{-2}[HR] - k_2[H][R] \tag{4}$$

The rate of change of the labeled hormone–antibody complex, H*R, is

$$\frac{d[H^*R]}{dt} = k_1[H^*][R] - k_{-1}[H^*R] = -\frac{d[H^*]}{dt} \tag{5}$$

The rate of change of unlabeled hormone–antibody complex, HR, is

$$\frac{d[HR]}{dt} = k_2[H][R] - k_{-2}[HR] = -\frac{d[H]}{dt} \tag{6}$$

These differential equations are subject to the following constraint equations:

$$H^*{}_{total} = [H^*] + [H^*R] \tag{7}$$

$$H_{total} = [H] + [HR] \tag{8}$$

$$R_{total} = [R] + [H^*R] + [HR] \tag{9}$$

The differential equations for the labeled and unlabeled free hormone concentration or the equations for the hormone–antibody complex together with the constraint equations could be solved to determine the dynamics of these concentrations at *any* specified time after the initiation of the reaction. We could estimate the ratio of the molar concentrations of labeled free and antibody-bound hormone, $[H^*]/[H^*R]$, and thus estimate the total unlabeled hormone concentration H_{total}. Alternatively, we could let the reaction reach equilibrium and derive an equilibrium (steady-state) relationship for the unknown total unlabeled hormone concentration H_{total} in terms of the total antibody concentration R_{total} and the total labeled hormone concentration H^*_{total} and the properties of the antibody. We will pursue the latter alternative in order to explore the steady-state behavior of the hormone–antibody interaction.

At steady state, all derivatives must be equal to zero:

$$\frac{d[H]}{dt} \equiv \frac{d[H^*]}{dt} \equiv 0$$

therefore, the differential equations for free hormone (Eqs. 3 and 4) become

$$0 = k_{-1}[H^*R] - k_1[H^*][R] \tag{10}$$

$$0 = k_{-2}[HR] - k_2[H][R] \tag{11}$$

Now writing the respective equilibrium constants, we have

$$\frac{[H^*R]}{[H^*][R]} = \frac{k_1}{k_{-1}} = K^*_{eq} \tag{12}$$

and

$$\frac{[HR]}{[H][R]} = \frac{k_2}{k_{-2}} = K_{eq} \tag{13}$$

Since H* and H have identical physical-chemical properties and participate in the reactions identically (assumption 5),

$$K^*_{eq} = K_{eq} \tag{14}$$

Therefore,

$$\frac{[H^*R]}{[H^*][R]} = \frac{[HR]}{[H][R]} \tag{15}$$

Now, we would like to find a relationship between the ratio of the molar concentrations of hormone–antibody complex (bound hormone *B*) and the free hormone *(F)*, *B/F*.
By definition,

$$\frac{B}{F} = \frac{[HR]}{[H]} \tag{16}$$

and

$$\frac{B^*}{F^*} = \frac{[H^*R]}{[H^*]} \tag{17}$$

Now multiplying Eq. 15 by [R], we obtain

$$\frac{[H^*R]}{[H^*]} = \frac{[HR]}{[H]} = K_{eq} * [R] = K_{eq}[R] \tag{18}$$

Applying the definition of B^*/F^* and B/F we obtain

$$\frac{B^*}{F^*} = \frac{B}{F} \tag{19}$$

We have obtained the important result that the ratio of labeled hormone bound to antibody B^* to labeled free hormone F^* at steady state is equal to the unlabeled B/F ratio. Assuming that bound hormone can be perfectly separated from free hormone (assumption 7) and that labeled hormone can be detected by a suitable counter, we can estimate $[HR]/[H] = B/F$ for each tube.

Now we seek an expression relating B/F (which can be perfectly measured) and the design parameters of the competitive protein binding assay:

$$H^*_{total} = [H^*] + [H^*R] \quad \text{(known)} \tag{7}$$

$$H_{total} = [H + HR] \quad \text{(usually unknown)} \tag{8}$$

$$R_{total} = [R] + [H^*R] + [HR] \quad \text{(known)} \tag{9}$$

$$K_{eq} = \frac{[HR]}{[H][R]} \quad \begin{array}{l}\text{(property of antibody that is}\\ \text{known or can be estimated)}\end{array} \tag{13}$$

After substitution of Eq. 7, 8, 9, 13, 16, and 17 into Eq. 18 and considerable rearrangement, we obtain the desired expression:

$$\left(\frac{B^*}{F^*}\right)^2 + \frac{B^*}{F^*}(H^*_{total}\,K_{eq} - R_{total}\,K_{eq} + H_{total}\,K_{eq} + 1) - R_{total}\,K_{eq} = 0 \tag{20}$$

This quadratic equation can be solved for B^*/F^* and, since B^*/F^* can be directly estimated, we can solve for the only unknown, $[H]_{total}$.

This equation is the basic mathematical model of an equilibrium competitive protein binding assay.

The procedure for a competitive protein binding assay based on this analysis is as follows:

1. Use samples with known concentrations of H_{total} to find B^*/F^* for several concentrations of hormone (standard curve).
2. Run quality control samples, measure B^*/F^*, and compare with previous assays.
3. Run samples with unknown H_{total}, estimate B^*/F^*, and interpolate to estimate H_{total}.

EXPRESSION OF THE DATA

Several methods of expressing the data resulting from competitive protein binding assays are used for routine analysis of unknowns, as well as for assay optimization. We shall discuss three such methods and mention several others.

THE SCATCHARD PLOT

The solution of Eq. 20 derived above can be approximated by the following equation first postulated for small molecules binding to plasma proteins by Scatchard (1):

$$\frac{B}{F} = K_{eq}\,(R_{total} - B) \tag{21}$$

This equation is of the form

$$y = mx + b \tag{22}$$

that is, it is the equation of a straight line with intercept b and slope m. Therefore, a plot of B/F versus B (a Scatchard plot) will have intercept $K_{eq}R$ and slope $-K_{eq}$. Note that B/F and B are assumed to be measured independently, with B/F the dependent and B the independent variable. Examination of Eq. 21 suggests that

1. As $B \to 0$, $B/F \to K_{eq}R_{total}$.
2. As $B \to R_{total}$, $B/F \to 0$.
3. As R_{total} increases, the slope remains unchanged and the intercept increases. Thus, B/F increases for a particular B.
4. As $R_{total} \to 0$, $B/F \to 0$.
5. As K_{eq} increases, the slope increases but the intercept remains unchanged. Thus B/F increases for a particular B.
6. As $K_{eq} \to 0$, $B/F \to 0$.

COUNTS (FREE OR BOUND) VERSUS
LOG DOSE

In this representation, the raw free or bound counts are plotted against the logarithm of the hormone concentration. Bound counts will be maximal in the absence of unlabeled hormone and fall toward zero when the concentration of unlabeled hormone is increased. The shape of the resulting curve will be sigmoidal. Free counts will be low in the absence of unlabeled hormone and rise toward an upper threshold as the unlabeled hormone concentration is increased. The advantage of this method of data representation is its simplicity; however, its disadvantage is that it makes comparisons between assays for quality control or optimization very difficult.

B/B_0 VERSUS LOG DOSE

This method of data representation normalizes the standard curve of each assay to facilitate interassay comparisons, but preserves the sigmoidal shape of the response curve inherent in the raw count data. The following response variable is computed for each assay tube:

$$\frac{B}{B_0} = \frac{(B' - NSB)}{(B'_0 - NSB)} \tag{23}$$

where B' is the number of labeled hormone–antibody complex counts (cpm), B_0' is the number of labeled hormone–antibody complex counts in the absence of unlabeled hormone (cpm), NSB is the nonspecific binding (cpm). Thus, B/B_0 takes on numerical values between 0 and 1 and is commonly multiplied by 100 and expressed as the percentage bound. We see that:

$$B/B_0 \rightarrow 1 \quad \text{as} \quad B' \rightarrow B_0'$$
$$B/B_0 \rightarrow 0 \quad \text{as} \quad B' \rightarrow NSB.$$

B/B_0 is plotted on a linear scale against the hormone concentration on a logarithmic scale. The resultant response count is thus corrected for changes in initial binding B_0 and NSB so that response curves from many different assays can be easily compared. B/B_0 begins at 1 in the absence of unlabeled hormone and decreases sigmoidially toward zero as the concentration of unlabeled hormone increases.

LOGIT B/B_0 VERSUS LOG DOSE

This widely used representation of the data usually results in a linear response curve and is the basis of most computer analysis programs for competitive binding assays. The following response variable is computed for each assay tube:

$$\text{logit}\left(\frac{B}{B_0}\right) = \log_e\left[\frac{B/B_0}{1 - B/B_0}\right] \tag{24}$$

where B/B_0 is as defined in Eq. 23. This response variable is plotted on a linear scale against the hormone concentration on a logarithmic scale. For most assays, this logarithmic transformation of the normalized bound counts usually results in a linear response curve. Thus, a straight line can be fit to these data and the standard curve can be completely characterized by the resulting slope and intercept. This provides another basis for quantitative interassay comparison. Many gamma counters currently available contain microprocessors that perform these computations.

OTHER FORMS OF DATA REPRESENTATION

Many other methods of data representation have been proposed and have gained a following. Some of these are: B/T, F/B, B/F, B_0/F_0, F/T, and $H*R$.

PERFORMANCE CRITERIA

Competitive protein binding assays can be judged using several different and often conflicting performance criteria. Rather than trying to argue for an optimal or best single performance criterion, we will propose four criteria to be considered when optimizing a particular assay.

The first criterion is the *least detectable dose*, that is, the lowest total hormone concentration that results in a displacement equal to twice the standard deviation of the B_0 (initial bound) point. If the data are expressed as B/B_0 or logit B/B_0 versus log dose and the standard deviation of the B_0 point is $\sigma\%$, the least detectable dose is the hormone concentration corresponding to $[(100-2\sigma\%)/100]\ B/B_0$. The second criterion is the *steepness* of the slope and the *position* of the intercept on the response axes. Here we want to maximize the slope, to position it within the range of hormone concentration of primary interest, and we want to maximize the initial binding.

The third criterion of performance is the *half-maximal dose*, that is, the hormone concentration that displaces the response variable to one-half its initial value. If the logit B/B_0 − log dose data representation is used, the x intercept (logit $B/B_0 = 0$) corresponds to $B/B_0 = 0.5$. The lower this hormone concentration, the greater the sensitivity (Δ response/Δ hormone concentration) of the assay. However, the half-maximal concentration should be within the range of interest. The fourth criterion is the *coefficient of variation* at several hormone concentrations. The variance (and its square root, the standard deviation) is not uniform over the range of operation of competitive protein binding assays; in fact, it is inversely related to the hormone concentration (this is termed *heteroscedasticity*). In order to minimize this error over the concentration region of interest, we want to minimize the coefficient of variation (standard deviation/mean) at low, medium, and high hormone concentrations. The weight given to each of these performance criteria is dictated by the particular assay, its purpose (e.g., least detectable dose or minimized error), and the state of its development.

COMPUTATIONAL AND STATISTICAL ANALYSIS

We now consider practical implementation of the computational and statistical analysis of the results of a competitive protein binding assay. We will discuss a state-of-the art implementation of these techniques. First, an overall outline will be presented, followed by more detailed discussion.

1. Enter and store assay identification and title, total number of tubes, NSB, total, and B_0 counts in the computer or calculator.
2. Compute B/B_0 for each tube.
3. Compute response variable, Logit B/B_0, for each tube.
4. Compute logarithm of the hormone concentration for the standard curve tubes.
5. Perform linear regression (unweighted and weighted by 1/variance) and compute the slope, intercept, and correlation coefficient.
6. Compute 95% confidence envelope about regression line.
7. Compute least detectable dose.
8. Estimate concentration and response variable of quality control samples and accept or reject assay.
9. Estimate concentration ±95% confidence limits for unknown samples.

The first step informs the computer which of several stored assay programs will be used and allows the computation of B/B_0 from the raw bound counts for each assay tube. Then the logit B/B_0 and logarithm of hormone concentration are computed. At this stage, the use of a computer not only facilitates estimation of the hormone concentrations of the unknown samples but also allows the computation of an objective fit to the standard curve and the generation of error bounds on the estimated concentrations. Although the human eye is excellent at fitting straight lines to unweighted experimental data, the fact that the residual variance about the standard curve is nonuniform requires the use of both an unweighted and a weighted regression analysis of the standard curve data. First, the standard curve raw counts are read and an unweighted regression line is fit to the data by treating all data equally, and a slope intercept and correlation coefficient about the regression line are computed. Then the unweighted estimates of the slope and intercept are used as initial guesses for the computation of a weighted regression line in which each data point is weighted by 1/variance. Thus, the data points with the most scatter (low concentrations) are given a smaller weight and make a smaller contribution to the residual sum of the squared error than data points with less scatter (middle and high concentrations). The residual sum of the squares error, RRS, is given by

$$\text{RSS} = \sum_{i=1}^{N} (y_i - \bar{y})^2 \tag{25}$$

where $\bar{y}_i$ is the experimentally observed response variable at a particular hormone concentration, y is the corresponding predicted response variable at the same hormone concentration, and N is the total number of standard curve tubes.

The computer starts with initial guesses for the slope and intercept and computes a regression line and the corresponding RSS. Then the initial guesses of the slope and intercept are adjusted, a new line is computed, and a hopefully smaller RSS is computed. This process continues until no further significant improvement (as measured by a previously specified tolerance) in the RSS is obtained. A correlation coefficient about the final regression line is computed, and the final estimate of the slope and intercept and the correlation coefficient are printed. For most competitive protein binding assays, the results of the weighted regression will be superior (measured by a smaller RSS and a higher correlation coefficient) to the results of the unweighted regression. It has become standard practice to compute both regression lines and to use the results of the weighted regression during analysis of the unknown samples. Next, a 95% confidence envelope is computed around the regression line by adding and subtracting the product of the standard deviation and the value of Student's t at several concentrations of hormone. The envelope is constructed by connecting these 95% confidence limits at several different hormone concentrations. The least detectable dose is then computed and stored in memory so that any response variable above the value corresponding to this hormone concentration will result in the printing of a message such as "cannot read this sample."

Then the raw counts of the quality control samples are read, the response variables are computed, and the estimated hormone concentrations are interpolated from the standard curve regression line:

$$\text{logit } (B/B_0) = M[\log H] + C$$

or

$$\log [H] = \frac{1}{M} \left(\text{logit } \left(\frac{B}{B_0} \right) - C \right) \tag{26a}$$

or

$$[H] = \text{Antilog} \left[\frac{1}{M} \left(\text{logit } + \left(\frac{B}{B_0} \right) - C \right) \right] \tag{26}$$

where $[H]$ is the estimated hormone concentration, M is the slope of the standard curve regression line, and C is the intercept of the standard curve regression line.

The response variables (logit B/B_0) and the estimated hormone concentration of each quality control sample are compared to the running average of the results of previous assays, and the assay is rejected if they are not in close agreement (with $\pm$SD of the running average). If the assay is rejected, all processing should be halted and a message printed. If, on the other hand, the quality control samples are within normal limits, the assay is accepted and the estimated hormone concentration of each unknown sample is computed using Eq. 26. In addition, the 95% confidence limits of each unknown hormone concentration can be computed by using the boundaries of the 95% confidence envelope about the standard curve. For example, suppose that at an insulin concentration of 1 ng/ml the 95% confidence envelope is $\pm$0.2 ng/ml. Then an unknown sample with a logit B/B_0 equal to that of the 1 ng/ml standard would be reported as 1 ng/ml $\pm$ 0.2 ng/ml. Each unknown will be estimated in turn until all samples have been processed, thus completing the routine processing procedure for a competitive protein binding assay.

EXAMPLE: INSULIN ASSAY PERFORMED IN THE DEPARTMENT OF PHYSIOLOGY AT NORTHWESTERN UNIVERSITY

The assay consisted of rat insulin standard, a guinea pig antibody, and ^{125}I-labeled porcine insulin in phosphate buffer containing protein. The reaction volume was 800 μl, and the assay was incubated at 4°C for 96 hours. Unknown, standard, or pool samples of rat insulin (100 μl), antibody, and buffer were added to tubes and incubated at 4°C for 24 hours. Then 100 μl of ^{125}I-labeled insulin was added to each tube, and all tubes were well mixed and returned to 4°C to incubate for the remaining 72 hours. Free hormone was separated from bound hormone using charcoal. After aspiration of the supernatant (containing bound hormone), the free fractions were counted to 10,000 counts in order to maintain the counting error at 1% or less. After each tube was counted, the tube number, counting time, and counts were printed on a Teletype and simultaneously entered into an input file on a LSI 11/23 microcomputer system.

After completion of the counting of all the tubes in the assay, data processing proceeded in two stages. First, the standard curve was computed and the slope and intercept of the linearized curve were determined. Next, the insulin concentration in each pool or unknown tube was estimated. If the pool values were within acceptable ranges, the assay was accepted and the assay results were processed and printed.

The input file for computation of the standard curve was as follows:

Standard Curve for Assay G269

0.962	1.946	1.079
(total counts average counting time)	(F_0 initial free average counting time)	(NSF counts average counting time)

35	10.000
(total of STD tubes)	(preset counts)

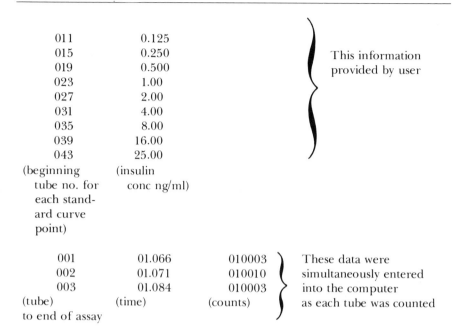

011	0.125		
015	0.250		This information
019	0.500		provided by user
023	1.00		
027	2.00		
031	4.00		
035	8.00		
039	16.00		
043	25.00		
(beginning tube no. for each standard curve point)	(insulin conc ng/ml)		

001	01.066	010003	These data were
002	01.071	010010	simultaneously entered
003	01.084	010003	into the computer
(tube) to end of assay	(time)	(counts)	as each tube was counted

After creation of this input file, a one-line command resulted in the computation of both the unweighted and weighted standard curves. The output of the standard curve program was:

STD Curve for Assay G269

VALUES IN TIME:
TOTAL = 0.962
F_0 = 1.946
NSF   = 1.079
NO OF TUBES = 35
PRESET COUNTS = 10000
VALUES IN CPM
TOTAL = 10395
F_0 = 5139
NSF   = 9268

Data were entered in tube number—counting time format:

TUBE NO	COUNTS	CONC	LOGIT
11	5345.	0.125	2.947
12	5355	0.125	2.897
13	5517	0.125	2.293
14	5555.	0.125	2.188
15	5685	0.250	1.881
17	5566.	0.250	2.159
18	5625.	0.250	2.013
19	5966	0.500	1.384
20	5825.	0.500	1.613
21	5855.	0.500	1.562
22	5743	0.500	1.764
23	6310.	1.000	0.927
24	6269.	1.000	0.975
25	6277.	1.000	0.966
26	6179	1.000	1.088
27	6556.	2.000	0.649
28	6731	2.000	0.465
29	6626.	2.000	0.574
30	6650	2.000	0.549
31	7227.	4.000	−0.023
32	7444	4.000	−0.234
33	7398	4.000	−0.189
34	7324	4.000	−0.117
35	7628	8.000	−0.417
36	7713	8.000	−0.504
37	7634	8.000	−0.423
38	7669.	8.000	−0.459
39	7993.	16.000	−0.806
40	7809	16.000	−0.604
41	8061.	16.000	−0.885
42	7937	16.000	−0.743
43	8213	25.000	−1.070
44	8305.	25.000	−1.190
45	8423	25.000	−1.358
46	8261	25.000	−1.131

UNWEIGHTED REGRESSION:

SLP   = -1.598
YINT =   1.051
RS   =   0.96

WEIGHTED REGRESSION:

SLP   = -1.623 (slope)
YINT =   1.046 (y intercept)
RS   =   0.980 (correlation coefficient)
CN   = 35   (number of standard curve tubes used)

Then a second input file was created to compute the estimated insulin concentration of the pool and unknown samples:

ASSAY G269 CONTAINS EXPT   SI 121

0.926 (TOTAL time)	1.946 (F_0 time)	1.079 (NSF time)	-1.623 (slope)	1.046 (y intercept)	
323 (no. of tubes)	2 (duplicates should be averaged)	10 000 (preset counts)			Provided by the user

001	01.066	010003	
002	01.071	010010	Already in the computer
003	01.084	010003	

to the end of the assay.

Again a simple command directed the computer to calculate the insulin concentration in each assay tube and to compute the average concentration of duplicates. Some of the output for assay G269 is shown below:

ASSAY G269
TOTAL CPM   = 10395
F_0 CPM   = 5139
NSF CPM   = 9268
SLOPE   = -1.623
INTERCEPT   = 1.046
NO OF TUBES = 323   REPLICATES = 2

TUBE NO	COUNTS	LOGIT	CONC	AVG	
QUALITY CONTROL POOL			(ng/ml)	(ng/ml)	
47	7925	−0.730	12.42		
48	7686	−0.477	8.68	10.55	Pool 1:2
49	7205	−0.001	4.42		
50	7395	−0.186	5.74	5.08	Pool 1:4
51	6659	0.540	2.05		
52	6590	0.612	1.85	1.95	Pool 1:8
53	6227	1.027	1.03		
54	6428	0.790	1.44	1.23	Pool 1:16
55	5931	1.438	0.57		
56	5833	1.598	0.47	0.52	Pool 1:32
UNKNOWNS					
83	7051	0.148	3.58		
84	7017	0.181	3.41	3.49	
85	6335	0.897	1.24		
86	6365	0.862	1.30	1.27	
87	6410	0.810	1.40		
88	6405	0.816	1.39	1.39	
89	7486	−0.276	6.52		
90	7437	−0.227	6.09	6.30	

These programs together with automated data entry from the counter allow the processing of a 1000-tube competitive protein binding assay in 20–30 minutes. If the counter data must be entered into the input file manually, the computation will require approximately 3–4 hours.

NONIDEAL BEHAVIOR

Although the basic mathematical model for a competitive protein binding assay and the analysis presented above are adequate to explain the general response characteristics and to optimize most assays, in many experimental situations significant deviations from theoretical predictions occur. Most of these deviations are due to the fact that often the hormone and the antibody are not single homogeneous species. Indeed, several types of multicomponent behavior may account for these deviations: a population of antibody-binding sites, each with different equilibrium constants; more than one molecule of hormone may bind to the same binding site; the binding of hormone to a binding site may affect subsequent hormone binding (cooperativity); or labeled and/or unlabeled hormone may be a population of closely related ligands. The most important multicomponent effect to be included in analysis of the competitive protein binding assay is the presence in the assay system of multiple species of hormones and antibody-binding sites. The extension of the simple model to include these cases has been carried out by Ekins and co-workers (2,3), Berson and Yalow (4), and Feldman et al. (5,6).

First, consider the case of a single homogeneous hormone and multiple species of n antibody-binding sites. The reaction may now be written as

$$H + R_i \rightleftharpoons HR_i \qquad i = 1, \ldots, n \tag{27}$$

Where R_i is the binding site of the ith species.

Then at equilibrium,

$$\frac{[HR_i]}{[H][R_i]} = K_{eq_i} \tag{28}$$

Then, the constraint equations become

$$H_{total} = [H] + \sum_i^n [HR_i] \tag{29}$$

$$R_{total_i} = [R_i] + [HR_i] \tag{30}$$

and

$$\frac{B}{F} = \sum_i^n \frac{[HR_i]}{[H]} \tag{31}$$

Substitution of Eqs. 29 and 30 into Eq. 31 yields the following expression for $(B/F)i$.

$$\frac{B}{F}i = \frac{[HR_i]}{[H]} = \frac{K_{eq_i} R_{total_i}}{\dfrac{K_{eq_i} H_{total}}{1 + B/F} + 1} \tag{32}$$

Summing over the n binding sites,

$$\frac{B}{F} = \sum_{i=1}^n \frac{R_{total_i}}{\dfrac{H_{total}}{1 + B/F} + \dfrac{1}{K_{eq_i}}} \tag{33}$$

or

$$\sum_{i=1}^n \left(\frac{\dfrac{R_{total_i}}{B/F} \dfrac{1}{B/F} + 1}{\dfrac{H_{total}}{B/F} + \dfrac{1}{B/F K_{eq_i}} + \dfrac{1}{K_{eq_i}}} \right) = 1 \tag{34}$$

Equation 34 represents a generalized version of Eq. 20 for the multibinding site competitive protein binding assay. The intercept on the B/F axis is given by

$$\frac{B}{F}(B = 0) = \sum_{i=1}^n K_{eq_i} R_{total_i} \tag{35}$$

This analysis indicates that, for a mixture of binding sites, the slope of the response curve is proportional to a weighted average of the binding constants with the weights given by $K_{eq_i} R_{total_i}$. Further details of this analysis may be found in Ekins et al. (2).

Now, consider the case where we have m hormones, $H_i, \ldots, H_m$ (some containing label), and n antibody binding sites, $R_i, \ldots, R_n$. At equilibrium we have mn equations of the form

$$K_{eq_{ij}} = \frac{[H_i R_j]}{[H_i][R_j]} \qquad \begin{array}{l} i = 1, \ldots, m \\ j = 1, \ldots, n \end{array} \qquad (36)$$

Now

$$H_{total} = \sum_{i=1}^{m} [H_i] + \sum_{i=1}^{m} \sum_{j=1}^{n} [H_i R_j] \qquad (37)$$

$$R_{total} = \sum_{j=1}^{m} [R_j] + \sum_{i=1}^{m} \sum_{j=1}^{n} [H_i R_j] \qquad (38)$$

Combining these equations, Feldman, Levine, and Rodbard (5) have derived the following expression for the multicomponent assay at equilibrium.

$$\frac{B}{F}_i = \frac{H_{total_i} - H_i}{H_i} = \sum_{j=1}^{m} \left[\frac{K_{eq_{ij}} R_{total_j}}{1 + \sum_{a=1}^{m} K_{eq_{aj}} H_a} \right], \quad i = 1, \ldots, m \qquad (39)$$

where $(B/F)_i$ is the bound/free ratio for H_i.

This expression can be used in three ways: (1) It can be solved for the response variable $(B/F)_i$ as a function of assay design parameters to simulate the competitive protein binding assay; (2) it can be solved for the parameters K_{eq_i}, H_i, and R_i in terms of the experimental variables $(B/F)_i$, H_{total_i}, R_{total_i}; or (3) it can be differentiated to yield the slope of any standard curve of interest. The latter two applications can be used to optimize the maximum slope or the least detectable dose of the multicomponent assay. Further details of the application of this equation to analysis of the behavior of the multicomponent competitive binding assay can be found in Feldman and Rodbard (4).

Other types of nonideal behavior sometimes observed in the response of competitive protein binding assays (e.g., cooperativity, "hooking" of standard curves) occur because the actual hormone antibody reaction occurring is not well modeled by the law of mass action and the simplified kinetic behavior it predicts. These effects can be simulated using more complex theoretical models of the antigen–antibody reaction; however, the simple analysis presented here is usually adequate for the development, optimization, and computation of the results of most competitive protein binding assays.

NONEQUILIBRIUM ASSAYS

A very interesting and widely used modification of the equilibrium assay (discussed above) is the nonequilibrium assay. The differential equations for the rate of change of H^* and H (Eqs. 3 and 4), which were derived from the law of mass action, are adequate to predict the behavior of a competitive protein binding assay in which *(1)* equilibrium is not attained, *(2)* all reagents are not added simultaneously, and *(3)* labeled and unlabeled hormones react at different rates. The typical application of a nonequilibrium assay is to increase the sensitivity of the assay at low hormone concentrations. Antibody and unknown (or standard or pool) samples are combined, and the assay is incubated for a short period (4–24 hours). Labeled hormone is then added to the reaction volume, which is mixed, and then the incubation is continued. This procedure usually results in a lower least detectable dose and a steeper slope of the standard curve in the low-hormone-concentration region.

PROCEDURE FOR OPTIMIZATION OF COMPETITIVE PROTEIN BINDING ASSAY

After the completion of routine assay processing, several additional computational steps are required to optimize a particular competitive protein binding assay. First, the equilibrium constant K_{eq} of the antibody and the total concentration of antibody binding sites are estimated using Scatchard or Lineweaver–Burke analysis. In the Scatchard analysis B^*/F^* ratios are experimentally determined for each standard curve tube. The unlabeled bound hormone concentrations *(B)* are calculated by multiplying each known total hormone concentration by the initial B^*/F^* ratio. The resulting B^*/F^* data are plotted against B, and a straight line is fitted to these data as predicted by Eq. 21. The equilibrium constant of the antibody is the negative of the slope of the resulting linear regression line, and the total concentration of antibody binding sites R_{total} is the B^*/F^* intercept divided by K_{eq}. These antibody parameters, together with the total concentration of labeled hormone in the reaction mixture H^*_{total}, allow eq. 20 to be completely specified for the particular assay under study.

However, a straight-line fit of the B/F versus B data occurs only if a single species of antibody-binding site is present or if hormone binding to multiple binding sites is dominated by a subpopulation of binding sites (e.g., a large number of sites with a specific K_{eq} and smaller number of other sites with other K_{eq} values.) Since there is usually more than one population of binding sites, Odell and co-workers (7,8) have suggested an alternate method of estimating the *average* equilibrium (affinity) constant of an antibody preparation. This method is based on the Michaelis–Menten formulation of an enzyme-catalyzed reaction. Consider the reaction

$$E + S \underset{k_{-1}}{\overset{k_1}{\rightleftharpoons}} ES \overset{k_2}{\to} P + E \tag{40}$$

where enzyme (E) combines with substrate (S) to form an enzyme substrate complex (ES) which spontaneously decomposes yielding product (P) and unaltered enzyme (E). The Michaelis constant is defined as

$$K_m = \frac{k_{-1} + k_2}{k_1} \tag{41}$$

The Michaelis constant is numerically equal to the substrate concentration corresponding to a half-maximal rate of product formation. When applied to the hormone–antibody reaction, k_2 is assumed to be zero. This is because after generation of the hormone–antibody complex no further product is formed. Thus, if saturation (binding) curves for the antibody preparation are experimentally obtained, the concentration of free hormone that corresponds to 50% binding may be used to estimate the *average* association constant.

The procedure is to add varying amounts of labeled or unlabeled hormone to a fixed concentration of antibody preparation. The amount of hormone bound to the antibody (the HR or H*R complex) is determined as a function of the amount of hormone added to the reaction. These data are best represented graphically using a Lineweaver–Burke plot which linearizes the Michaelis–Menten model of enzyme–substrate interactions. The Lineweaver-Burke equation is

$$\frac{1}{V} = \left(\frac{K_m}{V_{max}} \right) \frac{1}{[S]} + \frac{1}{V_{max}} \tag{42}$$

where V is the rate of complex formation and V_{max} is the maximal formation rate. This equation is of the form of the equation of a straight line:

$$y = mx + b$$

where m is the slope and b is the y-intercept. Therefore, if the reciprocal of the amount of bound hormone is plotted against the reciprocal of the amount of hormone added in the saturation experiment, the slope of the curve will be K_m/V_{max}, and when $1/V = 0$, the $1/S$ intercept will be $-(1/K_m)$. Thus, K_m can be determined experimentally. From the definition of K_{eq} (Eq. 13) $K_{eq} = k_1/k_{-1}$, and from the definition of K_m (Eq. 43) $K_m = k_{-1}/k_1$.

We can derive a relationship between the average affinity constant, $\overline{K}_{eq}$ and K_m.

$$\overline{K}_{eq} = \frac{1}{K_m} \tag{43}$$

Once an estimate of K_{eq} is obtained by either method, various performance criteria such as least detectable dose, half-maximal dose, and initial binding are computed for this particular assay. These criteria are compared to the desired values if known or past values with previously optimized assays. Simulation studies using Eq. 20 and systematic variation of assay design parameter are then performed to find values for H^*_{total} and R_{total} that will maximize assay performance with respect to the selected criteria.

Alternatively, the optimal assay conditions can be calculated by solving a "sensitivity" equation for the conditions that maximize the sensitivity of the assay. Sensitivity has been defined as the maximum slope of the standard curve (Yalow and Berson) or the least detectable dose (Ekins). Yalow and Berson argue that maximizing the slope of the standard curve determines the maximum potential sensitivity independent of experimental error, and they suggest that the least detectable dose is a function of both the slope of the standard curve and the magnitude of the experimental error. Yalow and Berson (9-11) have examined the conditions that yield maximum sensitivity (maximal slope of the standard curve), assuming that experimental error is random and independent of the assay conditions.

Beginning with the simplest representation of the competitive protein binding assay,

$$\frac{B}{F} = \frac{b}{1-b} = K_{eq} (R_{total} - bH_{total}) \tag{44}$$

where b is the fraction of bound hormone and equals B/T. The slope of the standard curve db/dH is computed (9,10):

$$\frac{db}{dH_{total}} = \frac{-K_{eq} b (1-b)^2}{1 + KH_{total} (1-b)^2} \tag{45}$$

From this equation, they noted that db/dH_{total} approaches a maximum as $H_{total} \rightarrow 0$.

The maximal slope is found by setting $db/dH_{total} = 0$ and taking the derivative of the resulting equation with respect to b. Thus,

$$0 = -K_{eq} b (1-b)^2 \tag{46}$$

Now taking the derivative with respect to b,

$$\frac{d}{db} (-K_{eq} b (1-b)^2) = -K_{eq} (1-b)^2 + 2K_{eq} b (1-b) = 0. \tag{47}$$

Two solutions exist for this equation:

$b = \frac{1}{3}$ which corresponds to a maximum

$b = 1$ which corresponds to a minimum

Substituting $b = \frac{1}{3}$ into Eq. 45 yields

$$\frac{db}{dH} = -\frac{4}{27} H_{total} \tag{48}$$

To find the optimal concentration of antibody, we substitute $b = \frac{1}{3}$ into Eq. 44

$$\frac{B}{F} = K_{eq} (R_{total} - \frac{1}{3} H_{total}) \tag{49}$$

In the absence of unlabeled hormone

$$H_{total} = H^*_{total} + H_{total} = H^*_{total} \approx 0$$

and

$$\frac{B}{F} = \frac{b}{1-b} = \frac{\frac{1}{3}}{\frac{2}{3}} = 0.5$$

Thus,

$$0.5 = K_{eq} R_{total}$$

or

$$R_{total} = 0.5/K_{eq} \tag{50}$$

Based upon this analysis, the slope increases for any value of B/T as $H_{total} \rightarrow$ 0 and reaches a maximum value of

$$\frac{d\,(B/T)}{dH_{total}} = \frac{-4}{27} K_{eq} \qquad \text{when } B/T = \frac{1}{3}$$

This implies that the maximal sensitivity (maximal slope) can be obtained by using an antibody with a very large K_{eq} at a concentration of $0.5/K_{eq}$ together with a sufficiently high specific activity of the labeled hormone so that H^*_{total} can be as small as possible with an initial $B/T = \frac{1}{3}$.

Ekins and his colleagues (3) define assay sensitivity as "the quantity of unlabeled hormone that will change the distribution of radioactivity by an amount equal to the standard deviation of the experimental determination of B^*/F^* in the absence of unlabeled hormone"; in other words, the least detectable dose. The total experimental error (in addition to counting errors) can be estimated from the amount and specific activity of the tracer and errors in the separation method. The slope of the standard curve can also be computed as a function of antibody properties and hormone concentrations. Ekins then combines these two expressions to estimate the least detectable hormone concentration for any given values of binding site and labeled hormone concentration, equilibrium constant, specific activity of the tracer, and reaction volume. The optimal concentrations of antibody and labeled hormone concentrations can be determined by taking the partial derivative of this expression and solving for the values that optimize assay sensitivity. The result of this analysis was that, in the case of no experimental error (other than counting error) for maximum sensitivity to be obtained:

$$
\begin{aligned}
R_{total} &= 3/K_{eq} \\
H^*_{total} &= 4/K_{eq} \\
B_0/F_0 &= 1 \qquad \text{(or } B/T = 0.5\text{)}.
\end{aligned}
\tag{51}
$$

With the above concentrations of antibody and labeled hormone, the least detectable dose is given by

$$\Delta H = \frac{5.66}{(K_{eq}\,SVT)^{\frac{1}{2}}} \tag{52}$$

where K_{eq} is the equilibrium constant of the antibody, S is the specific activity of the labeled hormone (cpm/unit weight), V is the reaction volume (milliliters), T is the total counting time for both free and bound fractions (minutes), and ΔH is the least detectable dose.

Therefore, this analysis yields three important results:

1. Maximum sensitivity is obtained when the reaction mixture in the absence of unlabeled hormone has $B^*/F^* = 1$.

2. The optimal concentrations of tracer and of binding protein are independent of the specific activity of the labeled hormone.
3. The least detectable dose is inversely proportional to the square root of the specific activity of the tracer, the binding constants, the reaction volume, and the counting time.

When the analysis was extended to include experimental errors (pipetting, incomplete separation of bound and free hormone, etc.), the following results were obtained:

1. As the experimental error or the specific activity of the labeled hormone increase or K_{eq} decreases, the optimal concentrations of R_{total} and H^*_{total} decrease sigmoidially from the zero error values of $3/K_{eq}$ and $4/K_{eq}$ toward $1/K_{eq}$ and 0, respectively.
2. Increases in the maximum theoretical sensitivity due to increases in specific activity and $1/K_{eq}$ are significantly reduced as experimental error increases. In general, experimental error increases the least detectable dose.
3. With non-zero experimental error, labeled hormone with a binding constant slightly higher than that of the unlabeled hormone yields the highest sensitivity.

The approaches to optimization of the competitive protein binding assay taken by Yalow and Berson and by Ekins and co-workers differ in the definition of sensitivity, the scope of the analysis, and which mathematical model of the competitive protein binding assay was used. These differences in approach account for some of the differences in the results of these analyses. Ekins has chosen to determine under what conditions the least detectable dose will be minimized, taking into account specific activities of labeled hormone, the reaction volume, and the counting time. He has used the complete model of the basic competitive protein binding assay that was derived above (Eq. 20) rather than the more simplified Scatchard representation used by Yalow and Berson. However, although different models of the competitive protein binding assay and different definitions of sensitivity were used, the resulting optimal conditions are more similar than different:

	B_0/T_0	B_0/F_0	R_{total}	H^*_{total}
Yalow and Berson	0.333	0.5	$0.5/K_{eq}$	0
Ekins et al.	0.50	1.0	$3/K_{eq}$	$4/K_{eq}$

These results can be used as starting conditions for the optimization of a particular assay. If it is desired to measure the lowest possible hormone concentration, the conditions of Ekins would be selected, whereas if it were more important to maximize the slope of the standard curve, the conditions proposed by Yalow and Berson would be used. However, it is important to remember that a particular competitive binding assay should be optimized with respect to the performance criteria most appropriate for its anticipated use.

ESTIMATION OF ASSOCIATION AND DISSOCIATION RATE CONSTANTS

When it is desired to use the differential equations (Eqs. 3 and 4) derived above for labeled and unlabeled hormone to optimize the competitive protein binding assay, estimates of the association and dissociation rate constants are required. This approach is the only one valid for nonequilibrium assays. In order to estimate these constants, experiments must be performed in which the rate of binding of labeled hormone to the antibody-binding site (association) or the rate of displacement of previously bound hormone from the antibody-binding site by the addition of unlabeled hormone (dissociation) are estimated. These kinds of experiments are commonly used to quantitate the binding of hormones to receptors. In order to estimate the association rate constant, antibody and hormone are mixed together in the same buffer used in the assay. After a short period of incubation, free and bound hormone are separated and the free or the bound hormone–antibody complex is measured. The experiment is then repeated at different incubation times. The amount of labeled hormone remaining or the amount of labeled hormone–antibody complex is then plotted as a function of the incubation time. The rate of disappearance of H* or the rate of appearance of H*R is then estimated by fitting these data with a single exponential function. For the disappearance of H*, we use

$$y = y(0) \, e^{-at} \tag{53}$$

where y is the amount of H* remaining at time t, $y(0)$ is the amount of H* added at time $t = 0$, a is the association rate constant $(1/t)$, and t is the time of incubation for the appearance of H*R, use

$$g = c \, (1 - e^{-at}) \tag{54}$$

where g is the amount of H*R measured at time t, c is the steady-state concentration of H*R, and a is the association rate constant.

If the equilibrium constant K_{eq} and the association rate constant k are known, the dissociation rate constant can be calculated from Eq. 13:

$$K_{eq} = \frac{k_1}{k_{-1}}$$

or

$$k_{-1} = k_1 / K_{eq} \tag{55}$$

In order to estimate experimentally the dissociation rate constant, labeled hormone and a large concentration of antibody are mixed together in assay buffer and allowed to come to equilibrium. Under these conditions, most of the labeled hormone (>95%) is bound to the antibody. An excess of unlabeled hormone is then added, and free and bound hormone are separated and either the labeled free hormone (assumed to be produced by the dissociation of H*R) or the bound hormone–antibody complex is measured. The experiment is then repeated at different times after the addition of unlabeled hormone. These data are plotted as a function of time and are fitted by a single exponential function. If the disappearance of H*R is plotted, then Eq. 53 is used, where $y(0)$ is the initial bound hormone–antibody complex counts and a is the dissociation rate constant, whereas if the appearance of H* is plotted, then Eq. 55 is used.

These experiments are designed to estimate the association rate constant k_1 and the dissociation rate constant k_{-1} of the reaction of labeled hormone to the antibody represented by Eq. 3. The same assumptions used in the derivation of Eq. 3 are required for the estimation of these rate constants. Once we have obtained estimates of k_1 and k_{-1}, we assume that $k_2 = k_1$ and $k_{-2} = k_{-1}$ based on the assumption that H* and H have identical physical-chemical properties and participate in the reactions identically (assumption 5) and the following identities:

$$K_{eq}{}^* = K_{eq}$$

$$\frac{k_2}{k_{-2}} = \frac{k_1}{k_{-1}} \tag{56}$$

Given these estimates of the association and dissociation rate constants k_1, k_2, k_{-1}, k_{-2} and the initial values of $[H^*]_0 = H^*{}_{total}$, $[H]_0 = H_{total}$, and $[R]_0 = R_{total}$, we can solve Eqs. 3 and 4 for both the free labeled and unlabeled hormone concentration at any specified time. These solutions may then be used to predict the responses of labeled and unlabeled hormone and to optimize a nonequilibrium competitive binding assay. The performance criteria discussed above are applicable to a nonequilibrium assay, and simulation studies with different initial combinations of the assay design parameters should lead to the optimal assay for the desired application.

REFERENCES

1. Scatchard G: The attractions of proteins for small molecules and ions. *Ann NY Acad Sci* 51:660, 1949.

2. Ekins RP, Newman GB, O'Riordan, JHL: in Haynes RL, Goswitz FA, and Murphy BEP (eds): Theoretical aspects of "saturation" and radioimmunoassay. *Radioisotopes in Medicine: In Vitro Studies.* Oak Ridge, US atomic energy commission, 1968, pp 59–100.

3. Ekins RP, Newman GB, O'Riordan JHL: Saturation Assays, in: McArthur JW, Colton J (eds): *Statistics in Endocrinology.* Cambridge, MIT Press, 1970, pp 345–378.

4. Berson SA, Yalow RS: Quantitative aspects of the reaction between insulin and insulin-binding antibody. *J Clin Invest* 38:1996, 1959.

5. Feldman H, Levine D, Rodbard D: Theory of complex ligand-binding system: Applications to radioimmunoassay and plasma steroid-protein equilibria. 10 Reunion Annual de la Societad Mexicana de Nutricion y Endocrinologia, Mexico, D.F. 615, 1970.

6. Feldman H, Rodbard D: Mathematical theory of radioimmunoassay, in Odell WD, Daughaday WH (eds): *Principles of Competitive Protein-Binding Assays*. Philadelphia, J.B. Lippincott Co, 1971, pp 158–203.

7. Odell WD, Abraham G, Raud HR, et al: in: Diczfalusy E (ed): Influence of immunization procedures on the titer, affinity & specificity of antisera to glycopeptides. *First Karolinska Symposium in Reproductive Endocrinology*. Copenhagen, Bogytrykkerikt Forum, 1969, p 64.

8. Abraham G, Odell WD: in Peron FG, Caldwell BV (eds): Solid-phase radioimmunoassay of serum estradiol-17β: A semi-automated approach. *Immunological Methods in Steroid Determination*. New York, Appleton-Century-Crofts, 1970, p 87.

9. Berson SA, Yalow RS: Principles and Methodological Considerations in Radioimmunoassay, in *Proceedings of the 9th Japan Conference on Radioisotopes*. Tokyo, 1969, p 643.

10. Yalow RS, Berson SA: *Proceedings of Symposium on "In vitro" Procedures with Radioisotopes in Clinical Medicine and Research*. Vienna, IAFA, SM-124-106, 1970, p 455.

11. Yalow RS, and Berson SA: Introduction and General Considerations, in Odell WD, Daughaday WH (eds): *Principles of Competitive Protein-Binding Assays*. Philadelphia, J.B. Lippincott, 1971, pp 1–24.

CHAPTER 9

PITFALLS IN PEPTIDE RADIOIMMUNOASSAYS

Paul Franchimont
Jean-Claude Hendrick
Jean-Pierre Bourguignon
Aimée-Marguerite Reuter

Various nonspecific factors may alter the reaction between the antigen to be measured and the antibody or may interfere with complete separation of free labeled antigen from that bound to antibody. Among these nonspecific factors, one must consider damage to labeled antigen leading to alterations in its physical and immunochemical properties, as well as interferences due to ionic concentration, to the presence of certain serum proteins, and to marked pH changes. Further, several polypeptide hormones are characterized by polymorphism. In the presence of a given immunologic substance, certain of these forms may not be detected or, on the other hand, may cause complete or incomplete cross-reaction with the standard hormone preparation. Definition of the forms of an antigen measured by a particular system is essential for knowledge of whether the results obtained correspond to measurement of the hormone monomer or, on the other hand, to the sum of the hormone, its precursors, and its metabolites.

EFFECT OF TRACER DAMAGE

Labeled antigen may be damaged during incubation as a result of various processes: decay catastrophe resulting from a change in the antigen when a radioiodine atom undergoes decay; chemical alterations induced by oxidizing or reducing radicals arising as a result of the absorption of ionizing radiation by the water molecules of solution containing radioactive substances; and actions of proteolytic enzymes (1).

As a rule, the greater the amount of serum added to the incubation medium, the greater the percentage of labeled hormone damaged. Furthermore, protein molecules labeled with a large number of radioactive iodine atoms are particularly fragile and are readily damaged during incubation. Finally, they are more likely to be deiodinated during incubation when the specific activity is high and there is resulting chemical instability.

Damaged molecules lose some of their chemical and immunochemical properties (see review of [2]). Thus, some damaged molecules aggregate, and others bind nonspecifically to normal serum proteins and to immune complexes such as those formed by the double-antibody separation method. Others are broken down into small peptide fragments. The damaged products do not retain their property of reacting with ion-exchange resins as does unlabeled antigen. Finally, their reactivity with antibody is reduced or lost. The degree of tracer damage can thus be assessed by measuring the percentage of radioactivity that, in the absence of antibody,

- migrates from the point of application to the paper when submitted to chromatoelectrophoresis for hormones of molecular weight less than 10,000
- does not bind to charcoal or silicates as do labeled and unlabeled antigens of molecular weight less than 10,000 [calcitonin, parathormone, (PTH), insulin, glucagon, β-endorphin]
- does not react with ion exchangers that normally bind it
- absorbs to precipitating immune complexes or to the double antibody solid phase (DASP) used for the separation of free labeled antigen from that bound to antibody
- is precipitated by organic solvents such as alcohol, dioxane, and propylethylene glycol

The degree of damage can also be assessed from the percentage of labeled hormone that cannot be bound by excess antibody before and after incubation. Nevertheless, the assessment of damage by the use of excess antibody is a less useful method than others, because it is known that even damaged antigen may still react with antibody when the latter is present in large amounts.

It is therefore always necessary to run controls, that is, measurement of the amount of tracer that in the absence of antibody behaves in the same way as the labeled antigen–antibody complex. Assays in which tracer damage exceeds 10% must be regarded as quantitatively imprecise and should be discarded.

Incubation damage may be reduced by a series of precautions: incubation carried out at low temperature, lower serum protein concentration in the incubation medium, the presence of reducing substances (iodacetamide) or proteolytic enzyme inhibitors, and late addition of the labeled hormone.

Among the enzyme inhibitors, Trasylol (Bayer) may be mentioned; it neutralizes competitively the protease and esterase activities of kallikrein and other enzymes such as plasmin, trypsin, and chymotrypsin. Soybean trypsin inhibitor has a powerful antiprotease activity. Benzamidine chlorhydrate is a strong enzyme inhibitor. EDTA complexes ionized calcium which is a cofactor in a number of enzyme reactions, particularly those involving carboxypeptidases.

NONSPECIFIC INTERFERENCE

With certain antisera, the antigen–antibody reaction may be affected significantly by the nature and concentration of the buffer, of salts, and of proteins present in the plasma, urine, or tissue extract. Likewise, the pH of the incubation medium may lead to lower binding of the antigen to the antibody (3).

EFFECT OF pH

Antigen–antibody complexes are dissociated at extremes of pH. It is therefore useful to define for each system the pH region in which the antigen–antibody reaction is not affected (Table 1). A buffer should therefore be used in the incubation medium that ensures an optimal antigen–antibody reaction and avoids pH changes.

The results of gonadotrophin assays are not changed under the usual conditions of urinary pH (Fig. 1).

Table 1. Effects of pH of the Incubation Medium on the Reaction Between Labeled LH and Anti-LH Antibody[a]

pH of Incubation Medium	$\dfrac{Bound}{Total} \times 100 \pm SD$
4.2	13.5 ± 0.4
4.8	17.7 ± 0.7
5.3	21.5 ± 0.6
6.1	26.7 ± 0.4
6.5	29 ± 0.5
6.9	28.5 ± 0.4
7.5	29.8 ± 0.9
8.2	28.4 ± 0.4
10.1	21.1 ± 0.2

[a]In this system, the immunologic reaction is stable between pH 6.5 and 8.2.

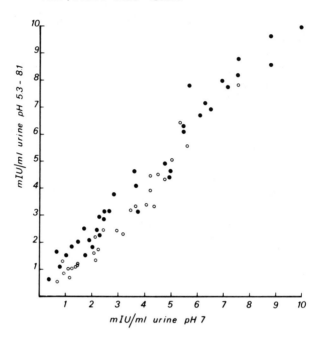

• LH
○ FSH

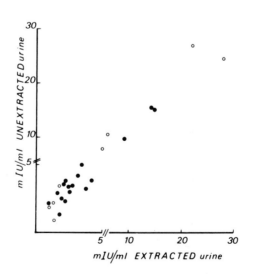

Table 2. Effect of Osmolality on the Binding of Labeled LH to Anti-LH Antibody

Concentration of Incubation Medium (osmoles/liter)	$\frac{Bound}{Total} \times 100 \pm SD$
0.1	29.3 ± 0.9
0.2	29.6 ± 0.7
0.4	28.5 ± 0.4
0.6	28.4 ± 0.5
0.8	28.2 ± 1.1
1	26.4 ± 0.4
2	23.4 ± 0.6

EFFECTS OF OSMOLALITY

With certain antibodies, the antigen–antibody reaction may be changed by the ionic concentration of the incubation medium. In this situation, serum dilutions, as a result of the reduced osmolality, give values different from those found in undiluted or slightly diluted serum.

Heparin also appears to inhibit the antigen–antibody reaction with certain antisera, probably because of its strongly polyanionic nature.

On the other hand, certain antisera show little sensitivity to changes in osmolality in a region which it is thus convenient to establish (Table 2). These antisera once selected, can be used to measure antigens in biologic

Figure 1. Correlation between FSH (●) and LH (○) values measured by radioimmunoassays in several urine samples using different conditions of pH and urine extraction. On the bottom is shown the correlation between values determined in unextracted samples and acetone extracts of the same urine specimens. A highly significant correlation ($p < .001$) was found for both FSH and LH. This correlation was also observed for very low gonadotrophin concentrations as seen in prepubertal children, that is, values below 5 mIU/ml urine. On the top is shown the correlation between values determined in unextracted urine at various pH values and after previous neutralization of urine. For both gonadotrophins, a highly significant correlation ($p < .001$) was obtained between values measured at different urinary pH values. This suggests that pH variations of urine within normal limits do not influence the radioimmunoassays of gonadotrophins in unextracted urine in the experimental conditions of these radioimmunoassays. (With permission from Bourguignon JP, Vanderschueren-Lodewyckx, M, Reuter Am, et al: Radioimmunoassays of unextracted gonadotrophins in timed fractions of 24 hours urine: Morning increase of gonadotrophin excretion, a sleep–wake pattern in relation to puberty. *Horm Res,* 1980, in press.)

fluids such as urine (Fig. 1) in which changes in pH (5.1 to 8.2) and osmolality (100–800 mosmoles/liter) are known to occur under normal circumstances.

EFFECTS OF SERUM PROTEINS

All radioimmunoassayists are aware of the nonspecific effect of serum on the inhibition curve of the labeled antigen–antibody reaction. Serum proteins usually reduce the binding of labeled antigen to antibody in the absence of unlabeled antigens and displace the curve downward. Under exceptional circumstances, the presence of serum proteins increases the reaction between labeled antigen and antibody.

This effect, often inhibitory and rarely stimulatory, on the immunologic reaction, can be exerted on the first antigen–antibody reaction and/or on the immunologic reaction used for separation, as occurs with the double-antibody or DASP method. In order to establish on which reaction the serum proteins have their effect, one must compare the percentage binding of labeled antigen to antibody in the absence of antigen-free serum or in its presence, added at the beginning of the incubation or at the same time as the separation system. Reuter et al. (4) showed that the effect of serum on the primary immunologic reaction was due to steric inhibition by certain serum proteins, particularly IgM globulin and α_2-macroglobulin.

PRACTICAL CONSIDERATIONS

These nonspecific effects depend on particular antigen–antibody systems and should be evaluated for each system.

In all cases, care must be taken that the inhibition curve obtained with known quantities of the reference antigen are established under conditions as close as possible to those used to assay biologic media: qualitative and quantitative identity of the proteins present, the same pH, and the same ionic concentration. Ideally, the standard curve should thus be established in the presence of the same biologic fluid free of the antigen (antigen-free serum, urine, organ extract).

COMPLETE SEPARATION OF FREE ANTIBODY-BOUND LABELED ANTIGEN

The separation method must be controlled precisely, as errors may arise at this step of the assay (see Chapter 16).

The separation method must be adapted to the antigen to be measured. Thus, chromatoelectrophoresis is particularly suitable for small polypeptides such as ACTH, insulin, glucagon, and PTH. On the other hand, for glycoprotein hormones such as human chorionic gonadotrophin (HCG) and thyroid-stimulating hormone (TSH) chromatoelectrophoresis should not be used, as the free labeled hormone does not remain absorbed at the site of application.

The experimental conditions must be carefully chosen to ensure complete separation. This is the case for the double-antibody technique which is used for the radioimmunoassay of practically all peptide hormones. The procedure depends on precipitation of the labeled antigen–antibody complex by anti-γ-globulin antibody. The conditions for precipitation should be in the zone of equivalence between the γ-globulins (i.e., those involved in the soluble immune complex of the labeled antigen–antibody) and the anti-γ-globulin antibody. This zone of equivalence must be determined by changing the γ-globulin concentration and the amount of anti-γ globulin antiserum. Likewise, the use of organic solvents such as dioxane and polyethylene glycol (PEG) requires that the optimal concentration that leaves the free labeled antigen in solution and precipitates all that is antibody-bound be established.

Serum proteins may interfere in the separation method. Thus, they may carry free labeled antigen from its site of application when chromatoelectrophoresis is used. Likewise, they can prevent absorption of free labeled antigen to silicate (kaolin, talc) and to charcoal or, on the other hand, they may lead to precipitation of free labeled antigen by organic solvents. They may also lower the binding of the labeled antigen–antibody complex to the DASP. Thus, validation of the radioimmunoassay method always requires a study of the effect of the biologic fluids, particularly of serum and plasma, on the method of separation.

The quality of the tracer affects the efficiency of the separation method. Damaged labeled antigen does not behave like undamaged tracer: It does not bind to charcoal, it leaves the point of application in chromatoelectrophoresis, it adsorbs nonspecifically to the DASP and to the immune complexes in the double-antibody system, and it is precipitated by organic solvents.

POLYMORPHISM OF PEPTIDE HORMONES

It has been shown over the past 10 years that many protein and polypeptide hormones exist in several forms both in their gland of origin and in the plasma (see reviews in [5] and [6]); such heterogeneity was established by radioimmunologic studies. For example, the heterogeneity of PTH was de-

Table 3. Causes of the Heterogeneity of Protein
and Polypeptide Hormones

Precursors
Isohormones
Polymers
Protein-bound hormones (?)
Subunits
Metabolites
Artifacts of extraction and purification
Tumor or adenoma hormone analogues

scribed first by Berson and Yalow (1968) (7), who noted a dissociation between the immunologic activity of plasma PTH and the hormone in glandular extracts with one antiserum, whereas with another antiserum there
was no difference. This indicated that the first antiserum contained antibodies against antigenic groups present in the PTH molecule extracted
from the gland but absent or altered in their binding affinity in the plasma
PTH molecule. The other antisera contained only antibodies directed
against antigenic groups present on the PTH molecules both in plasma and
in the gland extract.

The heterogeneity of plasma and urinary peptide hormones has been
evaluated by radioimmunoassay of eluates from gel filtration or of fractions obtained from samples subjected to ultracentrifugation. Heterogeneity of charge is evaluated by radioimmunoassay of eluates from paper
strip or starch gel electrophoresis or from isotachophoresis (8). The advantage of starch gel electrophoresis is that it separates proteins on the basis of
their size and charge (9).

Striking examples of the heterogeneity of plasma hormones and hormones in glandular extracts have been found with insulin, ACTH, PTH,
thyrocalcitonin, gonadotrophins, glucagon, thyroid-stimulating hormone
(TSH), gastrin, growth hormone, and prolactin.

This heterogeneity of protein and polypeptide hormones may be due to
one or more of the causes listed in Table 3. The theoretical possibility of a
carrier protein is represented in the table, but it has not been established
that any circulating peptide hormone is bound to serum proteins.

BIG FORMS

For the majority of peptide hormones, radioimmunoassay has demonstrated the existence of one or more forms with a molecular weight greater
than that of the commonly recognized highly purified hormone obtained
from glandular extracts (5). In certain cases, treatment with 4–8 M urea

dissociated these "big" or "big-big" hormones into monomeric forms, whereas under other circumstances they were not affected by urea or guanidine treatment. One must suspect polymerization, aggregation, or binding to other proteins in the first case, whereas the second raises the possibility of the existence of a prohormone or even of a pre-prohormone. This hypothesis is more likely, as these big forms differ in charge as well as in size from the conventional small forms; trypsin treatment converts them to substances with the characteristics of the known small forms. In cerebrospinal fluid, three peaks of β-endorphin-like material have been identified, the first probably corresponding to pre-pro-opiomelanocortin, the second to β-lipotrophin, and the third to β-endorphin itself.

Ectopic hormones may also have specific forms and charges, as is the case for big ACTH produced by cancer of the lung and for big calcitonin produced by medullary thyroid carcinoma, the behavior of which on isotachophoresis is different from that of the circulating forms in normal subjects (8).

SMALL FORMS

These forms of lower molecular weight correspond either to the constituent subunits or to hormonal fragments. This is the situation in the assay of PTH when an anti-C-terminal antiserum is used. The immunoreactivity of PTH is then mainly due to the fragments derived from the 34–84 sequence which has a long half-life (10). Likewise, it is known that the four glycoprotein hormones, follicle-stimulating hormone (FSH), luteinizing hormone (LH), TSH, and HCG are made up of two nonidentical polypeptide subunits designated α and β. These exist in the free state in serum and urine and are found particularly in cases of hypersecretion of the intact hormone: pregnancy for HCG, hypothyroidism for TSH, and menopause or the luteinizing hormone-releasing hormone (LH-RH) stimulation test for the gonadotrophins. Figure 2 shows the presence of free HCG α and β subunits in the serum of pregnant women, and Figure 3 the presence of free α subunit, LH β subunit, and fragments of free β subunit in the concentrated urine of menopausal women.

Depending on whether the antiserum used reacts with an antigenic determinant present and accessible on all circulating forms or only on some of them, certain of the values obtained on the same sample will be different. Certain fragments may cross-react completely and thus give inhibition curves that are superimposable on that obtained when the purified antigen is used as a standard. In contrast, fragments may give only an incomplete cross-reaction and the criterion of parallelism of inhibition curves is not fulfilled. Under these circumstances, it must be concluded that the standard and endogenous forms of the hormone in the unknown sample do not

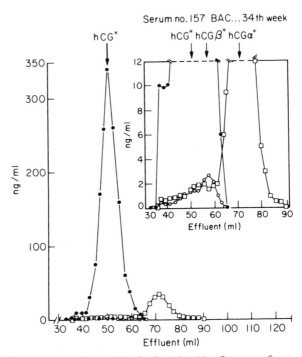

Figure 2. Chromatography on Sephadex G-100 of serum from a woman at 34 weeks of pregnancy. Each 2-ml fraction of the eluate was assayed for HCG, HCGα, and HCGβ. The arrows indicate where labeled native HCG, HCGα, and HCGβ subunits are eluted. The inset shows a magnified version of the effluent fractions containing α and β subunits. •, HCG; □, HCGα; ○, HCGβ. In late pregnancy, β-subunit immunoreactivity still shows two distinct peaks, the first coinciding with maximum elution of HCG and the second in the elution area of the β subunit. The α subunit immunoreactivity shows essentially one peak in the position of monomeric α subunit. (With permission from Reuter AM, Gaspard UJ, Deville, JL, et al: Serum concentrations of human chorionic gonadotrophin and its alpha and beta subunits: 1. During normal singleton and twin pregnancies. *Clin Endocrinal* 13:305, 1980.)

Figure 3. Sephadex G-100 chromatography of concentrated urinary gonadotrophins and assays of FSH, LH, α subunit, and LHβ subunit. One peak of urinary immunoreactive FSH was found to be eluted in a volume similar to that of labeled pituitary FSH. In contrast, urinary immunoreactive LH was eluted in two fractions. The first was eluted in the same volume as pituitary LH, whereas the second was more retarded. The urinary LH fragment was retarded on Sephadex to a position beyond that of the LHβ subunit and between the elution volumes of PTH and calcitonin, suggesting that its moelculare weight was near 5,000. The α subunit is eluted in a volume similar to that of labeled LHα subunit. This α subunit material does not seem to cross-react in FSH and LH radioimmunoassay. Three elution

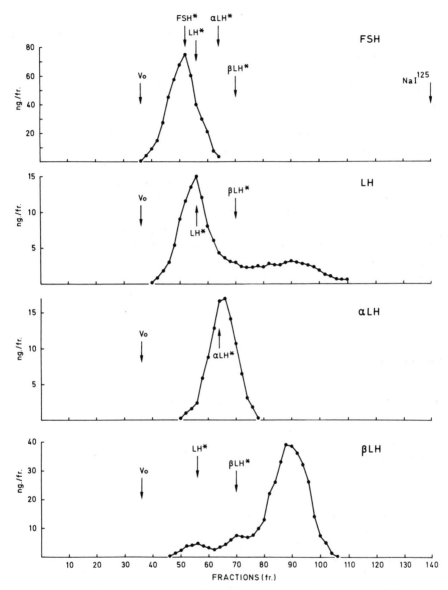

peaks of immunoreactive LHβ subunit material are detected: the first in the elution zone of native LH, the second where LHβ subunit is eluted, and the third (the most important) in a more retarded region. This experiment suggests that urinary immunoreactive FSH is similar to pituitary FSH, whereas urinary LH, like immunoreactive material, appears heterogeneous and likely to contain an immunoreactive fragment smaller than LH and LHβ subunit. There is a complete cross-reaction between LHβ subunit and this small LH fragment indicating a close immunolgical similarity between them.

behave identically. An antiserum must then be found with which the standard preparation and the circulating endogenous forms react equally.

At the present time, it is not possible to assign a physiological significance to every cause of heterogeneity of protein and polypeptide hormones. Nevertheless, the emerging concept of prohormones for peptide hormones, either in the form of higher-molecular-weight precursors or in the form of lower-molecular-weight subunits, suggests strongly that prohormones have some function. In the case of nonhormonal proteins such as pancreatic proteases, the proenzyme is inactive and thus prevents self-digestion. The connecting peptide in proinsulin ensures the proper folding necessary for formation of the disulfide bridges of insulin. Prohormones may have a role in the postsynthetic transport and storage of hormone in the cell. Another possibility is that the conversion of prohormone to hormone provides an additional point for the control of hormone secretion, as seems to be the case for pro-PTHs.

Obviously many years of research will be needed before the significance and possible function of all the causes of hormone heterogeneity are determined.

REFERENCES

1. Berson SA, Yalow RS: In *Methods in Investigative and Diagnostic Endocrinology.* Edited by Berson, Yalow (eds): New York, American Elsevier, 1973.
2. Franchimont P: Les principes géneraux des dosages radioimmunologiques. *Ann Biol Clin* 28:3, 1970.
3. Yalow RS, Berson SA: Problems of validation of radioimmunoassays, in Odell WD, Daughaday, WH (eds): *Principles of Competitive Protein-Binding Assays.* Philadelphia, JB Lippincott, 1971, p. 374.
4. Reuter AP, Hendrick JC, Sulon J, Franchimont P: Interference by serum proteins with LH radioimmunoassay using immunosorbent. *Acta Endocrinol,* 72:235, 1973.
5. Berson SA, Yalow RS: Heterogeneity of peptide hormones in plasma as revealed by radioimmunoassay, in *Endorinopathies et Immunologie.* Paris, Masson, 1971, p. 239.
6. Franchimont P, Gaspard U, Reuter, A, et al: Polymorphism of protein and polypeptide hormones. *Clin Endocrinol* 1:315, 1972.
7. Berson, SA, Yalow RS: Immunochemical heterogeneity of parathyroid hormone in plasma. *J Clin Endocrinol Metab* 28: 1037, 1968.
8. Heynen G, Gaspar S, Gysen, PH, Franchimont P: Démonstration de formes multiples de calcitonine immunoréactives (CTi) dans le sérum humain par isotachophorèse. Résultats préliminaries, 1980 (in press).
9. Legros, JJ, Crabbe, J: Serum neurophysins in familial central diabetes insipidus. *J Clin Endocrinol Metab* 47:1065, 1978.
10. Bouillon R, Koninckx PH, De Moor P: A radioimmunoassay for human serum parathyroid hormone: Methods and clinical evaluation, in *Radioimmunoassay and Related Procedures in Medicine.* Vienna, Int. Atomic Energy Agency, 1:353, 1974.

CHAPTER **10**
RADIOIMMUNOASSAY OF STEROIDS

Renzo Malvano

The radioimmunoassay (RIA) of steroids in biologic fluids is complicated by several factors, including the structural similarity of steroid molecules, their wide concentration ranges, the presence in most cases of interacting plasma proteins and of conjugated metabolites (i.e., steroid sulfates and glucuronides), and the nature of the steroid–antibody bond.

Preliminary concentration–purification operations provide an obvious tool for meeting the sensitivity and specificity requirements. Thus, in its most general design, the determination of a steroid implies a three-step analytical procedure where RIA is preceded by solvent extraction and chromatographic purification.

Both proteins potentially competing with steroid antibody and water-soluble steroid catabolites possibly competing with the analyte are eliminated in the first step. Extraction itself could be effective to some extent in increasing the overall selectivity of measurement through enrichment of the steroid analyte (see the example in Fig. 1*a*).

Intersteroid specificity is mainly achieved with the chromatographic step (see the example in Fig. 1*b*). Chromatography can furthermore help in removing lipophilic substances known largely to affect the steroid–antibody interaction. A variety of procedures have been proposed; among them column chromatography using Celite (1) or LH-Sephadex (2) has been of particular interest.

The preliminary operations, although minimizing the need for optimal RIA conditions, can entail experimental difficulties in routine steroid determinations. Much effort has therefore been oriented in recent years toward simplifying the assay scheme. This has resulted in several cases in the elimination of time-consuming, cumbersome chromatographic purifications thanks to the availability of highly specific antisera, and in some cases even in the direct assay of unextracted samples, though further complications arising from the presence of nonextractable interferences still limit the wide applicability of such methodologic simplifications. Other attempts have been directed toward improving the experimental ease of the RIA itself; among these, of greatest practical importance are the replacement of

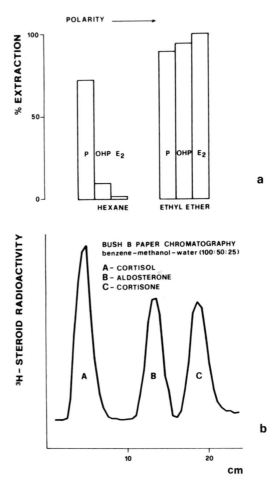

Figure 1. Examples of selectiveness potential of preliminary operations. (*a*) Extraction of progesterone, 17-hydroxyprogesterone, and estradiol with solvents with different polarity: Hexane improves assay specificity for progesterone; ethyl ether would be better used for group extraction and assay with highly specific antisera. (*b*) Purification by paper chomatography of some corticosteroids.

tritiated ³H-labeled steroids by γ-emitting tracers and the development of simpler and safer techniques for the separation of antibody-bound and free fractions.

Rather than being an exhaustive review of analytical techniques and results, this contribution is to be regarded as a tentative definition of some general aspects of steroid RIA in terms of assay practicability. Some recent developments of simplified procedures—as well as the peculiar features of steroid antisera and their analytical implications—will be used as a guideline in discussing what extent methodologic simplifications may be accepted and which problems the elimination of preliminary sample treatments still leaves, or even introduces, in the optimization of steroid RIA.

For the sake of brevity and simplicity the examples reported here are all derived from our own experience in setting up and optimizing steroid RIAs.

SPECIFICITY OF ANTISERA AND ASSAY SIMPLIFICATION

Any simplification of the prepurification procedures, and even more so their full elimination, demand as a necessary condition that antiserum specificity be adequately increased.

In this context the preparation of steroid immunogens according to a strategy aimed at maintaining the molecular identity of the haptens by

ESTRADIOL COUPLING POSITION FOR IMMUNOGEN PREPARATION	% CROSS – REACTION	
	ESTRONE 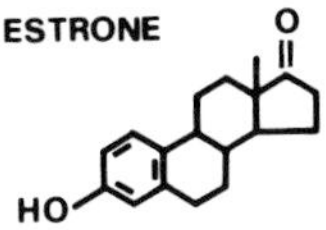	ESTRIOL 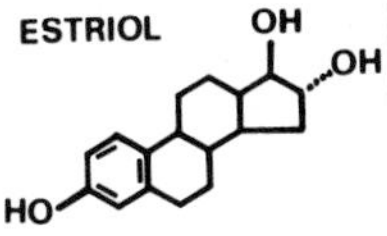
$n = 3$, 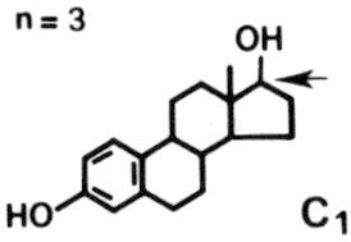 C_{17}	48 ± 8	5.0 ± 1.8
$n = 3$, 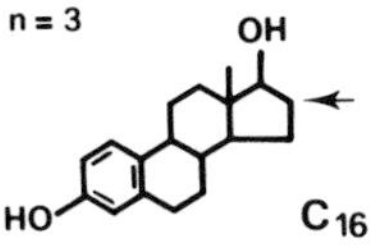 C_{16}	5.6 ± 2.0	40 ± 10
$n = 6$, 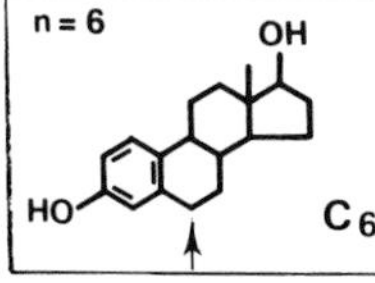 C_6	3.8 ± 1.2	0.48 ± 0.27

Figure 2. Specificity of estradiol antisera. Data refer to mean± SD.

TESTOSTERONE COUPLING POSITION FOR IMMUNOGEN PREPARATION	% CROSS - REACTION	
	DIHYDRO-TESTOSTERONE 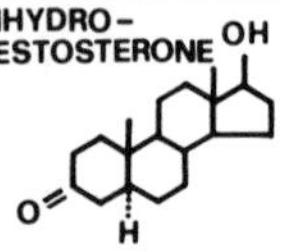	PROGESTERONE 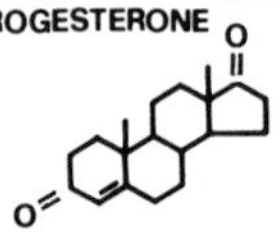
n = 4 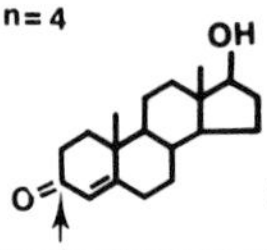 C3	62 ± 17	0.02 ± 0.01
n = 8 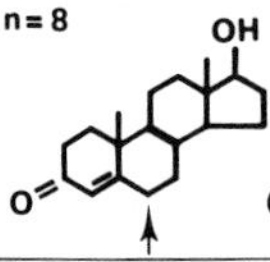 C6	47 ± 7	0.01 ± 0.005
n = 1 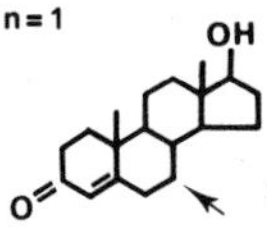 C7	43	0.02
n = 1 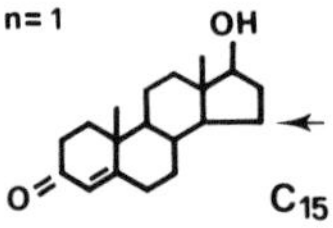 C15	2.2	1.5
n = 1 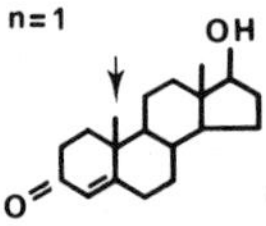 C19	10	0.01

Figure 3. Specificity of testosterone antisera. Data refer to groups of antisera (mean ± SD) or selected single antisera.

proper choice of the coupling position has proved critically important.* Thus high specificity has been conferred on antisera by selecting, in the immunogen preparation, a position on the steroid nucleus either different from those bearing any functional group or remote from the characterizing groups. Relevant examples are reported in regard to both approaches, for example, the use of progesterone-11 conjugates (3), C-6 or C-7 conjugates for Δ^4-3-oxosteroids (4), C-6 conjugates for estrogens (5–7), and C-15 and C-19 conjugates for testosterone (8,9), and coupling at C-3 for testosterone and progesterone (3), aldosterone (10), and cortisol (11). Most of the antisera obtained in these ways are now widespread in the routine RIA of dried plasma extracts.

*For details of conjugation techniques, also see Chapter 4 by Grover.

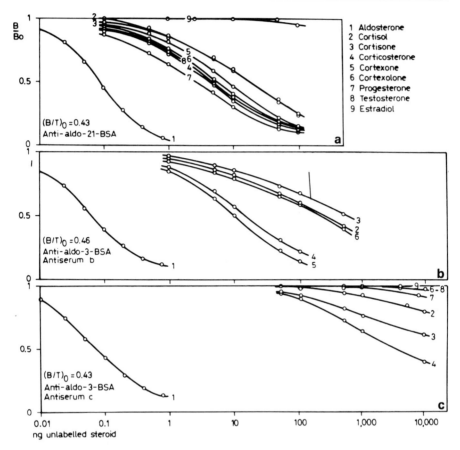

Figure 4. Multiple-titration curves of aldosterone antisera using as standards aldosterone and cross-reacting steroids (DCC, ^{3}H-labeled tracer). Data in (*a*) refer to pooled antisera, (*b*) and (*c*) to individual antisera.

How the choice of the coupling position can be effective in determining specificity can be illustrated by the example in Figure 2 relative to estradiol antisera [dextran-coated charcoal (DCC), ^{3}H-labeled tracer]. In this case, the extent of cross-reactivity of estrone and estriol is shown to be completely reversed when passing from C-17 to C-18 conjugates, as a consequence of the abolishment of either characterizing groups on coupling. The best specificity is expectedly obtained with C-6 derivatives.

The cross-reactivity data in Figure 3 well exemplify the problems possibly encountered when attempting a recognition of slight structural differences such as that involved in the discrimination of dihydrotestosterone in testosterone RIA (DCC, ^{3}H-labeled tracer). The inadequacy of the antisera raised against conjugates in the C-3, C-6, and C-7 positions is apparent. But when coupling through C-15, that is, far from the characterizing part of the molecules, the low cross-reaction resulting for dihydrotestosterone is counterbalanced by the loss of specificity for progesterone: the "shadow" effect of carrier protein around the D ring results in fact in attenuation of the difference between testosterone and progesterone. A compromise solution, allowing direct assay of plasma extracts to be performed for both men and women (9), is given by using C-19 testosterone derivatives for coupling.

Figure 4 indicates that, besides maintaining the integrity of the characteristic functional groups (like those borne by the C- and D-rings of corticosteroids), the individual variability of the immune response also remains a crucial point. In this figure, the analytical dose–response curves for aldosterone RIA and the multiple titration curves related to cross-reacting steroids are shown for a pool of antisera raised against a C-21 conjugate (Fig. 4a) and for two single antisera both obtained with a C-3 conjugate (Fig. 4b and c). The overall gain in specificity when changing from C-21 to C-3 immunogens is evident. Nevertheless, a comparison of Figure 4b and c points to the requirement for a proper selection among the individual antisera. Only with the high-quality antiserum c, in fact, is a reliable direct assay of crude plasma extracts feasible, as seen in Figure 5 from the correlation of parallel estimates with and without chromatographic purification.

The role of the individual response to immunization, hence the impor-

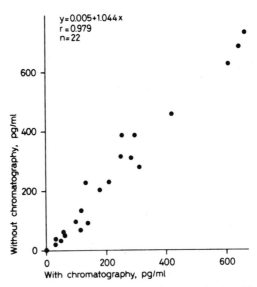

Figure 5. Correlation of plasma aldosterone estimates obtained by including and omitting a chromatographic purification (DCC, ^{3}H-labeled tracer). Data refer to antiserum in Figure 4c.

tance of obtaining highly specific antisera by immunizing an adequate number of animals, is further emphasized by the examples in Figure 6 and Table 1. In Figure 6 dramatic differences in specificity are indicated by the multiple titration curves obtained for three estriol antisera all elicited under identical conditions using a C-6 immunogen. The cross-reaction data listed in Table 1 for 14 antisera to a progesterone-11 conjugate show a large variability in both 17-hydroxyprogesterone and pregnenolone interference. As for the possibility of direct extract RIA, the antiserum in Figure 6a appears not to be adequate for a selective estriol measurement; progesterone antisera A to H in Table 1 should at least require the more selective hexane extraction to differentiate 17-hydroxyprogesterone contributions (see Fig. 1a).

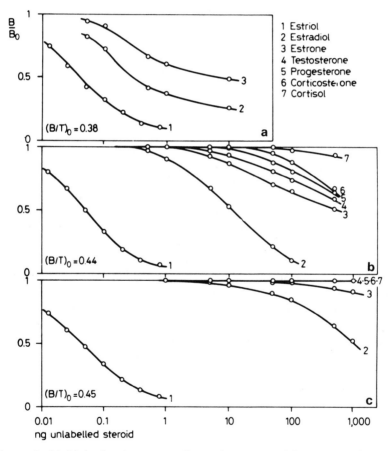

Figure 6. Multiple-titration curves for antisera to estriol-6–BSA, using as standards estriol and cross-reacting steriods (DCC, ³H-labeled tracer).

Table 1. Specificity of Some Individual Antisera Raised Against Progesterone-11-Succinyl—BSA[a]

Antiserum	Cross-Reaction (%)	
	17-Hydroxyprogesterone	Pregnenolone
A	4.7	1.8
B	4.0	1.5
C	2.3	4.0
D	2.3	3.0
E	1.3	1.3
F	1.2	0.40
G	1.0	3.8
H	0.92	0.69
I	0.75	0.45
J	0.50	0.49
K	0.40	0.60
L	0.32	0.16
M	0.15	1.0
N	0.14	0.35
$\bar{x} \pm$ SD	1.43 ± 1.37	1.40 ± 1.25

[a]DCC, ^{3}H-labeled tracer.

Not even exceptionally high specificity, such as that shown for estriol antiserum in Figure 6c, suffices to distinguish acceptably between estriol and estriol 3-sulfate, whereas the other main conjugate metabolite, estriol-16-glucuronide, is satisfactorily discriminated. These findings, illustrated in Figure 7, point to the limitations still inherent in differentiating slight structural changes around the steroid nucleus. An antiserum to estriol 2,4-conjugate was, however, recently reported to cross-react within limits with estriol 3-sulfate (12). In any case, the closeness of the coupling position to that involved in the structural change to be evidenced on the one hand, and the fact that we consistently failed to reproduce these results on the other, led us to conclude that a lucky accident had occurred rather than that a generalizable approach to the problem had been found.

Extreme specificity does not always imply an absolute advantage. Thus in RIA of primary bile acids a cumulative estimate of the tauro- and glycoconjugates of the same class is sought. A complete within-class cross-reactivity, together with an adequate between-class specificity, is readily obtained by coupling through the C-24 position in preparing the immunogens [see the example in Table 2 relative to polyethylene glycol (PEG) separation, ^{125}I-labeled tracer direct RIA, C-24 derivatives from glycoconjugates used in both cases].

Besides the steroid position for coupling to antigenic proteins, a relevant role in eliciting a specific immune response should be attributed to other

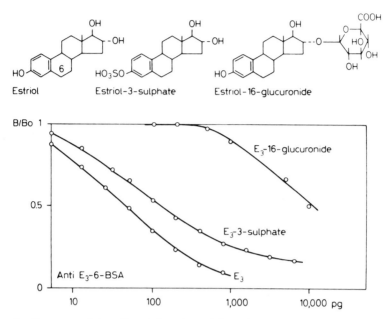

Figure 7. Cross-reactivity of estriol and estriol conjugates, using a highly specific antiserum (antiserum in Fig. 6c, DCC, ^{3}H-labeled tracer).

factors, including the number of steroid residues per protein molecule, the purity of the steroid derivatives, and seemingly the kind of hapten–protein chemical bridge. In the practice of steroid RIA, little is done to improve and control the antiserum specificity beyond proper preparation of immunogens and a careful selection from among the antisera obtained. Treatment of the antisera themselves could perhaps be of some interest. Though the heterogeneity of steroid antisera does not automatically imply the presence of antibody sites directed toward either the steroid analyte or the steroid-protein interface, this is apparently the case for the testosterone-15–bovine serum albumin (BSA) antiserum in Figure 8. The example in fact demonstrates how a neutralization procedure (13) is effective in increasing specificity toward progesterone interferences, thus allowing a direct assay of extracts even for female plasma (see the results in Table 3).

A marginal consideration, holding true in any RIA system, is worth being made concerning the effect of tracer–standard homology or heterology upon the apparent specificity of antisera. As seen in Figure 9 in the case of a testosterone-3–BSA antiserum, the extent of testosterone and dihydrotestosterone cross-reactivity is reversed on changing from testosterone to dihydrotestosterone ^{3}H-labeled tracer, with the practical consequence of allowing a sensitive assay for both steroids after a previous separation.

Table 2. Cross-Reactivity of Selected Antisera to Primary Bile Acids[b]

Bile Acid	Cross-Reaction (%)	
	Anti-CA[a]	Anti-CDCA[a]
Cholic	21	0.1
Glycocholic	100[b]	0.4
Taurocholic	98	0.5
Chenodeoxycholic	2.6	50
Glycochenodeoxycholic	8.3	100[b]
Taurochenodeoxycholic	3.8	102
Deoxycholic	0.1	<0.005
Glycodeoxycholic	0.6	<0.005
Taurodeoxycholic	0.8	<0.005
Ursodeoxycholic	<0.05	0.8
Lithocholic	<0.05	0.3
Glycolithocholic	0.5	1.6
Taurolithocholic	0.5	1.0

[a]CA = Cholic acid
CDCA = Chenodeoxycholic acid
[b]These assays used C-24 derivatives of glycoconjugates as an immunogen to prepare antisera, and ^{125}I-labeled tracers with polyethylene glycol as a separation reagent.

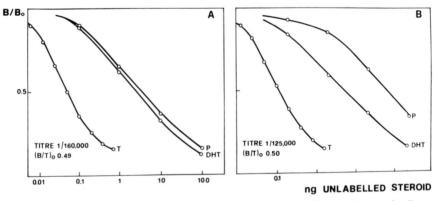

T-15-BSA ANTISERUM
A – UNTREATED
B – ADDED WITH
   0.25 mg/ml PROGESTERONE

Figure 8. Improvement of specificity of testosterone-15–BSA antiserum by "saturation" with progesterone (DCC, ^{3}H-labeled tracer). A 10-fold gain in specificity to progesterone is obtained when passing from situation (a) to (b), the cross-reactivity with dihydrotestosterone remaining unchanged.

170

Table 3. Testosterone Estimated by RIA
Using Anti-Testosterone-15–BSA[a]

Antisera Conditions	Testosterone (ng/ml)	
	Normal Men	Normal Women
Untreated	5.58 ± 1.98	0.76 ± 0.26
Progesterone Added	5.14 ± 2.07	0.46 ± 0.13

[a]DCC, ^{3}H-labeled tracer; $n = 25$. Each value is the mean ± SD.

METHODOLOGICAL IMPLICATIONS OF OTHER ANTISERUM CHARACTERISTICS

EFFECTS ASSOCIATED WITH THE NATURE OF THE STEROID–ANTIBODY BOND

Some aspects of the nature of the binding forces in the steroid–antibody interaction and their practical implications are worth considering when setting up a RIA procedure.

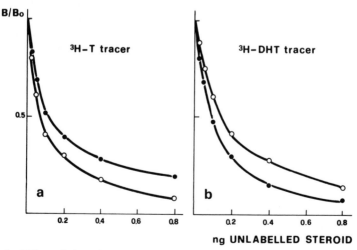

Figure 9. Effect of changing the tracer on testosterone–dihydrotestosterone cross-reactivity (testosterone-3–BSA antiserum, DCC,[3]H-labeled tracer).

Experimental evidence has been provided for the view that this interaction is mainly entropy-driven (14–18). Temperature proved in fact to have a limited effect on steroid binding; also, the incubation pH was found to exert only moderate effects, thus suggesting that the electrostatic forces play a minor role in stabilizing the antibody bond (17). As an example of the relative stability of steroid immunoreactivity under various conditions of pH and temperature, Table 4 reports the equilibrium constants derived by applying Sips' relationship (19) to the dose–response curves in the case of a cortisol–anticortisol system (^{3}H-labeled tracer, cellulose-coupled IgG separated from an anti-cortisol-21–BSA serum).

The slight temperature and pH dependence of steroid binding to antibody could be practically exploited in some instances for selective inhibition of interacting plasma proteins (see below). On the other hand, and more in general, the hydrophobic nature of the steroid–antibody bond could account for the susceptibility of the steroid RIA systems to interference from nonpolar substances. The modifications of the analytical response commonly found in the presence of dried residues of extraction solvents (solvent blank) or plasma extracts (sample blank) can be induced by substances of undefined origin left by solvents themselves, by lipids, or in general by lipophilic species coextracted with steroids from biologic fluids.

Table 5 and Figure 10 illustrate the variability of the solvent blank and of the effects associated with the sample blank within groups of antisera to the same steroids; a case of inaccuracy of estimation in the presence of lipoprotein extracts is shown in Table 6 (all the examples referring to DCC RIA and ^{3}H-labeled tracers). In particular in Figure 10 the uncorrected recovery of exogenous steroids accounts for the dose dependence of the blank, for positive and negative blanks (i.e., systematic overestimation or underestimation related to upward or downward shifts in binding values, respectively), as well as for crossing-over of the response curves in the absence and in the presence of the disturbing factors.

The impact of this nonsteroidal interference is expected to be especially important for less polar steroids (20). In fact, in our laboratory, the occurrence of unpredictable deviations in response in the presence of extracts and the incidence and extent of blank effects were found particularly to affect progesterone RIA.

A comprehensive, unequivocal explanation of the nature of these kinds of blanks remains difficult, as they probably originate from a complex interplay of several factors related to antibody bond stabilization, the characteristics of individual antisera, mechanisms of steroid entrapping in lipidic microemulsions, and the effects on bound–free separation (e.g., inhibitory action directed toward adsorbents).

In any case, blank effects have precise methodologic implications, not excluding a selection of antisera and methods according to wider selectivity

Table 4. Effect of pH and Temperature of the Affinity of Cortisol–Anticortisol Interaction[a]

| Reaction Conditions | | Equilibrium Constant, |
pH	Temperature (°C)	$K_0 \times 10^9 (M^{-1})$
3.5	4	2.47
3.5	20	1.79
3.5	30	1.39
4.7	20	2.52
7.4	20	3.39

[a]Cellulose-coupled anticortisol IgG.

Table 5. Solvent Blank in Steroid RIA: Dependence on Individual Antisera[a]

Antiserum		Solvent	Blank (pg/tube)
Anti-testosterone-3–BSA	a	Ethyl Ether	6.4 ± 2.1
	b		0
	c		8.2 ± 3.1
	d		1.2 ± 1.0
Anti-progesterone-11–BSA	a	Hexane	13.5 ± 3.5
	b		28.1 ± 7.3
	c		34.0 ± 5.0
	d		5.0 ± 3.5
	e		39.5 ± 5.1

[a]DCC, ^{3}H-labeled tracers.

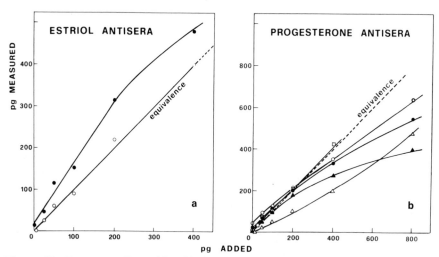

Figure 10. Recovery of steroids added to steroid-free plasma. Data refer to parallel experiments with different antisera (DCC, ^{3}H-labeled tracers).

Table 6. Effect of Lipoprotein
Extract on Estradiol RIA[a]

Estradiol Present	Estradiol Measured
60	42 ± 8
120	72 ± 6

[a]Mean values ± SD obtained with three different estradiol-6–BSA antisera by assaying known estradiol amounts in the absence and in the presence of dried ethyl ether extracts of 2 mg lipoproteins; DCC RIA, ^{3}H-labeled tracer.

criteria which account also for nonsteroid interferences. Careful choice and checks of the solvents and/or an assay structure including equalization of standard and sample conditions (e.g., preparation of calibration curves in the presence of dried solvent residues) are usually required to circumvent the errors arising from the solvent blank. More serious problems can be created by sample effects, for example, the occurrence of modifications of the assay response, which are difficult to anticipate and control, and the limited efficacy of the approaches used to obviate their cause (20) imply certain limitations for the general validity of steroid RIA in unpurified extracts, at least when high levels of accuracy are necessary.

IMPLICATIONS OF REACTION RATES AND IMMUNOCOMPLEX STABILITY

Kinetic factors governing steroid–antibody reactions are not usually taken into consideration to maximize the assay sensitivity, by working at equilibrium. However, no particular problem related to nonequilibrium is seemingly encountered in steroid RIA. Under the usual experimental conditions adopted in our laboratory, in fact, an apparent equilibrium was constantly reached after a relatively short time (i.e., 0.5–2 hours; see the examples in Figure 11).

Major practical implications, on the contrary, derive from the high dissociation rates found to characterize steroid immunocomplexes, resulting in a rapid exchange between free steroid and antibody-bound steroid and in a pronounced effectiveness of the separation agents in perturbing the bound-free equilibrium.

The role of exchange reactions in RIA appears to have been somewhat neglected. In fact, the rate of exchange of free steroid with preformed immunocomplexes determines the adequacy of procedures intended to improve sensitivity, such as sequential saturation (i.e., delayed addition of tracer) and techniques of premixing the RIA reagents, which are of some

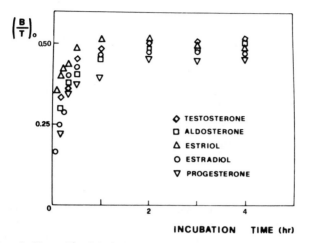

Figure 11. Binding of ^{3}H-labeled steroids to some antisera as a function of incubation time (40 ug/ml, pH 7.5 4°C, DCC RIA).

practical interest. Half-times of exchange ranging from a few minutes to less than 1 minute were observed for different steroid RIA systems, as exemplified in Table 7. Much lower exchange rates resulted instead for polypeptides and haptens other than steriods, as reported in the same table for comparison. Unlike these latter cases, therefore, in steroid RIA the counterbalancing effect of the high rate of exchange between free tracer and preformed "cold" immunocomplexes rapidly results in a complete re-equilibration of the system. Therefore, in practical terms (i.e., for time sequences compatible with large sample series), sequential saturation is of little or no help in steriod RIA. On the other hand, rapidly exchanging immunocomplexes allow antiserum and tracer to be premixed,

Table 7. Half-time of Exchange Between Free Labeled Ligand and Antibody-Bound Unlabeled Ligand[a]

Ligand	Bound–Free Separation Method	Half-time
Angiotensin II	DCC	60–70 hours
Triiodothyronine	GE	2 hours
Aldosterone	GE	2.5 minutes
Estradiol	GE	<2 minutes
Estradiol	DCC	8.5 minutes

[a]10 pg of the tracer (^{3}H for steroids) was added at equilibrium to a reaction mixture of antiserum and 100 pg native ligand; parallel experiments with tracer present since the beginning served as a reference. DCC results in an apparent lowering of the exchange rate (see Estradiol) seemingly for "cutoff" effects on more labile rapidly exchanging immunocomplexes.

Table 8. Effect of Delaying the Tracer Addition on Response Sensitivity[a]

RIA System	Tracer From Beginning		Tracer Addition Delayed[b]	
	Δ_{10}	Δ_{50}	Δ_{10}	Δ_{50}
Estradiol	13	110	11.5	105
Aldosterone	17	170	12	130
Testosterone	16	150	12	100
Progesterone	15	140	10	98
Angiotensin II	6.5	64	2.5	24
Insulin	40	280	12	110

[a]Expressed as picogram amounts corresponding to 10 and 50% of the initial binding (Δ_{10} and Δ_{50}, respectively). All data refer to DCC RIA; ^{3}H-labeled tracers used for steroid.

[b]Sequential incubations of 1 plus 1 hours for steroid and 18 plus 18 hours for polypeptides.

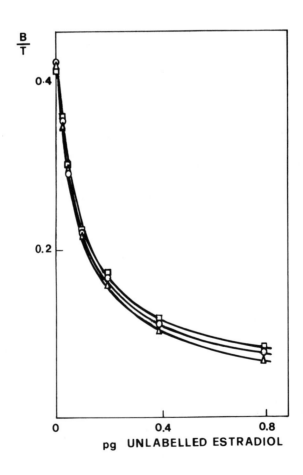

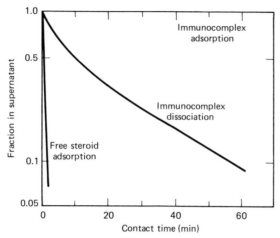

Figure 13. Effects of dextran-coated charcoal on the concentration of the species present at the equilibrium of an estriol RIA system. The data refer to 5 mg/ml DCC kept in suspension by continuous agitation at room temperature. The behavior of immunocomplexes toward adsorption was inferred by the constancy of the antibody site concentration kept in contact with DCC, as observed by antibody titration in supernatant. Immunocomplex dissociation was evaluated by resolving the complex kinetic curve corresponding to the evaluation of [3H]estriol radioactivity in solution, and the free estriol adsorption was separately confirmed in the absence of antiserum ([21]). All the data have been normalized to the initial concentration of the respective species (B - 60%, F - 40%). The presence of more than one class of immunocomplexes with different stability is indicated by the nonlinearity of the dissociation curve.

stored, and delivered together without significantly affecting sensitivity. Examples of these situations are given in Figure 12 for estradiol RIA, and Table 8 compares the sensitivity gain implied by sequential saturation for some steriods and polypeptide RIAs (DCC, ^{3}H-labeled tracers for steroids).

The bound-free equilibrium can be perturbed by many of the separation methods usually adopted, particularly by those based on irreversible adsorbents such as DCC (21). Figure 13 illustrates the situation occurring in an incubated estriol–antiestriol mixture kept in contact with DCC: A net

Figure 12. Effect of delaying the addition of tracer and of premixing tracer and antiserum on the slope of the response curve in estradiol RIA (^{3}H-labeled tracer, 4°C, DCC). O, two-hour incubation of the complete RIA mixture; Δ, 2 hour incubation in the absence of tracer followed by 2-hour incubation of the whole RIA mixture; □ 2-hour incubation in the absence of standard followed by 2-hour incubation of the whole RIA mixture.

Table 9. Dissociative Effects of Charcoal–Dextran on Steroid Immunocomplexes: Dependence on Individual Antiserum Characteristics[a]

	Initial Binding (%)			
Antiserum	5 minutes	10 minutes	15 minutes	20 minutes
Anti-estradiol-6–BSA	48.5 (1.10)	44.0 (1.00)	43.0 (0.98)	41.5 (0.94)
	43.7 (1.04)	42.1 (1.00)	41.9 (0.99)	42.0 (1.00)
	53.8 (1.38)	39.0 (1.00)	29.6 (0.76)	28.1 (0.72)
Anti-estradiol-6–BSA	46.5 (1.16)	40.0 (1.00)	38.5 (0.96)	37.5 (0.94)
	45.2 (1.10)	41.1 (1.00)	37.0 (0.90)	35.3 (0.86)
	48.2 (1.07)	45.1 (1.00)	43.7 (0.97)	43.3 (0.96)

[a]Data referring to different contact times with 1 mg/tube DDC; ^{3}H-labeled tracer. Figures in parentheses refer to normalization to binding at 10-minute contact time.

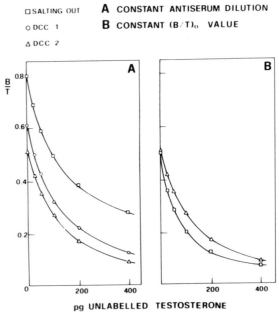

Figure 14. Effect of different separation techniques on the response curve in testosterone RIA, when keeping constant either the antiserum concentration or the initial binding (ammonium sulfate precipitation, 0.5 and 5 mg/tube of DCC, ^{3}H-labeled tracer).

decrease in the concentration of bound steroid, attributable only to dissociation of the immunocomplex, is apparent. The extent of the dissociative effects depends, among other factors related to the assay design (e.g., adsorbent kind and amount, contact time, temperature) on the individual characteristics of the antiserum used, as Table 9 indicates. However, in a general way, these effects are seemingly enhanced in steroid RIA as a consequence of the relative liability of steroid immunocomplexes. Different separation procedures, therefore, yield as a rule different classifications of the bound and free fractions. This is clearly demonstrated in Figure 14 by the dose–response curves obtained for the same testosterone–antitestosterone system, for which separation was achieved using salting out with ammonium sulfate and different amounts of DCC. The progressive dissociation resulting when passing from the nonperturbing precipitation method to the increasingly concentrated adsorbent suspensions is evidenced by lowering of the B/T and enhancement of the curve slope. Conversely, Figure 14b shows that, when the initial binding is kept constant, a steeper curve results for salting out than for charcoal. In fact, a larger concentration of antibody sites is used with the adsorbent to compensate for its dissociative action. Modifications of the response curves are also shown in Figure 15 for RIA of estrogens using DCC and gel equilibration (GE) (22), which is regarded in our laboratory as a reference nonperturbing method.

Besides affecting the slope of the response curve, that is, the response sensitivity, the use of dissociating agents can entail systematic errors. Typi-

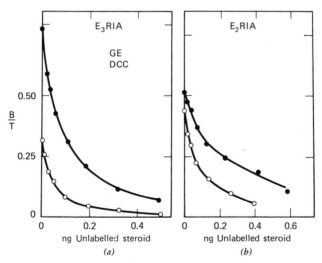

Figure 15. Effect of the separation method on the response curve for estriol and estradiol RIA (^{3}H-labeled tracers). Data refer to G and DCC (0.5 mg/tube).

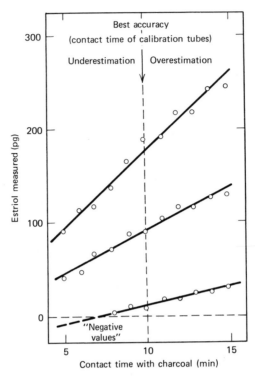

Figure 16. Effect of charcoal–dextran on the accuracy of estriol RIA (³H-labeled tracer). Conditions yielding a particular immunocomplex instability were used (room temperature, 2 mg/tube DCC). Replicates of three samples were sequentially treated with DCC during a time lapse of 10 minutes (15- to 5-minute contact time), and the resulting values of bound radioactivity were all refered to the calibration curve, for which a contact time of 10 minutes was allowed. See the occurrence of "negative" estimates for the low-estriol sample.

cal examples of inaccuracy arising from improper standardization of bound–free separation are shown in Figure 16 for an estriol RIA. In order to prevent such accuracy losses, separations based on steroid adsorption must be carefully designed for each antiserum in terms of adsorbent amount and contact time. The charcoaled RIA tubes can be allowed to stand for a period sufficient to reach a point at which dissociation of more labile immunocomplexes and settling of adsorbent minimize the time dependence of bound and free measurements (see Fig. 17). Particularly when a great number of samples are treated together, alternative expedients can be adopted, such as the use of devices allowing a simultaneous delivery of adsorbent, and the equalization of contact times with adsorbent by distributing it in a set of duplicate tubes symmetrically ranked.

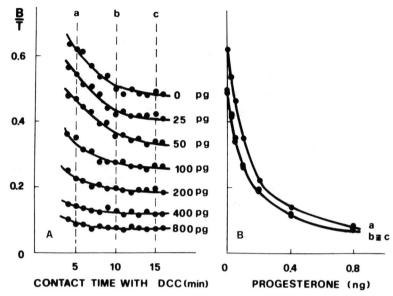

Figure 17. Variability of measurable bound levels with contact time with charcoal–dextran (*a*) and dose–response curves resulting for different contact time (*b*) for a progesterone RIA (^{3}H-labeled tracer). An acceptable stability of response is apparent beyond the 10-minute contact time.

ANTISERUM AFFINITY AND ASSAY SENSITIVITY

For the steroid antisera selected for RIA in our laboratory equilibrium constants ranging from 10^9 to 10^{10} M^{-1} were measured at 4°C.

Nonperturbing methods for evaluation of the bound and free fractions were used to compute binding parameters. In fact, dissociative techniques such as DCC adsorption can lead to incorrect estimations of both affinity and site homogeneity of antisera, particularly when large proportions of rapidly dissociating immunocomplexes are formed, as is apparently the case for steroids. Evidence for the inadequacy of this technique in assessing the characteristics of steroid antisera can be derived from the measured binding data reported in Table 10, which quantify and generalize the situation illustrated in Figures 14 and 15.

The apparent enhancement of the affinity constant and the lowering of both site concentration and of degree of heterogeneity with increasing amounts of DCC account in all cases for a progressive dissociative action mainly directed toward lower-affinity complexes.

The presence in steroid antisera of antibody populations with different characteristics implies a dose dependence of the average affinity constant

Table 10. Binding Data for Steroid–Antibody Interactions as Evaluated Using Different Bound–Free Separation Procedures [a]

Interacting System	Bound–Free Separation Procedure		Apparent Binding Parameter		
			Antibody Site Concentration, $Ab_0 \times 10^{-10}, M$	Average Affinity Constant $K_0 \times 10^9, M^{-1}$	Heterogeneity Coefficient, α
Estradiol—anti-estradiol-6–BSA	GE		10	0.53	0.65
	DCC	0.5 mg/tube	4.5	1.3	0.86
		1 mg/tube	1.7	4.3	0.93
		5 mg/tube	1.1	5.1	1.0
		10 mg/tube	1.1	5.2	1.0
Estriol—anti-estriol-6–BSA	GE		19	0.38	0.62
	DCC	0.5 mg/tube	5.0	2.9	0.70
		5 mg/tube	2.9	6.8	0.98
Testosterone—anti-testosterone-3–BSA	Salting out		17	0.38	0.60
	DCC	0.5 mg/tube	4.9	2.7	0.75
		5 mg/tube	3.0	4.8	1.0

[a] ^{3}H-labeled tracers.

K_0. This is exemplified by the data in Table 11 referring to an estradiol–antiestradiol system (Sepharose-coupled anti-E$_2$ IgG, ^{3}H-labeled tracer). The progressive involvement in the reaction of lower-affinity antibody sites with increasing doses is reflected in a sharp lowering of the measured K_0 values and enhancement of the degree of heterogeneity. To allow direct comparison of data related to different methods, the intervals of hapten concentration were therefore kept constant.

Table 11. Dose Dependence of Measurable Binding Parameters (Estradiol RIA)[a]

Dose Range (pg/tube estradiol)	Binding Parameters		
	Heterogeneity Coefficient, α	Average Affinity Constant, $K_0 \times 10^9 (M^{-1})$	Antibody Site Concentration $Ab_0 \times 10^{-10} (M)$
10–25	0.85	7.2	1.3
10–35	0.80	4.7	1.6
10–110	0.75	3.0	1.9
10–210	0.70	2.2	2.1
10–610	0.65	1.5	2.4

[a] Sepharose-coupled anti-estradiol-6–BSA IgG, ^{3}H-labeled tracer.

Table 12. Assay Sensitivity of Steroid Antisera Routinely Used[a]

Antiserum	Initial Binding, $(B/T)_0$ %	Sensitivity $(pg/tube)$[b]	n
Anti-aldosterone-3–BSA	42.8 ± 3.4	3.1 ± 1.0	21
	45.9 ± 3.2	4.3 ± 1.2	21
	51.0 ± 4.1	2.4 ± 0.8	6
Anti-progesterone-11–BSA	38.2 ± 4.4	7.5 ± 2.1	10
	46.9 ± 5.0	2.5 ± 0.5	6
Anti-testosterone-3–BSA	48.5 ± 3.5	6.0 ± 2.7	6
	44.1 ± 3.6	2.1 ± 0.9	6
Anti-testosterone-6–BSA	45.0 ± 2.9	2.0 ± 0.8	6
	50.3 ± 3.3	2.1 ± 0.6	5
Anti-estradiol-6–BSA	46.5 ± 4.3	3.8 ± 1.2	10
	42.8 ± 2.9	6.0 ± 3.0	9
	45.1 ± 3.0	2.2 ± 1.0	5
	50.6 ± 4.8	0.7 ± 0.3	6
Anti-estriol-6–BSA	43.9 ± 4.3	2.6 ± 0.5	20
	45.2 ± 2.8	1.9 ± 0.8	10

[a]DCC RIA using ³H-labeled tracers.

[b]Assumed as corresponding to the steroid amount causing a $(B/T)_0$ lowering of 5%.

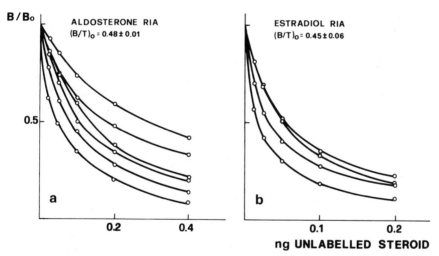

Figure 18. Variability of affinity characteristics within groups of steroid antisera obtained under the same immunization conditions (different slope of the response curves with the same initial binding, DCC, ³H-labeled tracers).

The dependence of the measurable immunologic properties of steroid antisera on both the separation method and steroid dose makes us aware that any generalization and comparison based on binding parameters must be regarded with caution. In any case, the equilibrium constants of steroid–antibody reactions seem to be not extremely high as compared to polypeptide RIA. Therefore proper selection of steroid antisera on the basis of assay sensitivity is necessary to allow minute amounts of steroid to be measured without the need for large sample volumes. Table 12 lists the actual sensitivity levels that resulted for some antisera routinely used in our laboratory, and the variability of the immunoresponse also as concerns affinity is illustrated by the different steepnesses of the RIA curves in Figure 18, which once again stress the requirement for a careful antisera selection (DCC RIA, ^{3}H-labeled tracer).

ANTIBODY PHYSICAL FORMS AND ASSAY QUALITY

Solid-phase methods based on insolubilized antibodies are gaining acceptance in steroid RIA. However, it is noted that modifications of the original immunologic properties can accompany insolubilization, thus preventing the sensitivity potential of a given antiserum to be fully exploited. Evidence for affinity losses in cases of solid-phase steroid RIA can be found in the literature (15,23,24).

More information emerges from the data in Table 13 relative to a Sepharose–antiestradiol IgG immunoadsorbent. The IgG/matrix mass ratio appears to be critical in determining the behavior of insolubilized antibodies: Both affinity and number of reactive sites per IgG weight unit are shown to decrease when the IgG/matrix ratio is progressively increased, negligible losses of immunoreactivity taking place for ratios as low as 0.1 nmoles/mg. A dependence on the IgG/matrix ratio was furthermore observed for the time required to reach the equilibrium of the immune reaction, as depicted in Figure 19.

These findings, which seem to be consistent with preliminary observations concerning physical antibody adsorption on plastic surfaces (Malvano, unpublished data), suggest that increasing values of surface density of the antibody molecules result in reduced accessibility of hapten to binding sites. The formation of superficial clusters of IgG molecules, favored by the higher protein concentrations, may support this hypothesis.

A minimal loss of immunoreactivity, if any, was reported to occur as a result of coupling to CNBr-activated cellulose whole antisteroid serum (25). This was later confirmed by our own experience, as shown by the examples in Table 14. Also, these results can be rationalized in light of the results in Table 13. In fact the presence in immune sera of proteins other

Table 13. Effect of IgG/Matrix Ratio on the Immunologic Properties of Immunoadsorbents (Sepharose-Coupled Anti-estradiol-6–BSA IgG)

IgG/Sepharose (nmoles/mg)	Average Equilibrium Constant $K_0 \times 10^9$ (M^{-1})	Number of Combining Sites[a] $Ab_0 \times 10^{-11}$ (M)	Residual Immunoreactivity $K_0 Ab_0/(K_0 Ab_0)_{sd}$ sol[b]
0.1	4.6	4.8	0.97
1.0	4.3	4.3	0.77
1.4	4.1	4.0	0.68
2.3	3.2	3.9	0.52
4.7	2.5	3.2	0.33
7.4	2.0	2.9	0.24
10.2	1.7	2.2	0.16

[a]Expressed as number of antibody sites per nanomole of IgG (MW 160,000).

[b]$_{sd}$sol = standardized solution (Normalized to the immunoreactivity of the original IgG fraction in solution: $K_0 = 4.8 \times 10^9$ M^{-1}, $Ab_0 = 5.0 \times 10^{-11}$) (evaluated with GE).

than antibodies can exert a sort of protective action, reducing the probability of formation of IgG clusters.

Though further investigations seem necessary for a better definition of the mechanism involved, the data reported create the need for careful design and control of antibody insolubilization procedures, at least as far as sensitivity potential and analysis time are concerned. As for specificity, the experimental results in our hands (see the example in Fig. 20) do not allow

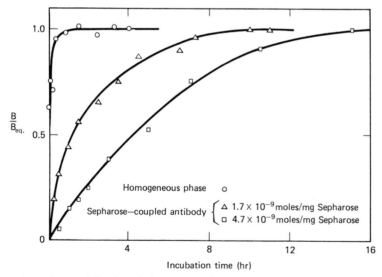

Figure 19. Binding kinetics of the system [³H]estradiol–antiestradiol IgG in solution and covalently bound to Sepharose with different substitution degrees.

Table 14. Binding Data of Whole Antisera in Solution (GE) and in Solid-Phase (Cellulose-Coupled)[a]

Binding Parameter	Solution		Solid-Phase	
	Cortisol	Testosterone	Cortisol	Testosterone
Affinity Constant, $K_0 \times 10^9$ (M^{-1})	2.9 ± 0.3	4.0 ± 0.2	3.1 ± 0.1	3.8 ± 0.2
Antibody Site concentration $Ab_0 \times 10^{-8}$ (M)	1.9 ± 0.2	2.9 ± 0.3	1.8 ± 0.2	2.1 ± 0.3

[a] ^{3}H-labeled tracers.

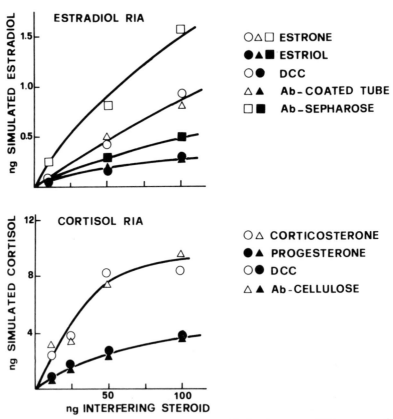

Figure 20. Interferences from competing steroids in the same RIA system (^{3}H-labeled tracers) in either a homogeneous (DCC) or heterogeneous phase (covalent linkage, physical adsorption).

a consistent picture to be derived as yet. It would appear that, during the insolubilization steps, alterations in antibody binding site conformation and accessibility may occur.

FURTHER SIMPLIFICATION OF STEROID ASSAYS

ELIMINATION OF EXTRACTION

The ideal steroid assay should not even require preliminary extraction. However, severe restrictions on direct assay arise from the possible spurious interactions of steroids under analysis with carrier proteins and of antibody sites with water-soluble steroid catabolites.

In fact, cases involving the absence of conjugated catabolites and analyte concentrations high enough to allow minimization of the protein effects by a simple sample dilution are relatively infrequent. This favorable situation

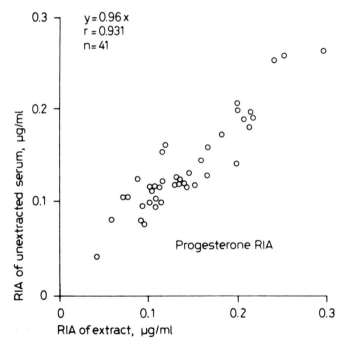

Figure 21. Correlation of progesterone estimates obtained in pregnancy serum (0.1%) using RIA of extracts and direct RIA of untreated samples (DCC, ^{3}H-labeled tracer).

is exemplified in Figure 21 by a progesterone RIA for pregnancy plasma (DCC, ^{3}H-labeled tracer, 0.1% sample concentration), where estimates on extracts and untreated samples demonstrated adequate consistency.

Competition of carrier proteins in the sample with the analytical antibody proteins disfavors the formation of immunocomplexes, although resulting in a higher overall proportion of protein-bound haptens. Therefore, depending on the separation method, misclassification of bound and free fractions may eventually occur. Methods such as GE and DCC adsorption, which do not distinguish between ligand complexes with antibodies and with carrier proteins, involve an enhancement of binding when plasma proteins are present. The opposite situation is encountered with methods, such as immunoadsorption and immunoprecipitation, that selectively recognize as bound only the immunocomplexed ligand. Underestimation (26) and overestimation (27) errors are thus respectively entailed

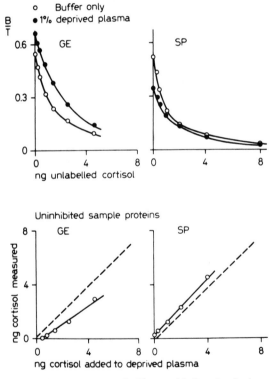

Figure 22. Effect of the presence of 1% steroid-deprived plasma on the response obtained for cortisol RIA with a gel equilibration (GE) and an immunoadsorbent (SP) procedure (^{3}H-labeled tracer). The displacement of the dose–response curve (top) and the systematic error resulting when referring to a calibration curve not corrected for protein effect (bottom) are shown.

when the sample response is referred to the calibration solution without considering the plasma effects. This is well illustrated by the case of cortisol RIA (^{3}H-labeled tracer) for which the response curves in the presence and absence of steroid-deprived plasma are compared in Figure 22 (GE and immunoadsorption) and Figure 23 (DCC adsorption).

Protein interferences must be obviated by re-establishing a standard–sample identity. This can be attempted in different ways, including protein degradation before the assay [heat denaturation (28,29), enzymatic proteolysis (30)], selective protein inhibition in the RIA incubation medium [use of chemical agents (31), addition of massive amounts of protein-interacting steroids that do not cross-react with antibodies (32–36), choice of proper incubation conditions (27,37,38)], and/or standard compensation with proteins (e.g., steroid-free plasma (26,32–36,39), as well as a combination of different approaches (40,41). Both protein inhibition and standard–sample equalization with proteins involve sensitivity losses (flatter response curves) because of parallel effects on the antibody interaction and an increase in the concentration of interacting sites, respectively (see the

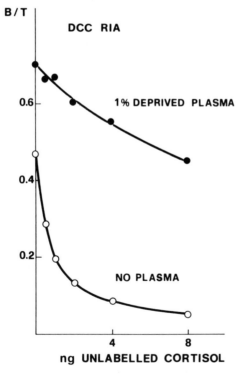

Figure 23. Plasma effect on the response of cortisol RIA using charcoal (^{3}H-labeled tracer).

curve slopes in Figs. 22 and 23 and the affinity data in Table 4). Again assuming as a model the solid-phase cortisol RIA, Figure 24 depicts the elimination of protein effects through preliminary heat denaturation and inhibition by incubating in a low-pH medium. With both procedures the RIA responses in the absence and presence of plasma are shown to coincide. In particular, selective inhibition of low pH should indicate a much more effective influence of the hydrogen ionic concentration in the medium on the interaction with carrier proteins than on the steroid–antibody interaction.

Once protein interferences have been accounted for, the risk of overestimation errors implied by nonextractable steroid catabolites remains a limiting factor for direct RIA. In principle, any definitive solution relies only upon the availability of adequately specific antisera, whose limits have been already mentioned (see the case of estriol and estriol 3-sulfate in Fig. 7). The data in Table 15 can be taken as an example of inaccuracies arising from steroid catabolites using an aldosterone direct RIA (^{125}I-labeled tracer, antibody-coated tubes), where protein effects have been effectively inhibited by using as standard diluent, steroid-deprived plasma. These results, which are consistent with some literature data (40,41), also demonstrate how the inaccuracy level depends on the specificity properties of individual antisera.

In conclusion, elimination of extraction introduces sources of systematic

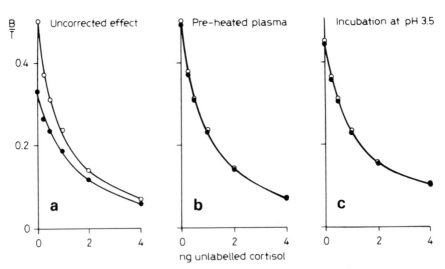

Figure 24. Effect of the presence of steroid-deprived plasma on the response curve of immunoadsorbent ^{3}H RIA for cortisol (a), and its correction through a preliminary 2-minute heating of samples at 60°C (b) and through protein inhibition by incubating at pH 3.5 (c). ○ No plasma; ● 1% deprived plasma.

Table 15. Correlation of Direct and Extracted Aldosterone RIA[a]

Antiserum	n	b	r
A	15	2.0	0.972
B	16	2.7	0.980

[a]Abcissa, ^{3}H DCC extract RIA; ordinate, ^{125}I coated-tube direct RIA.

errors whose extent and direction are dictated by a number of factors, including antiserum affinity and separation method (positive or negative protein-induced bias), antiserum specificity (overestimation from catabolite cross-reactions), and possibly the individual variability of samples. Therefore, fully adequate correction procedures are not easy, and any generalization appears risky.

USE OF RADIOIODINATED TRACERS

Advantages in the cost of counting and in counting time are achieved by replacing ^{3}H-labeled tracers with γ-emitting (or x-ray emitting) tracers. Among these, ^{125}I-radioiodinated steroid derivatives are increasingly gaining acceptance in RIA.

In ^{125}I-labeling operations, some choices concern the kind of derivative to be iodinated, the iodinatable residues, and the iodination procedure. The last point includes consideration of the adequacy of either direct iodination of derivatives or their condensation with preiodinated molecules (43). This latter approach, fully adequate for maintaining molecular integrity, was found particularly helpful with labile steroids such as aldosterone (preparation of ^{125}I-labeled tyraminyl-3-aldosterone).

More than the iodinatable compounds used (e.g., thyrosine, histamine, tyramine, tyrosine, methyl ester), practical implications are related to the identity of or differences in steroid derivatives with respect to those employed in preparing immunogens (homologous or heterologous tracers). Homologous iodinated derivatives have been initially preferred, as they yield higher antibody titers; however, some limitations to their general applicability are to be expected (43–45).

Some results we obtained for progesterone, estradiol, and testosterone RIA can be used as examples (DCC as separative agent). For progesterone, ^{125}I-labeled tyraminyl, prepared either through 11-succinyl or 6-(O-carboxymethyl) oxime derivatives, are compared in Figure 25 with the ^{3}H-labeled tracer taken as a reference when reacted with several antisera raised against a progesterone-11 conjugate. The antiserum dilution curves (Fig. 25a) show high titers and steeper slopes (indicating higher affinity) for the homologous tracer, and the heterologous tracer and [^{3}H] proges-

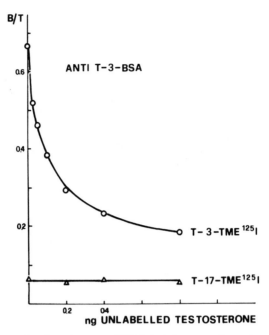

Figure 25. Effects related to the use of ^{125}I-labeled tracers homologous or heterologous in respect to the derivative used for immunogen preparation in testosterone RIA (DCC, same antiserum concentration).

terone behave similarly. These findings are confirmed by the apparent affinity constants in Table 16. The potential advantage of high titers, on the other hand, results in an actual sensitivity loss, that is, in much flatter dose–response curves for the homologous tracer; a sensitivity close to that related to the ^{3}H-labeled tracer is instead observed for the heterologous ^{125}I-labeled derivative (Fig. 25b). A similar picture is derived from Table 17 relative to a comparison of estradiol RIA with estradiol-6–BSA antisera, using homologous ^{125}I-labeled tyraminyl-6-estradiol, heterologous ^{125}I-labeled estradiol obtained by direct iodination, and reference [3H] estradiol. Conversely, Figure 26 shows that, in the case of a testosterone-3–BSA anti-

Table 16. Approximate Affinity Constants for the Progesterone—Anti-Progesterone 11–BSA Systems [a]

Tracer	Equilibrium Constant, $K \times 10^{-9}$ (M^{-1})
[3]H-Progesterone	3.8 ± 1.9
[125]I-labeled tyraminyl-11-progesterone	67 ± 16
[125]I-labeled tyraminyl-3-progesterone	4.7 ± 2.1

[a]The data ($\bar{x} \pm$ SD, $n = 11$) are merely indicative, as artifacts possibly involved in the DCC separation used and differences in antiserum concentrations were not accounted for.

Table 17. Effect of the Kind of Tracer on the Performances of Estradiol-6–BSA Antisera[a]

Tracer	Titer (reciprocal log)	Sensitivity [pg estradiol corresponding to 5% decrease in $(B/T)_0$]	Curve Slope [pg estradiol corresponding to 50% decrease in $(B/T)_0$]
[3]H-labeled estradiol	4.06 ± 0.70 (1.00)	3.6 ± 0.5 (1.00)	63 ± 34 (1.00)
[125]I-labeled tyraminyl-6–estradiol	5.41 ± 0.70 (29 ± 19)	6.5 ± 2.1 (2.2 ± 1.0)	490 ± 420 (10.2 ± 9.7)
[125]I-labeled estradiol (direct iodination)	4.13 ± 0.16 (1.5 ± 0.7)	4.6 ± 1.9 (1.4 ± 0.5)	113 ± 41 (2.4 ± 1.3)

[a]Mean ± SD obtained for eight antisera using approximately equimolar concentrations of each tracer. Figures in parentheses refer to normalization to the data resulting with ^{3}H-labeled tracer; in the case of titer the actual dilutions are used instead of their logarithms. DCC RIA.

serum, on changing from a homologous (C-3 derivative) to a heterologous (C-17 derivative) ^{125}I-labeled tyrosine methyl ester tracer any assay responsiveness is lost.

All these observations can be interpreted in light of the basic features of hapten RIA: (*1*) In principle, optimal sensitivity is reached when the identity of the affinity properties of native and labeled ligands allow a molecule-to-molecule competition to occur for antibody sites. (*2*) Affinity changes involve a competitive imbalance, hence a sensitivity loss in the RIA system; this is likely to take place when ^{3}H-labeled tracers, closely related to native

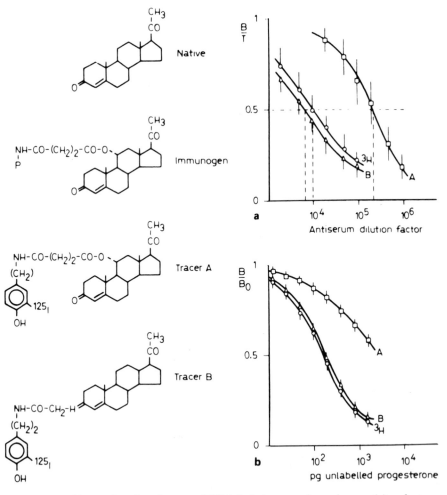

Figure 26. Effects related to the use of ^{125}I-labeled tracers homologous (*a*) or heterologous (*b*) in respect to the derivative used for immunogen preparation in progesterone RIA (DCC). The antiserum titration curves (*a*) and dose–response curve (b) are compared with those obtained with ^{3}H-labeled tracer. The values refer to the mean (± SD) recorded on 11 antisera to progesterone-11–BSA.

haptens, are replaced by radioiodinated tracers into which structural differences have been introduced during manufacture. (3) The presence in antisera of predominant antibody classes directed against the derivative employed in preparing the immunogens confers maximal affinity on a homologous tracer partly sharing the immunogen structure; thus, homologous immunogen–tracer systems result in high working titers, but the increased tracer affinity leads to reduced competitiveness of the native molecule. (4) Assay sensitivity can be re-established by balancing the [125]I-

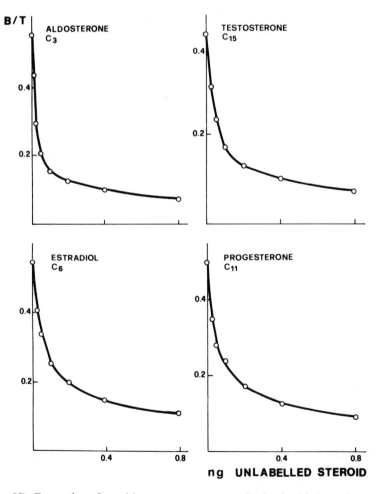

Figure 27. Examples of sensitive response curves obtained with homologous ^{125}I-labeled steroid tracers. All data refer to selected antisera.

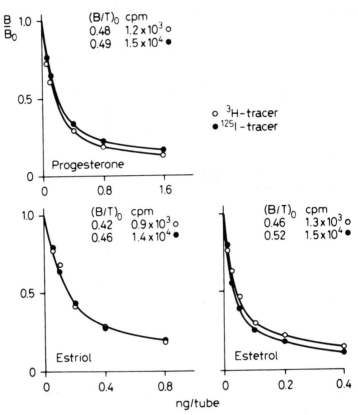

Figure 28. Dose–response curves obtained with heterologous ^{125}I-labeled tracers and ^{3}H-labeled tracers for some steroid RIA systems (anti-progesterone-11–BSA—^{125}I-labeled tyraminyl–3-progesterone; anti-estrogen-6–BSA—^{125}I-labeled estrogen by direct iodination; DCC RIA).

labeled tracer–native ligand competition by means of a controlled reduction in the radioligand affinity via heterologous derivation, while hindering any increase in titer. (5) However, precise limitations must be expected from a too drastic differentiation in the native ligand–immunogen–^{125}I-labeled derivative system, difficult to anticipate, which again can unbalance competition as a result of exceedingly low tracer affinity.

Points (2) and (3) could explain, besides the results in Figure 25 and Table 17, certain literature reports (43–48); it is noted that either heterology at the coupling position, as in the examples, or differences in the chemical bridge (48) could be effective in establishing assay sensitivity. Point (5) seemingly applies to both the examples in Figure 26 and to cases of inadequacy in heterologous systems previously described (44,46).

In any case, the complexity of factors governing the immunologic responses to hapten immunogens prevents oversimplified generalizations.

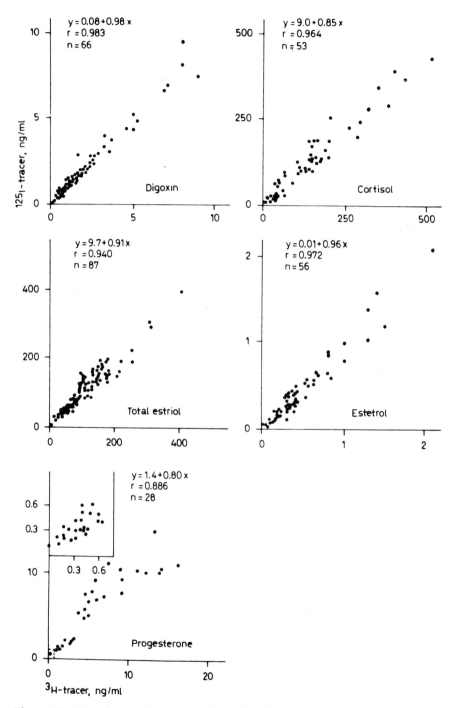

Figure 29. Correlation of estimates obtained with RIA of serum samples using ³H- and ¹²⁵I-labeled tracers for some steriods (DCC).

Better adequacy of heterologous ^{125}I-labeled tracers apparently holds in particular for progesterone and estrogen RIA; however, even in these cases the possibility of finding rare antisera with characteristics compatible with homologous derivatives does exist, as demonstrated by the response curves in Figure 27 (PEG plus double-antibody RIA), as well as by some literature data (42,49,50). This might explain apparently discrepant reports, as successful applications in homologous systems could possibly refer to single selected antisera. In fact, though fully suitable homologous ^{125}I RIA proved more readily obtainable for aldosterone, cortisol, and testosterone, all the data discussed suggest additional difficulties involved in the use of homologous tracers; the need for a proper antiserum selection is emphasized, not only in terms of specificity—as usually—but of sensitivity. The availability of suitable antisera is thus further restricted.

[125]I RIA procedures for different steroids (i.e., aldosterone, cortisol, digoxin, estradiol, estriol, estetrol, progesterone, testosterone) have been set up in our laboratory using either heterologous or homologous radioiodinated derivatives, both implying a 3- to 50-fold gain in specific activity in respect to ^{3}H-labeled tracers. As exemplified in Figure 28 for DCC RIA, essentially similar responses were obtained for ^{125}I and ^{3}H assays under standardized conditions. The results for some RIAs, applying the two tracers, show good agreement of estimates (Fig. 29). As far as specificity is concerned, no definite conclusion on the effect of tracer may be drawn

Table 18. Percent Cross-Reactivity of Some ^{3}H and ^{125}I RIA Methods (Charcoal–Dextran Separations)

		Cross-Reaction (%)	
RIA System	*Interfering Steroid*	[3]*H-Tracer*	[125]*I-Tracer*
Cortisol	Corticosterone	15	11
	Progesterone	6.0	6.5
Digoxin	Digitoxin	1.0	5.3
	Testosterone	5×10^{-3}	2×10^{-3}
Estradiol ($n = 3$)	Estrone	2.5 ± 0.7	1.3 ± 0.4
	Estriol	0.63 ± 0.19	0.34 ± 0.20
Estriol ($n = 4$)	Estradiol	0.30 ± 0.25	0.13 ± 0.09
	Estrone	≤ 0.003	≤ 0.008
Estetrol	Estriol	0.20	0.30
	Estradiol	0.002	0.001
Progesterone	17-Hydroxyprogesterone	4.0	5.9
	Pregnenolone	1.5	0.41
Testosterone	Dihydrotestosterone	75	61
	Androstenedione	0.22	0.80

from the experimental evaluation of cross-reactivity reported in Table 18. For completeness, the decreased stability on storage and the higher adsorbability of radioiodinated tracers as compared to ^3H-labeled tracers cannot be disregarded. Practical implications of these unfavorable features in standardization are obvious; economic considerations in routine assay management still favor ^{125}I label counting.

SIMPLIFICATIONS OF BOUND-FREE SEPARATION

In terms of RIA practicability and reliability, a critical role is played by the bound–free separation method adopted. Thus any improvement of this analytical step is of great importance. Chapter 7 deals with bound–free separation and also discusses aspects peculiar to steroids. Therefore this topic will not be further discussed beyond the examples previously given to demonstrate the impact of separation procedure on the assay quality.

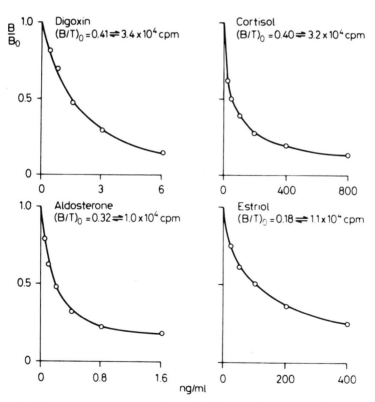

Figure 30. Dose–response curves obtained with coated-tube RIA for some steroids (^{125}I-labeled tracers, direct assay using steroid-free plasma as standard diluent).

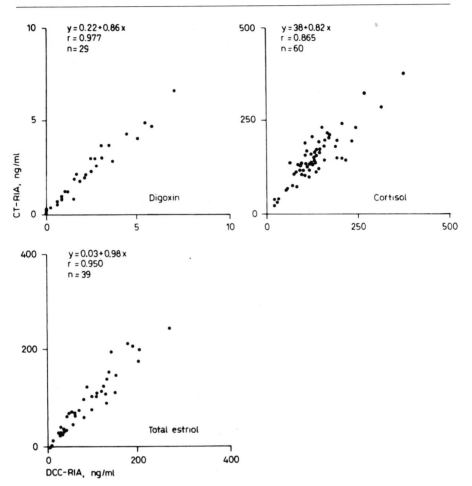

Figure 31. Correlation of estimates obtained with charcoal–dextran ³H RIA and coated-tube ¹²⁵I RIA for some serum steroids.

Brief mention, however, is due regarding extraction of free radioactivity into the scintillation solution (51) and the coated tube (CT) method. The former technique implies obvious practical advantages in the case of ³H RIA. CT methods, which largely help to simplify the assay scheme of any RIA, are particularly advantageous in the case of steroids when ¹²⁵I direct procedures are available.

Examples of dose–response curves for steroid coated tube RIA, using ¹²⁵I-labeled tracer and steroid-free plasma as standard diluent, are given in Figure 30. The correlations of estimates, with the reference RIA methods shown in Figure 31, indicate a quite acceptable consistency of the overall accuracy.

CONCLUSIONS

Complex mechanisms govern the steroid–antibody interaction, and a variety of factors concur in determining the response of steroid RIA. It seems therefore difficult to derive practical and general rules for assay optimization. However, even with the limitations implied by simplified models, such models provide a framework where empirical observations may be organized to avoid—or reduce—errors and difficulties through a better understanding of the effects from which they originate.

This holds in particular from the perspective of further simplification of steroid RIA, continuing the present trend toward increasing experimental ease. Elimination of preliminary operations and improvement of practicability set stricter requirements for a careful selection of immunoreagents and rigorous optimization of the assay in order to maintain an acceptable quality of measurement.

Not all the results reported and discussed here may be regarded as presently generalizable. Nor, on the other hand, is the need for simplified methodology the same for all routine measurements and for routine measurements and research. However, as far as increasingly simple steroid determinations are of interest in a clinical context, many of the methodologic approaches described look promising. More generally, the availability of adequate reagents, the specific experience and skill of each laboratory, and mainly the purpose for which any assay is intended remain the criteria based on which a procedure should be adopted.

REFERENCES

1. Abraham GE, Hopper K, Tulchinsky D, et al: Simultaneous measurement of plasma progesterone, 17-hydroxyprogesterone and estradiol-17β by radioimmunoassay. *Anal Letter* 4:325, 1971.
2. Carr BR, Mikhail G, Flickinger GL: Column chromatography of steroids on Sephadex LH-20. *J Clin Endocrinol Metab* 33:358, 1971.
3. Niswender GD, Midgley AR: Hapten-radioimmunoassay of steroids, in Peron FG, *Immunological Methods in Steroid Determination* Caldwell BV (eds): New York, Appleton-Century Crofts, 1970, p 149.
4. Lindner HR, Perel E, Friedlander A, Zeitlin A: Specificity of antibody to ovarian hormones in relation to the site of attachment of the steroid hapten to the peptide carrier. *Steroids* 19:357, 1972.

5. Weinstein A, Lindner, HR, Friedlander A, Bauminger S: Antigenic complexes of steroid hormones formed by coupling to proteins through position 7: Preparation from Δ^4-3-oxosteroids and characterization of antibodies to testosterone and androstenedione. *Steroids* 20:789, 1972.

6. Jeffcoat SL, Searle JE: Preparation of a specific antiserum to estradiol-17β coupled to protein through the B-ring. *Steroids* 19:181, 1972.

7. Kuss E, Goebel R: Determination of estrogens by radioimmunoassay with antibodies to estrogen-6-conjugates. *Steroids* 19:509, 1972.

8. Rao PN, Moore PH: Synthesis of sex steroid haptens for radioimmunoassay: (1) 15β-carboxyethylmercaptotestosterone-bovine serum albumin conjugate; measurement of testosterone in male plasma without chromatography. *Steroids* 28:101, 1976.

9. Rao PN, Moore PH, Peterson DM, Tcholakian RK: Synthesis of news steroid haptens for radioimmunoassay: (5) 19-0-carboxymethyl ether derivative of testosterone; a highly specific antiserum for immunoassay of testosterone from both male and female plasma without chromatography. *J Steroid Biochem* 9:539, 1978.

10. Bayard F, Beitins IZ, Kowarski A, Migeon CJ: Dosage radioimmunologique de l'aldosterone plasmatique à l'aide d'aldosterone tritiée, in *Techniques Radioimmunologiques* Paris, INSERM, 1971, p. 489.

11. Fahmy D, Read GF, Hillier SG: Some observations on the determination of cortisol in human plasma by radioimmunoassay using antisera against cortiso-3-BSA. *Steroids* 26:267, 1971.

12. Künzig HF, Geiger W: Radioimmunologic determination of plasma unconjugated estriol in normal and abnormal pregnancies with a specific antiserum to estriol. *Arch Gynäk* 216:387, 1974.

13. Franchimont P, Hendrick JC: Radioimmunoassay of glycoprotein hormones, in *Radioimmunoassay and Related Procedures in Medicine*. International Atomic Energy Bulletin, Vienna, IAEA, 1974, Vol I, p 195.

14. Abraham GE, Odell, WD: Solid-phase radioimmunoassay of estradiol, in Peron FG, Caldwell, BV: (eds): *Immunological Methods in Steroid Determination*. New York, Appleton-Century Crofts, 1970, p 87.

15. Malvano R, Rolleri E, Gandolfi C, Rosa U: Steroid radioimmunoassay: Properties of estradiol-antibody complexes formed in homogeneous and heterogeneous phase. *Horm Metab Res* (suppl) 5:12, 1974.

16. Kley R, Hansen W: Radioimmunologische Bestimmung von Testosterone. *Ärzte Lab* 20:202, 1974.

17. Comoglio S, Massaglia A, Rolleri E, Rosa U: Preparation of biospecific supports for affinity chromatography and immunoadsorption, in McFarlane AS, Bianchi R, Mariani G (eds): *Plasma Protein Turnover*. London, McMillan Press, 1976, p 295.

18. Keane PM, Walker WHC, Gauldie J, Abraham GE: Thermodynamic aspects of some radioassay. *Clin Chem* 22:70, 1976.

19. Nisonoff A, Pressman D: Heterogeneity and average combining constants of antibodies from individual rabbits. *J Immunol* 80:417, 1958.

20. Rash JM, Jerkunica I, Sgoutas DS: Mechanisms of interference of nonesterified fatty acids in radioimmunoassay of steroids. *Clin Chim Acta* 93:283, 1979.

21. Rolleri E, Malvano R, Gandolfi C, Rosa U: Effects of irreversible adsorbents of the dissociation of antigen-antibody complexes. *Horm Metab Res* 6:57, 1974.

22. Pearlman WH, Crepy O: Steroid-protein interaction with particular reference to testosterone binding by human serum. *J Biol Chem* 242: 182, 1976.

23. Arends J: Comparison between covalently bound and free antibodies used for radioimmunoassay. *Acta Endocrinol* 68:425, 1971.

24. Moore PH, Axelrod LR: A solid-phase radioimmunoassay for estrogens by estradiol-17β antibody covalently bound to a water insoluble synthetic polymer. *Steroids* 10:199, 1972.

25. Bolton AE, Hunter WM: The use of antisera covalently coupled to Agarose, cellulose and Sephadex in radioimmunoassay systems for proteins and haptens. *Biochim Biophys Acta* 329:318, 1973.

26. Connolly TM, Vecsei P: Simple radioimmunoassay of cortisol in diluted samples of human plasma. *Clin Chem* 24:1466, 1978.

27. Rolleri E, Zannino M, Orlandini S, Malvano R: Direct radioimmunoassay of plasma cortisol. *Clin Chim Acta* 66:319, 1976.

28. Foster LB, Dunn RT: Single-antibody technique for radioimmunoassay of cortisol in unextracted serum or plasma. *Clin Chem* 20:365, 1974.

29. Donohue J, Sgoutas D: Improved radioimmunoassay of plasma cortisol. *Clin Chem* 21:770, 1975.

30. Hasler MJ, Painter K, Niswender GD: An ^{125}I-labelled cortisol radioimmunassay in which serum binding proteins are enzymatically denatured. *Clin Chem* 22:1850, 1971.

31. Kane JW: Use of sodium salicylate as a blocking agent for cortisol-binding globulin in a radioimmunoassay for cortisol on unextracted plasma. *Ann Clin Biochem* 16:209, 1979.

32. Pratt JJ, Wiegman T, Lapphön RE, Woldring MG: Estimation of plasma testosterone without extraction and chromatography. *Clin Chim Acta* 59:337, 1975.

33. Jurjens H, Pratt JJ, Woldring MG: Radioimmunoassay of plasma estradiol without extraction and chromatography. *J Clin Endocrinol Metab* 40:19, 1975.

34. Khadempour MH, Laing I, Gowenlock AH: A simplified procedure for serum progesterone. *Clin Chim Acta* 82:161, 1978.

35. Pratt JJ, Boonman R, Woldring MG, Donker AJM: Special problems in the radioimmunoassay of plasma aldosterone without prior extraction and purification. *Clin Chim Acta* 84:329, 1978.

36. McGinley R, Casey JH: Analysis of progesterone in unextracted serum: A method using Danazol, a blocker of steroid binding to proteins. *Steroids* 33:127, 1979.

37. Former RW, Pierce CE: Plasma cortisol determination: Radioimmunoassay and competitive protein binding compared. *Clin Chem* 20:411, 1974.

38. Gomez-Sanchez C, Murry BA, Kem DC and Kaplan NM: A direct radioimmunoassay of corticosterone in rat serum. *Endocrinology* 96:796, 1975.

39. Zucchelli GC, Giannessi D, Piro MA, et al: Radioimmunoassay of unconjugated and total serum estetrol using a ^{125}I-iodinated tracer. *Hormone Res* 11:227, 1979.

40. Jowett TP, Slater JDH: Development of radioimmunoassay for the measurement of aldosterone in unprocessed plasma and simple plasma extracts. *Clin Chim Acta* 80:435, 1977.

41. Connolly TM, Tibor L, Gless KH, Vecsei P: Screening radioimmunoassay for aldosterone in preheated plasma without extraction and chromatography. *Clin Chem* 26:41, 1980.

42. Nars PW, Hunter WM: A method for labelling estradiol-17β with radioiodine for radioimmunoassay. *J Endocrinol* 57:67, 1973.

43. Allen RM, Redshaw MR: The use of homologous and heterologous ^{125}I radioligands in the radioimmunoassay of progesterone. *Steroids* 32:2335, 1978.

44. Cameron EHD, Scarisbrick JJ, Morris SE, et al: ^{125}I-iodohistamine derivatives as tracer for the radioimmunoassay of progestagens, in Cameron EHD, Hilliers SG, Griffiths K (eds): *Steroid Immunoassay.* Cardiff, Alpha Omega Publ, 1975, p 153.

45. Hunter WM, Nars PW, Rutherford FJ: Preparation and behaviour of ^{125}I-labelled radioligands for phenolic and neutral steroids, in Cameron EHD, Hilliers SG, Griffiths K (eds): *Steroid Immunoassay.* Cardiff, Alpha Omega Publ, 1975, p 141.

46. Cameron EHD, Scarisbrick JJ, Morris SE, et al: Some aspects of the use of ^{125}I-labelled ligands for steroid radioimmunoassay. *J Steroid Biochem* 5:749, 1974.

47. Scarisbrick JJ, Cameron EHD, Radioimmunoassay of progesterone: Comparison of $(1,2,6,7\,{}^{-3}H_4)$-progesterone and progesterone-(^{125}I) iodohistamine radioligands. *J Steroid Biochem* 6:51, 1975.

48. Niswender GD, Nett TM, Meyer DL, et al: Factors influencing specificity of antibodies to steroid hormones, in Cameron EHO, Hillier SG, and Griffiths K, (eds): *Steroid Immunoassay*. Cardiff, Alpha Omega Publ, 1975, p 165.

49. Lindberg P, Edqvist LE: A use of 17β-estradiol-6-(O-carboxymethyl) oxine-(^{125}I) tyramine as tracer for a radioimmunoassay of 17β-estradiol. *Clin Chim Acta* 53:169, 1974.

50. Hammond GL, Vinikka L, Vikko R: Automation for some sex steroids with the use of both iodinated and tritiated ligands. *Clin Chem* 23:1250, 1977.

51. Edwards CRW, Taylor AA, Baum CK, Kurtz AB: Evaluation of two new separation techniques for steroid radioimmunoassay, in Cameron EHD, Hillier SG, Griffiths K (eds): in *Steroid Immunoassay*. Cardiff, Alpha Omega Publ, 1975, p 229.

CHAPTER 11

RADIOIMMUNOASSAY OF THYROID HORMONES, THYROID HORMONE-BINDING INTER-α-GLOBULIN, AND THYROGLOBULIN

Delbert Fisher

Thyroid hormones and their analogues are iodine-containing amino acids synthesized within the thyroid gland by oxidative iodination of the tyrosyl residues on thyroglobulin, the thyroid storage protein (1). Two iodotyrosyl residues, monoiodotyrosine (MIT) and diiodotyrosine (DIT), appropriately situated sterically on the thyroglobulin molecule, couple to form the iodothyronines thyroxine (T4), triiodothyronine (T3), and reverse triiodothyronine (rT3) (Fig. 1). Thus the predominant intrathyroidal organic iodine compounds are MIT, DIT, T4, T3, and rT3, and the major secretory products are T4 and T3. All are released into the serum when colloid thyroglobulin is endocytosed and hydrolyzed by the thyroid follicular cell. Significant amounts of thyroglobulin also are released into the circulation (1). In peripheral tissues T4 can be monodeiodinated to T3 or rT3, and these compounds in turn can be progressively deiodinated to T2, T1, and finally noniodinated thyronine (T0) (Fig. 2). In addition, the alanine side chain of the iodothyronines can be progressively deaminated and/or decarboxylated to form iodothyroacetic and iodothyropropionic acid derivatives (Fig. 1). As a result, the circulating blood of most mammals contains varying concentrations of MIT and DIT, all the iodothyronines, and significant concentrations of the iodothyroacetic and iodothyropropionic acid derivatives of the iodothyronines.

The major iodothyronines in adult human blood are T4, T3, and rT3; mean concentrations approximate 8000 ng/dl (8 μg/dl), 130 ng/dl, and 40 ng/dl, respectively. Other iodothyronine analogues are present in concentrations of less than 10 ng/dl. All are bound with varying affinity to three species of circulating serum proteins, thyroid hormone-binding inter-α-globulin (TBG), albumin, and prealbumin. TBG is the most important of the binding proteins because it has the highest binding affinity (approximately 10^8 liters/mole) for the active analogues T4 and T3;

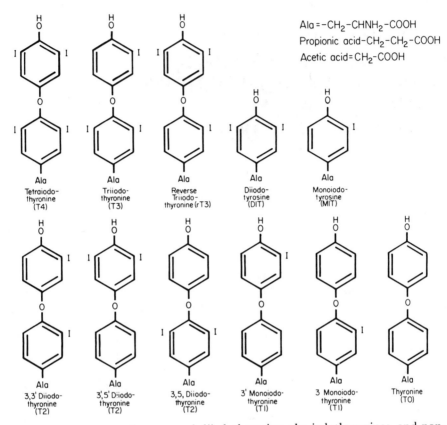

Figure 1. Structure of mono- and diiodothyrosine, the iodothyronines, and non-iodinated thyronine. Each substance is shown with an alanine (Ala) side chain, identified in the upper right corner. The alanine side chain can be modified to a propionic acid or an acetic acid derivative.

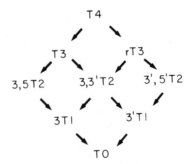

Figure 2. The pattern of progessive deiodination of thyroxine (T4) to the triiodothyronines (T3 or rT3), the diiodothyronines (3, 5T2, 3, 3'T2 or 3', 5'T2), the monoiodothyronines (3T1 or 3'T1) and finally T0. For structures of these analogues see Figure 1.

moreover it is present in a relatively high serum concentration (mean ~1.5 mg/dl).

The measurement of circulating thyroid hormone levels has been difficult. All except T4 are present in a relatively low concentration, and the analogues, as is true for the steroid hormones, are structurally similar and difficult to separate chemically. Until relatively recently the nonspecific protein-bound iodine (PBI) method or a modification was used for quantification (2). This approach took advantage of the fact that 95% of circulating PBI is T4. Specificity and sensitivity were increased with the introduction of the Murphy–Pattee protein binding method in which the binding protein, TBG, was utilized to set up a radioiodine-labeled ligand displacement radioassay system (2).

The modern era of thyroid hormone measurement began in 1970 with the introduction of radioimmunoassay (RIA) methods for the measurement of serum T3 levels by Brown et al. (3) and Gharib et al. (4). The T4 RIA was introduced by Chopra in 1971 and 1972 (5,6), the rT3 RIA by Chopra in 1974 (7), the 3,3'-T2 RIA by Wu et al. in 1976 (8), the 3', 5'-T2 RIA by Chopra et al. (9) and Burman et al. (10) in 1978, the 3,5'T2 RIA by Meinhold and Schurnbrand in 1978 (11), and the 3'-T1 RIA by Smallridge and colleagues in 1979 (12). RIA methods also were introduced for the measurement of serum MIT and DIT by Nelson and collaborators in 1976 (13,14), of tetraiodothyroacetic acid by Burger et al. in 1974 (15), of triiodothyroacetic acid and triiodothyroproprionic acid by Nakamura et al. in 1978 (16) and Gavin and colleagues in 1980 (17), of TBG by Levy and colleagues in 1971 (18), and of thyroglobulin by Roitt and Torrigiani in 1967 (19).

PRINCIPLES AND SPECIAL PROBLEMS OF
IODOTHYRONINE RADIOIMMUNOASSAY SYSTEMS

Most attention has been paid to the RIA of serum T4 and T3 levels, since these are the iodothyronines with biological activity (20–46). All the remaining analogues are inactive derivatives. Of the inactive analogues to date, most interest has focused on 3,3',5'-triiodothyronine or T3 (47–54). This analogue, like T3, is derived predominantly via monodeiodination of T4 in nonthyroid tissues, and circulating levels tend to reflect the tissue T4 monodeiodinase activity. However, several groups of investigators have reported studies of diiodothyronine and monoiodothyronine metabolism and/or levels in serum (55–59). The principles of all these iodothyronine RIA systems are essentially similar to those of other circulating hormone RIA methods. A high-specific-activity radioiodine-labeled ligand (in this case iodothyronine) is reacted with a high-affinity, specific antibody in the presence of the unknown (unlabeled) iodothyronine sample; the percentage of labeled hormone bound is then related to a standard curve (plotting percentage labeled hormone bound versus quantity of unlabeled iodothyronine) to quantify the concentration of iodothyronine in the unknown sample.

Several special problems exist for iodothyronine RIA systems. Serum TBG and other binding proteins interfere with antibody binding, so that the serum iodothyronine must be extracted or TBG binding of the iodothyronine must be selectively blocked before RIA. In addition, iodothyronines are subject to artifactual deiodination in dilute solution and during column and paper chromatographic procedures. Finally, several problems common to RIA procedures in general also plague iodothyronine RIA systems. Serum proteins in RIA systems produce artifacts by inhibiting the binding of labeled iodothyronine to antibody. Also, there is cross-reaction among the circulating iodothyronines for antibody binding. The latter usually is a minor problem when measuring T4, since other iodothyronines are present in much lower concentrations. When measuring T3, rT3, the T2's, and the T1's, however, antisera must be carefully screened and significant cross-reaction must be avoided, absorbed, or considered in the interpretation of results.

THE PROBLEM OF PLASMA PROTEIN BINDING OF IODOTHYRONINES

Plasma protein binding interference in iodothyronine RIA systems has been dealt with in several ways. Serum has been heated to 60°C to inactivate protein binding (33,41). This has the disadvantage of inconvenience as well as increasing the risk of artifactual deiodination, especially when measuring non-T4 derivatives. Denaturation of binding proteins also has been accomplished by the use of trichloroacetic acid–sodium hydroxide (45) or exposure to a pepsin solution (60). Iodothyronines can be extracted into methanol or ethanol, evaporated, and reconstituted in RIA buffer for assay (7,11,42), and column chromatographic separation of iodothyronines has been accomplished using Sephadex G-25 (26,43,61), or an ion-exchange resin (62).

Most investigators, however, have used a variety of chemicals to block preferentially iodothyronine binding to TBG (and not antibody binding). Sodium salicylate (23,28,31,40,57), merthiolate (4,9,24), tetrachlorthyronine (21), diphenylhydantoin (22), and 8-anilino-1-naphthalenesulfonic acid (ANS) (6,25,35,48,51–53,55,56,58) have been utilized. Of these, ANS probably is most commonly employed. ANS is a fluorescent dye with the general formula $C_6H_5NHC_{10}H_6SO_3H$ (49). It has been utilized for many

Table 1. ANS Effect on TBG Binding and Antibody Binding of [^{125}I] T4^a

Amount of ANS (μg)	T4 Equivalent (ng) in Displacement of [^{125}I] T4 from	
	TBG	T4 Antibody
1	None	None
10	4.4	None
100	18.0	None
1000	—	4.0

^{a}From Chopra [6].

years to study the binding properties of serum albumin. Dyes of the naphthalene and acridine series that possess anilino or substituted anilino groups fluoresce in aqueous solutions in the presence of (binding by) protein molecules such as those in serum. Green and colleagues (64) recently used ANS to study the TBG–iodothyronine binding site, and Chopra first utilized the compound to prevent binding protein interference during the RIA of T4 and T3 (6,25). The association constants of T4 and ANS for TBG are 2.35×10^{10} M^{-1} (at 23°C) and 2.09×10^6 M^{-1} (at 37°C) (64). In practice ANS is utilized in a $2–5 \times 10^3$ excess over the average T4 concentration for T4 or T3 RIA systems (7). However, the concentration in the RIA system must be carefully adjusted so that optimal TBG blockage is achieved with minimal inhibition of iodothyronine binding to antibody. Although ANS has about 50 to 100 times greater affinity for the T4 binding sites on TBG than for those on most antibodies, ANS binding to antibody binding sites may be significant (7) (Table 1).

PREPARATION OF ANTISERA

Antisera against iodothyronines have been produced in rabbits by injecting the natural iodothyronine–protein conjugate thyroglobulin or by conjugating the ligand of choice to an antigenic carrier protein. The carrier proteins most commonly employed have been bovine serum albumin (21–24,26,28,29,31,33), human serum albumin (24), hemocyanin (35,48), succinyl poly-L-lysine (3), and thyroglobulin (6,38). Thyroglobulin is highly antigenic when injected with complete Freund's adjuvant and regularly evokes antibody directed to T4 and T3 (65). Since T4 is present in serum in relatively high concentrations, cross-reaction with other iodothyronines is not a major problem for T4 RIA. Thus, thyroglobulin is most appropriately utilized to generate T4 antisera; it is less useful for developing T3 antisera. After immunization with thyroglobulin or other conjugates, it is desirable to screen for a T4 antiserum having less than 1% T3 or rT3 cross-reaction.

When developing antisera for T3, T2, or T1 RIA systems, conjugation to bovine serum albumin (BSA) or human serum albumin (HSA) is convenient and practical; with this approach, levels of contaminating cross-reacting species are minimized. Carbodiimide condensation has been successfully employed for these conjugations. Burke and Shakespeare have described a rapid procedure for the purification of T3 and T4 protein conjugates (66). Antisera, usually generated in rabbits, must be screened to minimize potentially significant cross-reactions.

Thyroglobulin or iodothyronine–protein conjugates usually evoke relatively low-titer antisera; 1:1000 to 1:20,000 final dilutions of first antibodies are common in iodothyronine RIA systems. High-titer antisera are occasionally encountered. Iodothyronine antisera can be partially purified by standard immunoglobulin purification methods or by affinity chromatography. Kruse has reported that charcoal adsorption of T4 antisera to remove endogenous iodothyronine increases antibody titer and RIA system sensitivity (67). In vitro monoclonal antibody production techniques applied to iodothyronines promise to minimize the cross-reaction problem and simplify iodothyronine RIA methodology.

PREPARATION OF IODINATED IODOTHYRONINES

For the past two decades the conventional method for radioiodine labeling of iodothyronines has been the iodide-exchange reaction described by Gleason (68). Exchange-labeled T4 and T3 have been commercially available and have been widely utilized for RIA. More recently the chloramine-T method for labeling peptides has been employed to label iodothyronines (69,70). This approach labels only the 3' and/or 5' positions. Radioiodination occurs by one or both of two mechanisms: either exchange or substitution for existing iodine atoms on the iodothyronine molecule or addition of new iodine atoms. A number of iodothyronine substrates have been utilized for the reaction, including T4; T3; rT3; 3,3'-T2; 3', 5'-T2; 3,5-T2; 3-T1; 3'T1, tetraiodothyroacetic acid, triiodothyroacetic acid, triiodothyropropionic acid, and 3,5-diiodothyropropionic acid (7,9,10, 69,70).

Radioiodine incorporated into iodothyronines during the chloramine-T reaction is separated from unreacted radioiodide by column chromatography using LH-20 Sephadex (69,70). The various radioiodothyronines produced can be purified in various ways depending upon the analogues to be separated. Descending paper chromatography in a hexane–*tert*-amyl alcohol–ammonia solvent system (69,70), Sephadex G-25 chromatography (12,71), ion-exchange chromatography (62), and thin-layer chromatography (hexane–*tert*-amyl alcohol–ammonia) have been utilized.

The production of inner ring 3- and/or 5-position-labeled iodothyronines can be accomplished by synthesis utilizing labeled tyrosines. A practical method was described by Sorimachi and Cahnman in 1977 (72).

VEHICLE FOR PREPARATION OF STANDARD CURVE

Serum tends to inhibit iodothyronine binding to first antibody. Thus, when iodothyronine RIA is conducted using whole serum or plasma, standard curves usually must be prepared using hormone-free serum or a suitable substitute. In some instances, especially when measuring T4 by RIA in small volumes of sera (<20 μl), a buffer standard curve may prove adequate. Usually, however, and particularly when the volume of unknown serum in the RIA system exceeds 50 μl, protein-matched standard tubes are necessary.

Iodothyronine-free serum can be readily prepared by charcoal (Norit A) adsorption (23). It is useful to add a tracer amount of the labeled analogue in question to the serum before charcoal is added. In this way, radioactivity in the adsorbed serum can be measured to ensure completeness of serum stripping; usually 99% of the iodothyronines are removed by this procedure. Amberlite IRA-400 also has been utilized to prepare iodothyronine-free pooled serum for standard tubes (6).

Alternatively a hypothyroid serum can be utilized to set up standard curve tubes. Chopra and colleagues have utilized hypothyroid sheep serum (20,25); sheep serum has TBG and albumin concentrations similar to those in human sera. Four percent HSA (22) also has been utilized as a serum substitute for standard curve tubes in iodothyronine RIA systems. Adequacy of the standard vehicle usually is indicated by relatively low blank values after separating bound and free labeled hormone, high recovery of hormone added to unknown sera, and parallelism of unknown serum dilutions and standard curve tube results.

SEPARATION OF BOUND AND FREE HORMONE

Bound and free radiolabeled iodothyronines in RIA systems have been separated by a variety of techniques. These include second antibody, usually goat anti-rabbit γ-globulin when rabbit antisera are utilized (6,8,20,22,25,30,34,38); dextran-coated charcoal (23,26,31); methycellulose–charcoal (24,39); QAE-Sephadex A-25 (35,48); polyethylene glycol (51,58); ammonium sulfate precipitation (51, 55), and resin sponges (54). Reusable Sephadex columns also have been utilized for T3 RIA (34).

Protein A, a major cell wall component of most strains of *Staphylococcus aureus*, has been utilized to precipitate first antibody in RIA systems (73,74). Protein A binds rapidly and with a high affinity to over 90% of the immunoglobulins in rabbit, human and guinea pig serum and has been found to be as effective as second antibody (goat anti-rabbit γ-globulin) for the separation of bound and free radioligand in RIA methods for prolactin, follicle-stimulating hormone (FSH), luteinizing hormone (LH), and β-endorphin (74). Mitchell et al. (74a) have reported using protein A to separate bound and free analyte in RIA of thyroid-stimulating hormone (TSH) and T₄ in dried blood.

SOURCES OF ARTIFACTUAL ERROR IN IODOTHYRONINE RADIOIMMUNOASSAY RESULTS

Artifactual error in the iodothyronine RIA system, as in other serum RIA systems, may arise from several sources. These include counting errors, in vivo or in vitro seasonal variation in iodothyronine levels, variation in potency of standards, variations in non-thyroid-binding serum proteins, variations in thyroid-binding serum proteins, and the presence of autoimmune iodothyronine antibodies in the unknown sera.

Counting errors may arise from inherent variations in gamma radiation counting equipment (75). Drift in counter sensitivity in large assays over a fairly long period of counting can be significant (76). The overall between-assay variance usually is one of the major sources of error and may range from 10 to 20% (23). Both these sources of error can be significantly reduced by utilizing adequate numbers of control tubes dispersed among the unknown RIA tubes (76). Optimum ease and benefit can be derived from computer analysis of the results.

Variations in potency of reference pool materials also occur. Because iodothyronines are relatively stable in stored serum or plasma, serum pools have been used for iodothyronine "house reference" material in order to reduce between-assay variance (77). In preparing such standards it is important to recognize that T4, T3, rT3, and TBG levels are higher in winter than in summer sera (about 15, 13, 9, and 8%, respectively) (77) and that serum iodothyronine concentrations decrease progressively with storage at rates between 1 and 5% per year (77).

The quality and quantity of non-thyroid hormone-binding serum proteins, as well as thyroid hormone-binding serum proteins, change among species and change with age within species. Thus it is important to match sera for standard tubes with the sera to be measured by RIA. Human serum pools are best for human iodothyronine RIA systems, and stripped human sera are best for standard curve tubes. If other materials are to be used (hypothyroid sheep sera, albumin, etc.) it must be demonstrated that this other material influences radioiodinated ligand binding to antibody similarly to human serum or plasma. Moreover, serum proteins vary qualitatively and quantitatively in fetal or newborn and adult sera. Thus, it is necessary to ascertain whether stripped adult serum and stripped cord or newborn serum react similarly in an iodothyronine RIA system before measuring cord sera relative to adult serum standard tubes. Sera from pregnant women also may react differently from nonpregnant adult serum, particularly if the concentration of ANS used in the RIA system is inadequate.

The presence of anti-T4 and anti-T3 antibodies has been demonstrated in the serum of human subjects (78,79). These sera produce artifactual results in iodothyronine RIA systems, the particular artifact depending on the RIA procedure and the bound–free separation method (78–80). In most patients the autoimmune antibodies bind both T3 and T4, but specific antibody may be observed (79).

Recently a family has been reported with an inherited abnormal thyroid hormone-binding protein that resulted in increased serum T4 measured by RIA (81). The protein migrated with albumin in reverse-flow protein electrophoresis and eluted with TBG during Sephadex A-50 column chromatography. T3 binding to the abnormal protein was weak, such that nearly normal serum T3 and rT3 uptake results were noted (81). One male child (9 years old) and the father were involved; the mother and a fraternal twin were not. This suggests an autosomal dominant inheritance pattern.

APPLICATION OF IODOTHYRONINE RADIOIMMUNOASSAY TO TISSUES AND NONHUMAN SPECIES

Iodothyronine RIA methods have been adapted to measurements in human thyroid tissue, amniotic fluid, and urine (82–86) and to tissues and/or serum in a variety of species including monkeys, rats, rabbits, woodchucks, dogs, sheep, chickens, and amphibia (87–110). The principles and techniques for such measurements and the sources of error are essentially similar to those described for human serum RIA systems. Careful matching of standard sera is important whether or not extraction is conducted. The same inhibitors of serum protein binding of iodothyronines in serum and the same separation systems for bound and free radiolabeled ligand are applied to both animal and human sera (87,93,95–97,102,103,106–110). Tissue iodothyronine RIA systems have utilized alcohol extraction, evaporation, and reconstitution in iodothyronine-free sera (89,94) or alcohol extraction with direct RIA of the alcohol extract (99,100,103). In the latter instance the protein concentration in the alcohol extract is low so that the use of buffer standard curves without blockage of protein binding is possible. A sequential butanol–chloroform–2 N NH$_4$OH extraction method was employed by Nejed et al. (96); Obregon et al. (105) used an ethanol extract of tissue with subsequent paper chromatography and RIA of a methanol extract from the paper.

OTHER APPLICATIONS AND INNOVATIONS—FREE HORMONE MEASUREMENTS, COMBINED RADIOIMMUNOASSAY SYSTEMS, AND ENZYME RADIOIMMUNOASSAY

FREE IODOTHYRONINE CONCENTRATIONS

The concentrations of free T4 and T3 are of primary importance in regulating the availability of active thyroid hormones to tissues. Since the proportion of circulating T4 or T3 present in free or dialyzable form is small, it has not been possible to measure free hormone levels directly. Rather, free T4 and T3 levels usually are estimated by measuring the fraction of radiolabeled T4 or T3 that is ultrafilterable or dialyzable through a semipermeable membrane such as cellophane. The product of the dialyzable fraction and the total T4 concentration provides an estimate of absolute free T4 (in ng/dl) or free T3 (in pg/d1). Two recent reviews of this methodology are available (111,112).

Recently several authors have published methods adapting iodothyronine RIA to the measurement of free T4 in serum. Jiang and Tue (113) have used the dialysis procedure and measured the dialyzed (free) T4 fraction directly in the dialysate by RIA. A second approach has employed direct RIA of the free T4 fraction in serum (112). This is exemplified by the Corning Immunophase free T4 RIA (112). In this method a T4 RIA is run in two tubes, A and B. Tube A contains a test serum or standard radioactive T4 and anti-T4 antibody immobilized on porous glass particles. Tube B contains all the reagents in tube A with the addition of a chemical (thiomerosal) to block T4 binding to serum binding proteins. The tube A result is presumed to reflect free T4, and the tube B result total T4. The radioactivity bound in tube A relative to total radioactivity in counts per minute (A/T_e) is considered proportional to free T4, and total T4 is determined from B. A standard curve is prepared by plotting $A/T_e \times$ total T4 against the free T4 levels in the standards; $A/T_e \times$ T4 in the unknown tubes is used to estimate free T4 (in ng/dl) from the standard curve (112).

NEWBORN SCREENING FOR HYPOTHYROIDISM

Mass population screening for congenital hypothyroidism was facilitated in 1973 by the introduction of a method for the RIA of T4 in filter paper blood spots (114). This approach adapted newborn thyroid screening to the ongoing programs for newborn phenylketonuria (PKU) screening and allowed convenient transport of newborn samples via the mail system. The original method of Dussault and Laberge (114) used 1/4-in. filter paper disks, ANS to block TBG binding, and a second antibody bound–free separation system. Larsen and Broskin (115) introduced a method employing two 1/8-in. filter paper disks; these investigators employed salicylate to block TBG binding and a charcoal separation of bound and free labeled T4. Mitchell (116) modified the Larsen–Broskin method to employ a weak ion-exchange resin (Amberlite IRD-58M) for bound–free labeled T4 separation and carried out the assay at 22°C rather than 4°C. These modifications simplified and shortened the procedure without compromising reliability.

SIMULTANEOUS RADIOIMMUNOASSAY SYSTEMS

Several authors have proposed conducting simultaneous RIA of T3 and T4 or of T4 and TSH (117–119). These methods combine a single extraction with separate T3 and T4 RIA (118) or dual labels in a single-tube procedure (117, 119).

ENZYME RADIOIMMUNOASSAY SYSTEMS

RIA systems have the disadvantages of requiring that the laboratory using the method introduce special isotope safety procedures, purchase counting equipment, and obtain special licensure. To obviate these problems enzyme-linked RIA systems have been introduced (120–122). These methods use stable enzyme labels instead of isotope labels. Conjugation of T4 to an enzyme results in the inhibition of enzyme activity. When thyroxine-specific antiserum binds to enzyme-labeled T4, the enzyme is reactivated, and when the enzyme is activated, the chemical reaction that occurs can be monitored spectrophotometrically. T4 in an unknown sample competes with the enzyme-labeled T4 for antibody-binding sites and thereby decreases the antibody-induced activation of the enzyme (120,121). Thus, enzyme activity is inversely proportional to the total concentration of T4 in the sample. These procedures can be automated and have been shown to produce results for serum T4 measurement comparable to T4 RIA results (121,122). The major disadvantage of this approach, at present, is limited sensitivity. Thus, the method is applicable to measurement of serum T4 concentrations and is not yet available for the other iodothyronines.

THYROID HORMONE/BINDING INTER-γ-GLOBULIN AND THYROGLOBULIN RADIOIMMUNOASSAY SYSTEMS

To complete the spectrum of iodothyronine-related RIA systems, methods for the measurement of TBG and thyroglobulin in serum have been published.

THYROID HORMONE-BINDING INTER-γ-GLOBULIN RADIOIMMUNOASSAY METHODS

Levy and colleagues (18) introduced the first RIA for human serum TBG in 1971. Subsequently, Gershengorn and colleagues (123) and Hesch, et al. (124) published similar methods using different purified human TBG. Since the concentrations of TBG in serum are high (mg levels/dl) serum must be diluted 100 to 200 times for RIA. Thus, serum protein interference is not a significant problem. Second antibody is used for the separation of bound and free labeled TBG. The mean serum TBG level in the Gershengorn et al. RIA method (1.48 mg/dl) is about half that in the Levy et al. method (3.6 mg/dl), presumably because of the greater purity of the TBG utilized by Gershengorn and colleagues (123). The mean level in the RIA of Hesch et al. was 0.97 mg/dl (124). These investigators further purified their radioiodine-labeled TBG by affinity chromatography (124). More recently Kagedal and Kallberg reported both a radial immunodiffusion and a RIA method of TBG determination (125). Mean TBG values in men and nonpregnant women were 1.38 and 1.54 mg/dl, respectively, by radial immunodiffusion. The correlation of immunodiffusion and RIA results in 84 sera was high (r = .984) (125). Glinoer and colleagues have developed a method for the measurement of TBG in rhesus monkey plasma using purified monkey TBG (126,107). The mean level in control animals in their system was 2.4 mg/dl. This RIA was similar to the human RIA method from the same laboratory (123).

Finally, Chopra et al. (127) introduced a competitive ligand-binding RIA system for TBG in 1972. This approach utilized a T3 RIA system with a fixed amount of T3, anti-T3 antibody, and a goat anti-rabbit second antibody. Increasing quantities of TBG in the RIA tubes decreased the binding of labeled T3 to the T3 antibody. Standard curves were set up from a pool of high-TBG serum from estrogen-treated women. The mean TBG in euthyroid normal human subjects using this RIA was 2.85 mg/dl, since the reference serum pool was standardized to the Levy et al. (18) assay method. This TBG RIA measurement approach has the advantage that it can be applied across species.

THYROGLOBULIN RADIOIMMUNOASSAY SYSTEMS

The measurement of thyroglobulin in human serum by RIA was introduced by Roitt and Torrigiani (19) in 1967. These authors, using a double-antibody system, achieved a sensitivity of 10 ng/ml. Van Herle and colleagues (128) in 1973 reported an improved RIA system. Using a more highly purified human thyroid thyroglobulin preparation with a rabbit first antibody and a goat antirabbit second antibody for separation of bound and free label Van Herle et al. achieved a sensitivity of 1–2 ng/ml. With this method these authors reported that thyroglobulin levels were measurable in 74% of normal subjects (128). Subsequently, other similar RIA systems have been developed for human and rat serum (129–133; and see review by Van Herle et al. 134). The measurement of human serum thyroglobulin has been utilized as a marker for thyroid carcinoma (130,134).

The major disadvantage of the human RIA is that circulating antithyroglobulin autoantibodies interfere in the RIA system (19,134,135). Bayer and Kriss (136) have recently reported a solid-phase sandwich-type immunoradiometric assay for human serum thyroglobulin that allows a fairly accurate assessment of serum levels even in the presence of antithyroglobulin autoantibodies (136). In this system thyroglobulin in the sample or standard is first bound to plastic cups coated with rabbit antithyroglobulin antiserum and then measured by the binding of rabbit radioiodine-labeled antithyroglobulin. The sensitivity is reported to be 2.5 ng/ml.

REFERENCES

1. Ingbar SH, Woeber KA: The thyroid gland, in Williams RH (ed): *Textbook of Endocrinology*, Philadelphia, Saunders, 1974, pp. 95–232.

2. Fisher DA: Advances in laboratory diagnosis of thyroid disease. *J Pediatrics* 82:1, 187, 1973.

3. Brown BL, Ekins RP, Ellis SM, et al: Specific antibodies to triiodothyronine. *Nature* 226:359, 1970.

4. Gharib H, Mayberry WE, Ryan, RJ: Radioimmunoassay for triiodothyronine: A preliminary report. *J Clin Endocrinol Metab* 33:865, 1971.

5. Chopra IJ, Solomon DH, Ho, RS: A radioimmunoassay of thyroxine. *J Clin Endocrinol Metab* 33:865, 1971.

6. Chopra IJ: A radioimmunoassay for measurement of thyroxine in unextracted serum. *J Clin Endocrinol Metab* 34:938, 1972.

7. Chopra IJ: A radioimmunoassay for measurement of 3, 3', 5' triiodothyronine (reverse T3). *J Clin Invest* 54: 583, 1974.

8. Wu, SY, Chopra, IJ, Nakamura Y, et al: A radioimmunoassay of 3, 3' diiodothyronine (T2). *J Clin Endocrinol Metab* 43:682, 1976.

9. Chopra IJ, Geola F, Solomon DH, et al: 3', 5' diiodothyronine in health and disease: Studies by radioimmunoassay. *J Clin Endocrinol Metab* 47:1198, 1978.

10. Burman KD, Wright FD, Smallridge RC, et al: A radioimmunoassay for 3' 5'T2. *J Clin Endocrinol Metab* 47:1059, 1978.

11. Meinhold H, Schurnbrand P: A radioimmunoassay for 3, 5T2. *Clin Endocrinol (Oxf)* 8:493, 1978.

12. Smallridge RC, Wartofsky L, Green BJ, et al: 3'-L-monoidothyronine: Development of a radioimmunoassay and demonstration of in vivo conversion from 3', 5' diiodothyronine. *J Clin Endocrinol Metab* 48:32, 1979.

13. Nelson JC, Weiss RM, Lewis JE, et al: A multiple ligand binding radioimmunoassay of diiodothyrosine. *J Clin Invest* 53:416, 1974.

14. Nelson JC, Palmer FJ, Lewis JE: Radioimmunoassay of serum monoiodotyrosine (MIT), in *Proc. 5th Int. Congr. Endocrinol.* Excerpta Medica, Congr Ser No 40, Abst 128, 1976.

15. Burger A, Schilter M, Sokoloff C, et al: A radioimmunoassay for serum tetraidothyroacetic acid (TA4), abstracted. *Clin Res* 22:336A, 1974.

16. Nakamura Y, Chopra IJ, Solomon DH: An assessment of the concentration of acetic acid and propionic acid derivatives of 3, 5, 3' triiodothyronine in human serum. *J Clin Endocrinol Metab* 46:91, 1978.

17. Gavin LA, Livermore BM, Cavalieri RR, et al: Serum concentration, metabolic clearance and production rates of 3, 5, 3' triiodothyroacetic acid in normal and athyreotic man. *J Clin Endocrinol Metab* 51:529, 1980.

18. Levy RP, Marshall JS, Velayo NL: Radioimmunoassay of human thyroxine binding globulin (TBG). *J. Clin Invest* 32:372, 1971.

19. Roitt IM, Torrigiani G: Identification and estimation of undegraded thyroglobulin in human serum. *Endocrinology* 81:421, 1967.

20. Chopra IJ, Solomon, DH, Beall GN: Radioimmunoassay for measurement of triiodothyronine in human serum. *J Clin Invest* 50:2033, 1971.

21. Mitsuma T, Nihei N, Gershengorn MC, et al: Serum triiodothyronine: Measurements in human serum by radioimmunoassay with corroboration by gas liquid chromatography. *J Clin Invest* 50:2679, 1971.

22. Leiblich J, Utiger RD: Triiodothyronine radioimmunoassay. *J Clin Invest* 51:157, 1972.

23. Larsen PR: Direct radioimmunoassay of triiodothyronine in human serum. *J Clin Invest* 51:1939, 1972.

24. Gharib J, Ryan RJ, Mayberry WE: T3 radioimmunoassay: A critical evaluation. *Mayo Clin Proc* 47:934, 1972.

25. Chopra IJ, Ho RS, Lam R: An improved radioimmunoassay of triiodothyronine in serum: Its application to clinical and physiologic studies. *J Lab Clin Med* 80:729, 1972.

26. Surks MI, Schadlow AR, Oppenheimer JH: A new radioimmunoassay for T3. *J Clin Invest* 51:3104, 1972.

27. Williams ES, Pharoah P, Lawton NF, et al: Serum triiodothyronine concentration in subjects from an area of endemic goiter. *Isr J Med Sci* 8:1871, 1972.

28. Docter R, Hennemann, A, Bernard H: A radioimmunoassay for measurement of triiodothyronine (T3) in serum. *Isr J Med Sci* 8:1870, 1972.

29. Nejad IF, Bollinger VA, Mitnick MA, et al: Importance of T3 (triiodothyronine) secretion in altered states of thyroid function in the rat. Cold exposure, subtotal thyroidectomy and hypophysectomy. *Trans Assoc Am Physicians* 85:295, 1972.

30. Patel YC, Burger HG: A simplified radioimmunoassay for triiodothyronine. *J Clin Endocrinol Metab* 36:187, 1973.

31. Hufner M, Hesch RD: Comparison of different compounds for TBG blocking in RIA of T3. *Clin Chim Acta* 44:101, 1973.

32. Shimizu T, Shishiba Y, Yoshimura S: A new radioimmunoassay method for serum triiodothyronine using sephadex G25 column. *Endocrinol Jap* 20:365, 1973.

33. Sterling K, Milch PO: Thermal inactivation of thyroxine binding globulin for direct radioimmunoassay of triiodothyronine in serum. *J Clin Endocrinol Metab* 38:866, 1974.

34. Alexander NM, Jennings JF: Radioimmunoassay of serum T3 on small reusable sephadex columns. *Clin Chem* 20:1353, 1974.

35. Burger A, Sokoloff C, Stacheli V, et al. Radioimmunoassay of T3 with and without a prior extraction step. *Acta Endocrinol (Copenh)* 80:58, 1975.

36. Burman KD, Wright FD, Earll JM, et al: Evaluation of a rapid and simple technique for the radioimmunoassay of triiodothyronine. *J Nucl Med* 16:662, 1975.

37. Premachandra BN: A simple and rapid radioimmunoassay of T3 in unextracted serum. *J Nucl Med* 17:411, 1976.

38. Beckers C, Cornette C, Thalasso M: Evaluation of serum T4 by radioimmunoassay. *J Nucl Med* 14:317, 1973.

39. Watson D, Lees S: Comparative study of T4 assays employing radio-ligand reagents. *Ann Clin Biochem* 10:14, 1973.

40. Larsen PR, Dockalova J, Sipula D, et al: Immunoassay of thyroxine in unextracted human serum. *J. Clin Endocrinol Metab* 37:117, 1973.

41. Dunn RT, Foster LB: Radioimmunoassay of thyroxine by a single antibody technique. *Clin Chem* 19:1063, 1973.

42. Rubenstein HA, Butler VP, Jr, Werner SC: Progressive decrease in serum triiodothyronine concentrations with human aging: Radioimmunoassay following extraction of serum. *J Clin Endocrinol Metab* 37:247, 1973.

43. Alexander NM, Jennings JF: Analysis for total serum T4 by equilibrium competitive protein binding on small, re-usable sephadex columns. *Clin Chem* 20:533, 1974.

44. Ratcliffe WA, Ratcliffe JG, McBridge AD, et al: The radioimmunoassay of thyroxine in unextracted serum. *Clin Endocrinol (Oxf)* 3:481, 1974.

45. Premachandra BN, Ibrahim II: A simple and rapid thyroxine radioimmunoassay (T4-RIA) in unextracted human serum; a comparison of T4-RIA and T4 displacement assay T4(D), in normal and pathologic sera. *Clin Chim Acta* 70:43, 1976.

46. Kruse V, Lind O: A rapid and precise sequential saturation radioimmunoassay for thyroxine. *Scand J Clin Lab Invest* 37:149, 1977.

47. Meinhold H, Wenzel KW, Schurnbrand PZ: Radioimmunoassay of 3, 3′, 5′ triiodo-L-thyronine (reverse T3) in human serum and its application in different thyroid states. *Z Klin Chem Klin Biochem* 13:571, 1975.

48. Nicod P, Burger A, Stacheli V, et al: A radioimmunoassay for 3, 3′, 5′ triiodo-L-thyronine in unextracted serum: Method and clinical results. *J Clin Endocrinol Metab* 42:823, 1976.

49. Ratcliffe WA, Marshall J, Ratcliffe JB: A radioimmunoassay of 3, 3′, 5′ triiodothyronine, (reverse T3) in unextracted human serum. *Clin Endocrinol (Oxf)* 5:631, 1976.

50. Griffiths RS, Black EG, Hoffenberg R: Measurement of serum 3, 3′, 5′ (reverse) T3 with comments on its derivation. *Clin Endocrinol (Oxf)* 5:679, 1976.

51. Burman KD, Read J, Dimond RC, et al: Measurements of 3, 3′, 5′ triiodothyronine (reverse T3), 3, 3′-L-diiodothyronine, T3 and T4 in human amniotic fluid and in cord and maternal serum. *J Clin Endocrinol Metab* 43:1351, 1976.

52. Gavin L, Castle J, McMahon F, et al: Extrathyroidal conversion of T4 to reverse T3 and T3 in humans. *J Clin Endocrinol Metab* 44:733, 1977.

53. Kaplan MM, Schimmel M, Utiger RD: Changes in serum reverse T3 with altered thyroid hormone secretion and metabolism. *J Clin Endocrinol Metab* 45:447, 1977.

54. Premachandra BN: Radioimmunoassay of reverse T3. *J Clin Endocrinol Metab* 47:746, 1978.

55. Burman KD, Strum D, Dimond RC, et al: A radioimmunoassay for 3, 3′-L-diiodothyronine (3, 3′). *J Clin Endocrinol Metab* 45:339, 1977.

56. Burger A, Sokoloff C: Serum 3, 3′diiodothyronine, a direct radioimmunoassay in human serum: Method and clinical results. *J Clin Endocrinol Metab* 45:384, 1977.

57. Maciel RMB, Chopra IJ, Ozawa Y, et al: A radioimmunoassay for measurement of 3, 5T2. *J Clin Endocrinol Metab* 49:399, 1979.

58. Galeazzi RL, Burger AG: The metabolism of 3, 3′ diiodothyronine in man. *J Clin Endocrinol Metab* 50:148, 1980.

59. Pangaro L, Burman KD, Wartofsky L, et al: Radioimmunoassay for 3, 5T2 and evidence for dependence on conversion from T3. *J Clin Endocrinol Metab* 50:1075, 1980.

60. Chau KH, Cummins LM: A new extractant for serum thyroxine by enzymatic digestion of thyroxine binding proteins. *J Clin Endocrinol Metab* 42:189, 1976.

61. Green WH: Separation of iodocompounds in serum by chromatography on sephadex columns. *J Chromatogr* 72:83: 1972.

62. Sorimachi K, Ui N: Ion exchange chromatographic analysis of iodothyronines. *Anal Biochem* 67:157, 1975.

63. Brown ML, Metheany J: Use of 8 anilino-1-naphtahline-sulfonic acid in radioimmunoassay of triiodothyronine. *J Pharm Sci* 63:1214, 1974.

64. Green AM, Marshall JS, Pensky J, et al: Thyroxine-binding globulin: Characterization of the binding site with a fluorescent dye as a probe. *Science* 175:1378, 1972.

65. Chopra IJ: Production of antibodies specifically binding T3 and T4. *J Clin Endocrinol Metab* 32:299, 1971.

66. Burke CW, Shakespeare RA: Rapid purification of T3 and T4 protein conjugates for antibody production. *J Endocrinol* 65:133, 1975.

67. Kruse V: Removal of endogenous ligands from a high-affinity antiserum for radioimmunoassay. *Scand J Clin Lab Invest* 39:533, 1979.

68. Gleason GI: Some notes on the exchange of iodine with thyroxine homologues. *J Biol Chem* 213:837, 1955.

69. Burger A, Ingbar SH: Labeling of thyroid hormones and their derivatives. *Endocrinology* 94:1189, 1974.

70. Nakamura Y, Chopra IJ, Solomon DH: Preparation of high specific activity radioactive iodothyronines and their analogues. *J Nucl Med* 18:1112, 1977.

71. Burman KD, Dimond RC, Wright FD, et al: A radioimmunoassay for 3, 3' 5' L-triiodothyronine (reverse T3): Assessment of thyroid gland content and serum measurements in conditions of normal and altered thyroidal economy and following administration of thyrotropin releasing hormone (TRH) and thyrotropin (TSH). *J Clin Endocrinol Metab* 44:660, 1977.

72. Sorimachi K, Cahnman HJ: A simple synthesis of 3, 5' ^{125}I-T2 and of 3, 5 ^{125}I-T4 of high specific activity. *Endocrinology* 101:1276, 1977.

73. Jonsson S, Kronvall A: The use of protein-A-containing staphylococcus aureus as a solid phase anti-IgG reagent in radioimmunoassays as exemplified in the quantitation of a-feto protein in normal human adult serum. *Eur J Immunol* 4:29, 1974.

74. Ying SY, Guillemin R: Dried staphylococcus aureus as a rapid immunological separating agent in radioimmunoassays. *J Clin Endocrinol Metab* 48:360, 1979.

74a. Mitchell ML, McKenna JJ, McIver J: Radioimmunoassay of thyrotropin and thyroxine in dried blood by use of staphylococcus aureus containing Protein A. *Clin Chem* 26:1140, 1980.

75. Lubran M: Quality control of gamma counters. I. Experimental evaluation of sources of error. *Ann Clin Lab Sci* 7:57, 1977.

76. Oddie TH, Klein AH, Fisher DA: Reduction in errors of measurement by the use of control tubes for radioimmunoassays. *Clin Chim Acta,* to be published.

77. Oddie TH, Klein AH, Foley TP, et al: Variation in values for iodothyronine hormones, thyrotropin and thyroxine binding globulin in normal umbilical cord serum with season and duration of storage. *Clin Chem* 25:1251, 1979.

78. Stacheli Y, Vallotton MB, Burger A: Detection of human anti-thyroxine and anti-triiodothyronine antibodies in different thyroid conditions. *J Clin Endocrinol Metab* 41:669, 1975.

79. Wu SY, Green W: Triiodothyronine (T3) binding immunoglobulins in a euthyroid woman: Effects on measurement of T3 (RIA) and on T3 turnover. *J Clin Endocrinol Metab* 42:642, 1976.

80. Premachandra BN, Ginsberg J, Walfish PG: Binding of reverse triiodothyronine to serum immonoglobulins in man and the rabbit. *J Clin Endocrinol Metab* 50:802, 1980.

81. Lee WNP, Golden MP, Van Herle, AJ, et al: Inherited abnormal thyroid hormone-binding protein causing selective increase in total serum thyroxine. *J Clin Endocrinol Metab* 49:292, 1979.

82. Chopra IJ, Fisher DA, Beall GN, et al: Thyroxine and triiodothyronine in human thyroid tissue. *J Clin Endocrinol Metab* 36:311, 1973.

83. Sack J, Fisher DA, Hobel, CJ, et al: Throxine in human amniotic fluid. *J Pediatr* 87:364, 1975.

84. Chopra IJ, Crandall BF: Thyroid hormones and thyrotropin in amniotic fluid. *N Eng J Med* 293:740, 1975.

85. Rogowski P, Siersback V, Nielsen K: Radioimmunoassay of thyroxine and triiodothyronine in urine using extraction and separation on sephadex columns. *Scand J Clin Lab Invest* 37:729, 1977.

86. Shakespeare RA, Burke CW: Triiodothyronine and thyroxine in urine. I. Measurement and application. *J Clin Endocrinol Metab* 42:494, 1976.

87. Fisher DA, Dussault JH, Erenberg A, et al: Thyroxine and triiodothyronine metabolism in maternal and fetal sheep. *Pediatr Res* 6:894, 1972.

88. Fisher DA, Chopra IJ, Dussault JH: Extrathyroidal conversion of thyroxine to triiodothyronine in sheep. *Endocrinology* 91:1141, 1972.

89. Abrams GM, Larsen PR: Triiodothyronine and thyroxine in the serum and thyroid glands of iodine deficient rats. *J Clin Invest* 52:2522, 1973.

90. Kojima A, Hershman JM, Azukizawa M, et al: Quantification of the pituitary-thyroid axis in pregnant rats. *Endocrinology* 95:599, 1974.

91. Hagen GA, Solberg LA: Brain and cerebrospinal fluid permeability to intravenous thyroid hormones. *Endocrinology* 95:1398, 1974.

92. Belshaw BE, Cooper TB, Becker DV: The iodine requirement and influence of iodine intake on iodine metabolism and thyroid function in the adult beagle. *Endocrinology* 96:1280, 1975.

93. Butler WPP, Krey LC, Espinosa-Campos J, et al: Surgical disconnection of the medical basal hypothalamus and pituitary function in the rhesus monkey. III Thyroxine secretion. *Endocrinology* 96:1094, 1975.

94. Gordon A, Spira O: Triiodothyronine binding in rat anterior pituitary, posterior pituitary, median eminence, and brain. *Endocrinology* 96:1357, 1975.

95. Dussault JH, Labrie F: Development of the hypothalamic-pituitary-thyroid axis in the neonatal rat. *Endocrinology* 97:1321, 1975.

96. Nejed I, Bollinger J, Mitnick MA, et al: Measurement of plasma and tissue triiodothyronine concentrations in the rat by radioimmunoassay. *Endocrinology* 96:773, 1975.

97. Chopra IJ, Sack J, Fisher DA: Circulating 3, 3', 5' triiodothyronine (reverse T3) in fetal and adult sheep: Studies of metabolic clearance rate, production rate, serum binding and thyroidal content relative to thyroxine. *Endocrinology* 97:1080, 1975.

98. Thommes RC, Hylka VW: Plasma iodothyronines in the embryonic and immediate posthatch chick. *Gen Comp Endocrinol* 32:417, 1977.

99. Chopra IJ: A study of extrathyroidal conversion of thyroxine to 3, 3', 5' triiodothyronine (T3) in vitro. *Endocrinology* 101:453, 1977.

100. Wu WY, Klein AH, Chopra IJ, et al. Alterations in tissue thyroxine 5' monodeiodinating activity in the perinatal period. *Endocrinology* 103:235, 1978.

101. Davison TF: The turnover of thyroxine in the plasma of the domestic cow. *Gen Comp Endocrinol* 36:380, 1978.

102. Tokagi A, Isozaki Y, Kurate K, et al: Serum concentrations, metabolic clearance rates, and production rates of reverse triiodothyronine, triiodothyronine and thyroxine in starved rabbits. *Endocrinology* 103:1434, 1978.

103. Chopra IJ, Wu SY, Nakamura Y, et al: Monodeiodination of 3, 5, 3' triiodothyronine and 3, 3' 5' triiodothyronine to 3, 3'-diiodothyronine in vitro. *Endocrinology* 102:1099, 1978.

104. Laurberg P: Non-parellel variations in the preferential secretion of 3, 5, 3' triiodothyronine (T3), and 3, 3', 5' triiodothyronine (rT3) from dog thyroid. *Endocrinology* 102:757, 1978.

105. Obregon MJ, Morreale de Escobar G, Escobar del Rey F: Concentrations of triiodo-1-thyronine in the plasma and tissues of normal rats, as determined by radioimmunoassay: Comparison with results obtained by an isotopic equilibrium technique. *Endocrinology* 103:2145, 1978.

106. Regard E, Taurog A, Nakashima T: Plasma thyroxine and triiodothyronine levels in spontaneously metamorphosing Rana Catesbeiana tadpoles and in adult anuran amphibia. *Endocrinology* 102:674, 1978.

107. Robbins J, Berman M: Thyroxine binding globulin metabolism in rhesus monkeys: Effects of hyper and hypothyroidism. *Endocrinology* 104:175, 1979.

108. Melmed S, Harada A, Murata Y, et al: Fetal response to thyrotropin-releasing hormone after thyroid hormone administration to the rhesus monkey: Lack of pituitary suppression. *Endocrinology* 105:334, 1979.

109. Chopra IJ, Hollingsworth D, Davis SL, et al: Amniotic fluid 3, 3' and 3', 5' diiodothyronine in fetal hypothyroidism in sheep. *Endocrinology* 104:596, 1979.

110. Young RA, Danforth E, Jr, Vangenakis AG, et al: Seasonal variation and the influence of body temperature on plasma concentrations and binding of thyroxine and triiodothyronine in the woodchuck. *Endocrinology* 104:996, 1979.

111. Yamamoto T, Doi K, Ichihara K, et al: Reevaluation of measurement of serum free thyroxine by equilibrium dialysis based on computational analysis of the interaction between thyroxine and binding proteins. *J Clin Endocrinol Metab* 50:882, 1980.

112. Chopra IJ, Van Herle AJ, Teco GNC, et al: Serum free thyroxine in thyroidal and nonthyroidal illness: A comparison of measurements by radioimmunoassay, equilibrium dialysis and free thyroxine index. *J Clin Endocrinol Metab* 51:135, 1980.

113. Jiang NS, Tue KA: Determination of free thyroxine in serum by radioimmunoassay. *Clin Chem* 23:1679, 1977.

114. Dussault JH, Laberge C: Thyroxine (T4) determination in dried blood by radioimmunoassay: A screening method for neonatal hypothyroidism. *Union Med Can* 102:2062, 1973.

115. Larsen PR, Broskin K: Thyroxine immunoassay using filter paper blood samples for screening neonates for hypothyroidism. *Pediatr Res* 9:604, 1975.

116. Mitchell ML: Improved thyroxine radioimmunoassay for filter paper discs saturated with dried blood. *Clin Chem* 22:1912, 1976.

117. Mitsuma T, Colucci J, Shenkman L, et al: Rapid simultaneous radioimmunoassay for T3 and T4 in unextracted serum. *Biochem Biophys Res Commun* 46:2107, 1972.

118. Werner SC, Acebodo, G, Radichevich I: A radioimmunoassay for both T4 and T3 in the same sample of serum. *J Clin Endocrinol Metab* 38:493, 1974.

119. Bluett MK, Reiter EO, Duckett GE, et al: Simultaneous radioimmunoassay of TSH and T4 in human serum. *Clin Chem* 23:1644, 1977.

120. Ullman EF, Blakemore J, Leute RK, et al: Homogenous enzyme immunoassay for thyroxine. *Clin Chem* 21:1011, 1975.

121. Galen RS, Forman D: Enzyme immunoassay of serum thyroxine with the "autochemist" multichannel analyzer. *Clin Chem* 23:119, 1977.

122. Plomp TA, Drost RH, Thyssen JHH, et al: Evaluation of the manual enzyme immunoassay (EMIT) procedure for the determination of serum thyroxine. *J Clin Chem Clin Biochem* 17:315, 1979.

123. Gershengorn MC, Larsen PR, Robbins J: Radioimmunoassay for serum thyroxine-binding globulin: Results in normal subjects and patients with hepatocellular carcinoma. *J Clin Endocrinol Metab* 42:907, 1976.

124. Hesch RD, Gats J, McIntosh CHS, et al: Radioimmunoassay of thyroxine in human plasma. *Clin Chim Acta* 70:33, 1976.

125. Kagedal B, Kallberg M: Determination of TBG in human serum by single radial immunodiffusion and radioimmunoassay. *Clin Chem* 23:1694, 1977.

126. Glinoer D, McGuire RA, Gershengorn MC, et al: Effects of estrogen on thyroxine-binding globulin metabolism in rhesus monkeys. *Endocrinology* 100:9, 1977.

127. Chopra IJ, Solomon DH, Ho RS: Competitive ligand-binding assay for measurement of thyronine-binding globulin TBG. *J Clin Endocrinol Metab* 35:565, 1972.

128. Van Herle AJ, Uller RP, Matthews NL, et al: Radioimmunoassay for the measurement of thyroglobulin in human serum. *J Clin Invest* 52:1320, 1973.

129. Ochi Y, Hachiya T, Yoshimura M, et al: Radioimmunoassay for estimation of thyroglobulin in human serum. *Endocrinol Jap* 22:351, 1975.

130. Schneider AB, Favas MJ, Stachura ME, et al: Plasma thyroglobulin in detecting thyroid carcinoma after childhood head and neck irradiation. *Ann Intern Med* 86:29, 1977.

131. Bodlaender P, Arjonilla JR, Sweat R, et al: A practical radioimmunoassay of thyroglobulin. *Clin Chem* 24:267, 1978.

132. Botsch H, Schulz E, Lochner B: Serum thyreoglobulinbestimmung zur verlaufskontrolle bei schilddrusenkarzinoma patienten. *Deutsche Med Wochensch* 104:1072, 1979.

133. Van Herle AJ, Klandorf H, Uller RP: A radioimmunoassay for serum rat thyroglobulin: Physiologic and pharmacological studies. *J Clin Invest* 56:1073, 1975.

134. Van Herle AJ, Vassart G, Dumont JE: Control of thyroglobulin synthesis and secretion. *N Eng J Med* 301:239, 307, 1979.

135. Schneider AB, Pervos R: Radioimmunoassay of human thyroglobulin: Effect of antithyroid autoantibodies. *J Clin Endocrinol Metab* 47:126, 1978.

136. Bayer MF, Kriss JP: Immunoradiometric assay for serum thyroglobulin: Semiquantitative measurement of thryoglobulin in antithyroglobulin positive sera. *J Clin Endocrinol Metab* 49:557, 1979.

CHAPTER **12**

RADIOIMMUNOASSAY OF PROSTANOIDS

Fernand Dray
Wolfgang Seiss*

Prostanoids belong to a family of oxygenated unsaturated C_{20} fatty acids, the eicosanoids. The polyunsaturated fatty acid precursors, which are released mainly from membrane phospholipids, can be oxygenated either by the cyclooxygenase complex to form cyclic products, prostanoids, to which the prostaglandins (PGs) belong, or by lipoxygenases to form noncyclic, hydroxylated derivatives. Figure 1 shows the structure of the principal eicosanoids, and Figure 2 their metabolic pathways. Prostanoids are local or regional hormones with, in many cases, a high biologic activity and a very short half-life. They are present in most biologic systems at low concentrations (10^{-9}–10^{-11} M), thus requiring extremely sensitive techniques of detection. Mass spectrometry coupled with gas chromatography (GC–MS) is a very specific physical technique which is precise (1) and fairly sensitive when capillary columns are used (2). The other analytical method is radioimmunoassay (RIA): It is less specific, but as precise and more sensitive than GC–MS and can be used to dose a large number of samples. Since the first description of a RIA for PGs (3), this technique has progressively been developed for all stable prostanoids (4–14) and recently for a nonprostanoic compound (15). There is a great diversity in the procedure and performance of PG RIAs, which may explain the variability of results obtained from different laboratories. This situation sheds doubt on the reliability of some prostanoid estimations using this technique. We will consider here, after presentation of the antisera, the means of increasing the sensitivity and the specificity of the RIAs of prostanoids, and the limitation of the quantitative analysis of prostanoids in biologic systems.

*Supported by German Research Council.

225

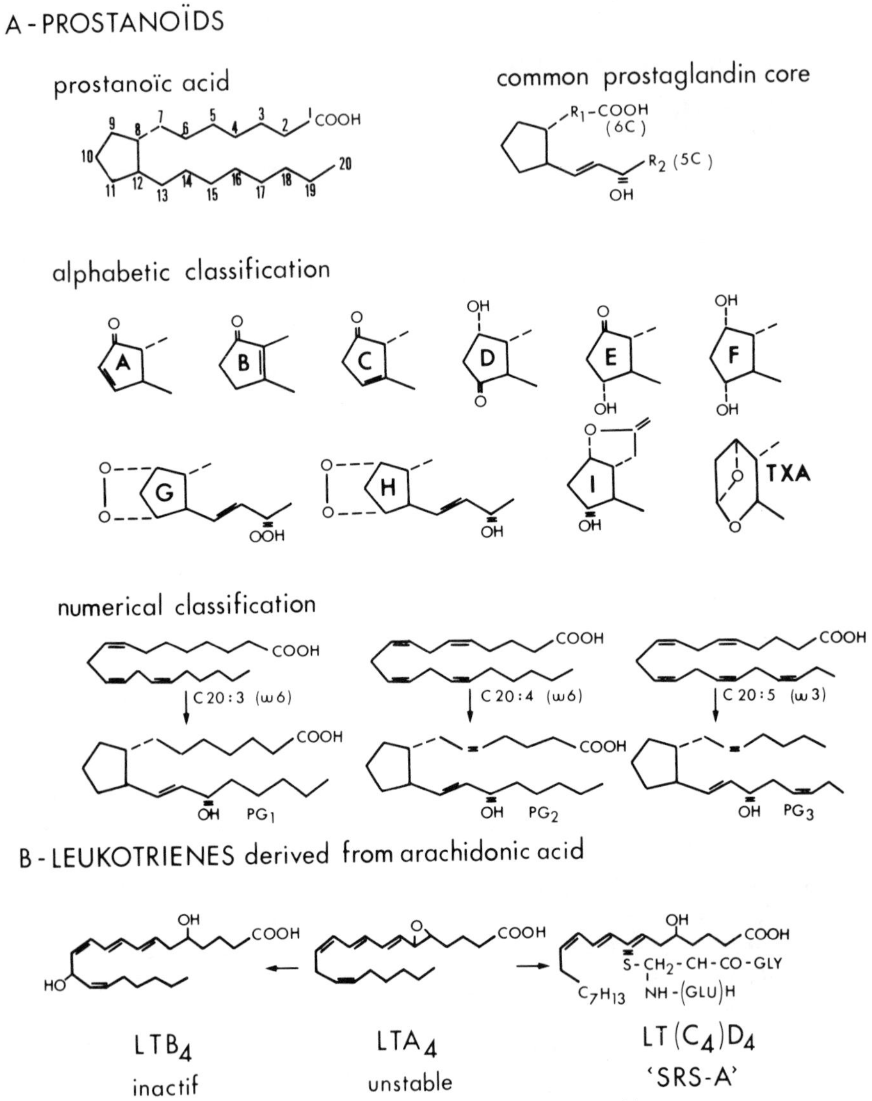
A-PROSTANOÏDS
prostanoïc acid
COOH
common prostaglandin core
R1-COOH (6C)
R2 (5C)
OH
alphabetic classification
A
B
C
D
E
F
G
H
I
TXA
OOH
numerical classification
C 20:3 (ω6)
C 20:4 (ω6)
C 20:5 (ω3)
PG1
PG2
PG3
B-LEUKOTRIENES derived from arachidonic acid
S-CH2-CH-CO-GLY
NH-(GLU)H
C7H13
LTB4
inactif
LTA4
unstable
LT(C4)D4
'SRS-A'

Figure 1. Structure of some eicosanoids.

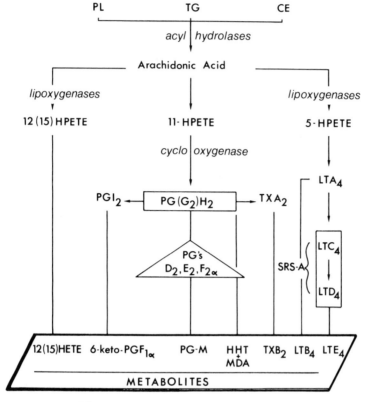

Figure 2. Metabolism of eicosanoids.

THE PRODUCTION AND CHOICE OF ANTISERA

PREPARATION OF IMMUNOGENS

This step concerns prostanoids as well as nonprostanoids. The eicosanoids (MW <400) are not immunogenic per se, but become so when covalently bound to an antigenic carrier, usually bovine or human serum albumin or thyroglobulin. This is generally done by forming a peptide bond between the free carboxyl group of the eicosanoid and an amino group of the protein. The reaction conditions depend on the solubility of the hapten and its stability at different pH values. Table 1 shows some examples of coupling procedures that are used successfully. The instability of certain substances (prostaglandin endoperoxides, thromboxane A, prostacyclin, hydro-

Table 1. Methods of Immunogen Preparation

Coupling Reagent [a]	Temperature (°C)	Buffer	pH	Time of Incubation (hours)
EDC	20	Na_2CO_3	5.5	16–24
Ethyl chloroformate triethylamine	4	Dioxane–0.1 M, $NaHCO_3$ (1:1)	7.0	2
EDC	20	DMF + distilled H_2O (1:20)	5.0–5.5	16–20
DCC–NHS	4	DMF–0.1 M, $NaHCO_3$ (1:5)	7.0	2–3

[a]EDC, N-ethyl-N'-(3-dimethylhylaminopropyl carbodiimide; DCC, N,N'-dicyclohexyl carbodiimide; DMF, N,N'-dimethylformamide; NHS, normal human serum. After coupling, the mixture is dialyzed against distilled H_2O.

peroxyeicosanoic acids, leukotriene A) makes this coupling impossible. Other substances, stable under biologic conditions, can be modified during the conjugation procedure, notably by dehydration; for example, PG derivatives of type E can be transformed to types A and B. This means that the structural integrity of the hapten must be verified before starting the immunization by studying the immunoreactivity of the conjugate against a corresponding standard antiserum or by identifying the noncoupled prostanoid.

IMMUNIZATION

The immunogen is administered to rabbits. Each animal receives 30 to 40 intradermal injections of the conjugate (0.2–1 mg) dissolved in 1 ml of physiologic buffered saline and emulsified in an equal volume of complete Freund's adjuvant (16). Booster injections, given 2–3 months after the primary injections, are carried out following the same schedule. Subsequent booster injections, using smaller amounts of antigen, are given when the antibody titer decreases again. Animals are bled every 10 days after the fourth week of immunization.

SELECTION OF ANTISERA

The course of the immune response is followed by measuring the titer of the antiserum, defined as the dilution giving 50% binding of the radioactive tracer. When the titer of the serum is high enough, the other binding

Table 2. Cross-Reactions of Prostaglandin Antisera

	Antisera									
Inhibitors	E_1	E_2	$F_{1\alpha}$	$F_{2\alpha}$	D_2	$DHKE_2$	$DHKF_{2\alpha}$	TXB_2	$6\text{-}KF_{1\alpha}$	$6,15\text{-}DKF_{1\alpha}$
E_1	100	15	0.2	<0.1	<0.05	<0.1	<0.1	<0.1	5.6	<0.3
E_2	3.0	100	<0.1	0.1	<0.05	0.1	<0.1	<0.1	2.2	<0.3
$F_{1\alpha}$	0.1	<0.1	100	7.0	<0.05	<0.1	<0.1	<0.1	18.0	<0.3
$F_{2\alpha}$	0.3	0.8	29	100	0.04	<0.1	4.0	<0.1	11.0	<0.3
D_1	<1.0	<1.0	<0.3	<0.3	16	<0.1	<0.1	<0.1	1.5	<0.3
D_2	<1.0	<1.0	<0.3	<0.3	100	<0.1	<0.1	0.15	0.5	<0.2
$DHKE_2$	<0.5	<0.5	<0.5	<0.5	<0.05	100	7.0	<0.1	<0.1	1.4
$DHKF_{2\alpha}$	<0.1	<0.1	<0.1	<0.1	<0.05	<0.1	100	<0.1	<0.1	3.5
TXB_2	<0.1	<0.1	<0.1	<0.1	0.9	<0.1	<0.1	100	<0.1	<0.1
$6\text{-}KF_{1\alpha}$	6.0	2.0	18	11	<0.05	<0.1	0.3	<0.1	100	<1.0
$6,15\text{-}DKF_{1\alpha}$	<0.3	<0.3	<0.3	<0.3	<0.1	<1.4	3.5	<0.3	<0.1	100

[a]Cross-reactivities are calculated on the basis of quantity (picograms) necessary for 50% tracer displacement.

parameters (affinity, specificity, dose–response curve) are tested. The best sera are kept separately or pooled. They are stored either at 4°C after dilution with 0.02% sodium azide or at −20°C after dilution in an equal volume of glycerol. Table 2 shows the relative specificity of some selected sera. All antibodies used for RIA of prostanoids have an apparent association constant above $10^9 \ M^{-1}$.

THE INCREASED SENSITIVITY OF RADIOIMMUNOASSAYS USING IODINATED TRACERS

PREPARATION OF PROSTANOIC DERIVATIVES

The first step in the preparation of iodinated prostanoid tracers is their coupling to substances into which ^{125}I can easily be introduced. Tyramine, tyrosyl methyl ester, and histamine have been compared, and similar binding parameters have been obtained (10). Table 3 shows the coupling procedure used for histamine. The derivative is purified and separated from the reagents by thin-layer chromatography (TLC) on silica gel. The addition of [^3H] histamine to the reaction mixture allows localization and identification of the derivative that is formed. After elution in methanol the derivative is divided into small fractions and lyophilized.

Table 3. Coupling of PGs to Histamine

Procedure	Reagent	Volume (ml)	Medium	Reaction Time
Step 1 (COOH activation)	PG (28.6 μmoles) plus EDCI[b] (52.0 μmoles)	0.5	Ethanol–water 1:1, v/v	1 hour
Step 2 (Coupling)	Plus histamine (90.0 μmoles) plus [³H] histamine (10 μCi)	0.5	Water	Overnight

[a]All reactions are carried out at room temperature. The products of the reaction are localized by radioactivity or colored tests (ninhydrin or Pauly).
[b]1-Ethyl-3-(3-dimethylaminopropyl) carbodiimide–HCl.

Table 4. Iodination Procedure[a]

Volume (μl)	Product	Concentration and Buffer
10	PG–histamine	1 nmole
10	Phosphate buffer	0.5 M, pH 7.4
2	Na^{125}I	100 Ci/ml
2	Chloramine-T	2.5 mg/ml in phosphate buffer

[a]Twenty seconds' reaction time; stopped with sodium metabisulfite (32 μg).

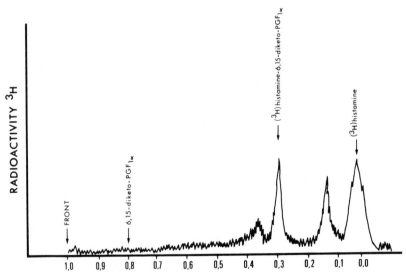

Figure 3. Purification of the coupled 6,15-diketo-PGF$_{1\alpha}$–histamine by TLC (solvent system, butanol–acetic acid–water, 75:10:25)

230

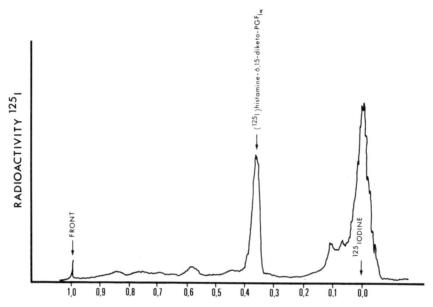

Figure 4. Detection by radioactivity and staining. Radiochromatographical purification of (^{125}I)-labeled histamine–6,15-diketo-PGF$_{1\alpha}$ on a silica gel plate (solvent system, chloroform–methanol–water, 80:20:2)

IODINATION PROCEDURE

The chloramine-T method (17) is used to incorporate ^{125}I into the imidazol ring of histamine (Table 4). The iodinated PG tracer is purified by TLC. Figures 3 and 4 illustrate the TLC migrations in the case of a metabolite of prostacyclin, 6,15-diketo-PGF$_{1\alpha}$.

BINDING PARAMETERS

With iodinated tracers the final dilution of antisera for different RIAs is always higher than with tritiated tracers, and the sensitivity is often increased (Tables 5,6). The cross-reactions of antisera with the inhibitors tested are not significantly different from those found when tritiated tracers are used. Using ^{125}I with a high specific activity (2000 Ci/mmole), a specific activity of the same order can be expected for the monoiodo derivative formed, that is, 10 to 20 times greater than that of tritiated tracers. Thus one can expect an increase in RIA sensitivity due to a greater dilution of the antiserum. In fact, the presence of two nonhomologous molecules, the labeled histamine–prostanoid and the unlabeled prostanoid, which are in

Table 5. RIA Procedures Using Tritiated or Iodinated Tracer

	Reagent	Quantity	Volume (ml)	Reagent	Quantity	Volume (ml)
Reaction	³H-labeled PG	~7,500 dpm	0.1	PG–¹²⁵I-labeled histamine	~14,000 dpm	0.1
	PG standard or biologic sample	—	0.1	PG standard or biologic sample	—	0.1
	Diluted antiserum	—	0.1	Diluted antiserum	—	0.1
Incubation	All reagents are diluted in phosphate-buffered saline, pH 7.4, 0.1 M NaCl 9%, gelatin 1% Overnight at +4°C			All reagents are diluted in phosphate-buffered saline, pH 7.4, 0.05 M, NaCl 9%, bovine γ-globulin 3% Overnight at +4°C		
Separation	Addition to each tube of 1 ml of coated dextran charcoal at +0°C, incubation for 12 minutes, and centrifugation at +4°C for 15 minutes at 2,000g.			Addition to each tube of 0.5 ml of polyethylene glycol 6000 (25 g/100 ml distilled water) at 0°C, mixing and centrifugation at +4°C for 15 minutes at 2,000g.		
Counting	The supernatant (bound fraction) is transferred to a vial for liquid scintillation counting			The supernatant is discarded and the pellet (bound fraction) counted in a gamma spectrometer		

Table 6. Sensitivities of PG RIAs Using Tritiated or Iodinated Tracer

Tracer	Antisera								
	E_1	E_2	$F_{1\alpha}$	$F_{2\alpha}$	$DHKE_2$	$DHKF_{2\alpha}$	TXB_2	$6\text{-}KF_{1\alpha}$	D_2
^{3}H-Labeled PG									
Sensitivity[a]	32	5	15	3.5	54	8	14	94	55
Specific radioactivity (Ci/mmole)	90	117	79	178	66	85	125	20	100
Final dilution of antiserum ($\times 10^{-3}$)	1:45	1:75	1:15	1:90	1:36	1:45	1:24	1:13.5	1:6
^{125}I-Labeled histamine–PG[b]									
Sensitivity[a]	18	2.5	29	7	33	5	8	15	20
Final dilution of antiserum ($\times 10^{-3}$)	1:300	1:150	1:25	1:105	1:15	1:150	1:45	1:168	1:12

[a] Quantity of Pg (picograms) necessary to give 50% displacement of B_0; for all assays, the final dilution of the antiserum was adjusted to obtain 40–50% initial binding.

[b] Specific radioactivity of ^{125}I-labeled histamine–PG tracers was estimated at 2000 Ci/mmole.

Table 7. Sensitivities of RIAs using PG or PG-ME as Inhibitor

	System					
Tracer and Inhibitor	PGE_1	PGE_2	$PGF_{1\alpha}$	$PGF_{2\alpha}$	$DHK\text{-}PGE_2$	$DHK\text{-}PGF_{2\alpha}$
PG–^{125}I-labeled histamine and PG	0.17	0.025	0.82	0.20	0.95	0.09
PG–^{125}I-labeled histamine and PG-ME	0.09	0.028	0.14	0.08	0.26	0.09

[a]Values are picomoles per milliliter required for 50% displacement of B_0. PG-ME, Prostaglandin–methyl ester.

competition for the same antibody site, makes it difficult to determine the performance of the RIA in advance. For example, the affinity of the tracer for the antibody site may be very important because of its structural resemblance to the haptenic determinant of the immunogen: Both form a peptide bond at the carboxyl end of prostanoids. Thus, a greater quantity of nonradioactive ligand will be necessary to displace it, rendering the RIA less sensitive. Because of the greater dilution of antisera this effect can be increased by the participation of antibody populations having a higher affinity for the tracer. However, it is possible to increase the structural resemblance of both competitors by modifying the structure of the ligand in a similar way (such as blockage of the carboxyl group by esterification) (Table 7 and reference 14). Thus, it is possible to ameliorate the level of detection of the ligand.

In all RIAs of prostanoids developed in our laboratory with iodinated tracers, we often observe a net increase in sensitivity and never a diminution. To this performance one can add the other advantages of iodinated tracers: less expensive analysis, less dangerous radioactive manipulation, procedure applicable to all eicosanoids, and independent of the industrial fabrication of tritiated tracers.

SPECIFICITY AND VALIDATION OF PROSTANOID RIAs

PROBLEM

It must be recalled that, like any radiocompetitive assay, the RIA of prostanoids is based on inhibition of the binding of a labeled antigen to its antibody site. This inhibition may be caused by the specific unlabeled antigen or by unspecific interfering material, such as lipids which may not only be

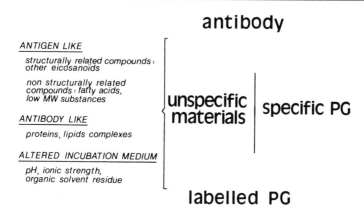

Figure 5. Problems of specificity of competitive RIAs.

present in important quantities in the biologic system but can also be concentrated during the purification of prostanoids (Fig. 5). The specificity of the RIA of prostanoids depends on (1) the binding parameters and conditions of the immunologic reaction, which can be controlled, and (2) the kind and amount of the nonspecific interfering material relative to the specific prostanoid, which varies with the biologic sample.

There are two ways of attenuating the unspecific factors: (1) Dilution of the sample, which is possible when the prostanoid concentration is very high. One can cite the case of TXB_2 in serum or in platelet-rich plasma after stimulation, and of certain prostanoids in human seminal fluid or in amniotic fluid during spontaneous labor. (b) Purification of the sample, the quality of which will determine the validity of the assay.

PURIFICATION PROCEDURES

Extraction

For the separation of proteins and aqueous soluble substances prostanoids can be extracted after acidification into organic solvents. The choice of the solvent (ether, chloroform, ethyl acetate) is primarily dependent on the polarity of the eicosanoid to be extracted. After extraction, the organic phase is evaporated under nitrogen or vacuum at 40°C. A recent method convenient for biologic fluids involves the extraction of prostanoids through an octadecylsilane column (18).

Chromatography Purification

The *silicic acid column method and TLC on silica gel* are very useful in the purification of prostanoids from other lipids and their separation into major classes. TLC has a better resolution but a lower recovery than the silicic

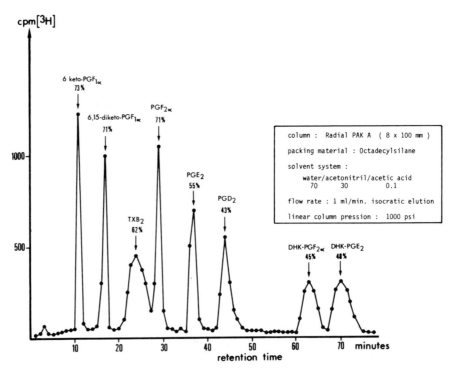

Figure 6. Separation of ³H-labeled PG standards by reversed-phase HPLC. The average recovery is shown for each compound (percentage of ³H-labeled PG injected).

acid column technique. TLC is not suitable as a final step before RIA, because it introduces a high blank value.

High-pressure liquid chromatography (HPLC) is a tool used increasingly for the purification of all eicosanoids and their derivatives (19). Figure 6 shows the separation and recovery of the main prostanoids. The reproducibility of this method is good, and the substances are obtained in a few milliliters of the eluting solvent, which are evaporated or lyophilized before the final quantification. The HPLC columns have good capacities and can be used several hundred times. Two HPLC systems are employed for the separation of eicosanoids, normal- and reversed-phase. Normal-phase HPLC is preferred for the separation of nonpolar eicosanoids because of the better resolution (i.e., for the metabolites of the lipoxygenase pathway), whereas reversed-phase HPLC is especially utilized for separation of the more polar metabolites of the cyclooxygenase (Table 8). Reversed-phase columns consist of a nonpolar phase chemically bonded to a silica surface such as octadecylsilane (ODS, C₁₈ μBondapak). In prostanoid RIAs HPLC should be used as the ultimate purification step before the RIA (20) and is imperative

Table 8. Separation of Eicosanoids by HPLC

		HPLC			
Phase	*Column*	*Solvent Composition*	*Flow (ml/min)*	*Elution*	*Eicosanoids*
Normal	Silicic acid (Porasil 7.8 × 300 mm)	Hexane, 2-propanol, acetic acid	3.5	Isocratic	Mono-OH and mono-OOH derivatives (see reference 19)
Normal	Silicic acid (Porasil 7.8 × 300 mm)	Methanol, chloroform, acetic acid	1	Gradient	Primary PGs and PG metabolites (see reference 20)
Reversed	Octadecylsilane (C_{18}) (radial pak A 8 × 100 mm)	Water, acetonitrile, acetic acid	1	Isocratic	Primary PGs and PG metabolites

for the control of specificity. The necessity for the use of HPLC as a purification step depends on the type of prostanoid to be dosed and the kind of biologic sample. This is illustrated in Figures 7 and 8. The comparison of the immunoprofiles of different plasma prostanoids shows that the use of HPLC is apparently more important for 6-keto-$PGF_{1\alpha}$ than for TXB_2 and PGE_2 (Fig. 7). On the other hand, the immunoreactive profiles of 6-keto-$PGF_{1\alpha}$ in various biologic systems show that a HPLC step is not always necessary. It is clear that for each prostanoid and for each biologic sample the necessity for using HPLC must be tested. Generally, it can be considered that, the lower the specificity of the antibody and the concentration of the prostanoid, the more important the purification on HPLC.

CONTROL OF SPECIFICITY AND VALIDATION OF RADIOIMMUNOASSAYS OF PROSTANOIDS

There are different ways of controlling the RIAs of prostanoids. Some of them will be mentioned here.

Comparison with Other Methods
A comparison with a quite different method of determination (GC–MS, bioassay, or radiometry) is the best way to evaluate RIA. However, in most

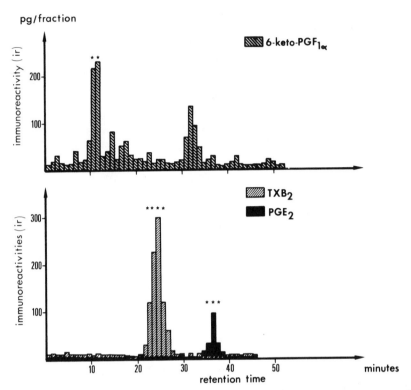

Figure 7. Immunoreactive profiles (ir) of 6-keto-PGF$_{1\alpha}$, TXB$_2$, and PGE$_2$ from human plasma after reversed-phase HPLC. Before separation, plasma was extracted and purified on a silicic acid column. Top: Ir obtained with 6-keto-PGF$_{1\alpha}$ antiserum. Bottom: ir obtained with TXB$_2$ and PGE$_2$ antisera. Asterisk indicates radioactivity of the corresponding tritiated tracer.

cases, these methods are not available or they are of value only for some prostanoids (bioassay) (21) or are much less sensitive (radiometry) (12).

Control of the Specificity of the Radioimmunoassay Itself

Blank Value. There are two kinds of blanks: the blank introduced by the purification procedure (acidification, organic solvents) and the biologic blank (the sum of all unspecific known and unknown materials deriving from the biologic sample). Whereas the former is easy to estimate, the only means of checking the latter is the inhibition of prostanoid synthesis by aspirin or indomethacin. However, this may be erroneous because of incomplete inhibition or the elimination of other possible cross-reacting prostanoids.

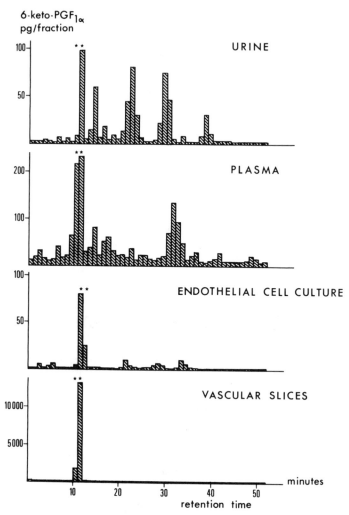

Figure 8. 6-keto-PGF$_{1\alpha}$ immunoreactive profiles (ir) after reversed-phase HPLC from various biologic systems. The samples for HPLC were prepared as described in Figure 7. Asterisks indicated radioactivity of the corresponding tritiated tracer.

Purification Procedure. Sequential purification steps make it possible to diminish the biologic blank and to control the specificity. This is achieved by comparing the values obtained before and after each purification step (Table 9). Because of its high resolution HPLC is a very important tool. Figure 9 shows the steps that should be followed when a RIA has to be developed and a simplification of the procedure is to be introduced.

Table 9. 6-Keto-PGF$_{1\alpha}$ and 6,15-Diketo-PGF$_{1\alpha}$ Concentrations in Plasma, Serum, and Urine before and after HPLC

	6-Keto-PGF$_{1\alpha}$ (pg/ml)		6,15-Diketo-PGF$_{1\alpha}$ (pg/ml)[a]	
	Before HPLC	*After HPLC*	*Before HPLC*	*After HPLC*
Pooled human plasma				
Men	74	5	—	<2
Women	71	6	71	<2
Pooled human serum				
Men	70	16	—	<2
Pooled rabbit plasma				
Arterial	61	24	26	<2
Venous	140	27	34	<2
Human urine[b]	300–3314	40–460	1662	192

[a][^{3}H]-6-keto-PGF$_{1\alpha}$ was used for recovery determination.
[b]$n = 4$.

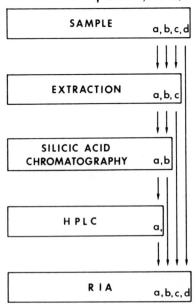

Figure 9. Purification procedure, diagram "à la carte."

Linear Graph of the Values.   A comparison of the values obtained with increasing volumes of the biologic sample must give equal increments in the prostanoid being dosed and a linear graph with a slope not equal to 1 is expected.

LIMITS OF THE SIGNIFICANCE OF QUANTITATIVE ANALYSIS OF PROSTANOIDS

We have demonstrated that the RIA of prostanoids is an extremely sensitive method when iodinated tracers are used and that its specificity may be greatly enhanced by HPLC purification of the biologic samples. Under these conditions, the RIA method because of its high sensitivity (1-10 pg/tube) may be superior to the GC–MS procedure.

There are several limitations to the quantitative analysis of prostanoids performed by RIA or GC–MS.

First, the chemical instability of many biologically active prostanoids (endoperoxides, thromboxane A, prostacyclin) excludes their quantitative determination by these methods. In this case one has the possibility of analyzing their respective metabolites. This is complicated by the existence of several metabolites of prostacyclin and by the possible nonenzymatic transformation of endoperoxides into PGD_1, $PGF_{1\alpha}$, or PGE_2.

Second, it is known that the experimental conditions under which the sample is handled can alter the prostanoid profile by causing either their synthesis or their degradation.

All these factors should be reduced to a minimum before the quantitative information obtained either by RIA or by GC–MS can be considered to have physiologic significance.

REFERENCES

1. Green K, Hamberg M, Samuelsson B: Quantitative analysis of prostaglandin and thromboxanes by mass spectrometric methods, in Samuelsson B, Paoletti: *Advances in Prostaglandin and Thromboxane Research.* New York, Raven Press, 1976, p 47.

2. Maclouf J, Rigaud M, Durand J, Chebroux P: Glass capillary columns applied to prostaglandins measurement: A useful tool for gas chromatography-mass spectrometry analysis. *Prostaglandins* 11:999, 1976.

3. Levine L, Van Vunakis H: Antigenic activity of prostaglandins. *Biochem Biophys Res Commun* 41:1171, 1970.

4. Caldwell BV, Burstein S, Brock WA, Speroff L: Radioimmunoassay of the F prostaglandins. *J Clin Endocrinol* 33:171, 1971.

5. Jaffe BM, Smith JW, Newton WT, Parker CW: Radioimmunoassay for prostaglandins. *Science* 171:494, 1971.

6. Dray E, Maron E, Tillson SA, Sela M: Immunochemical detection of prostaglandin with prostaglandin-coated bacteriophage T4 and by radioimmunoassay. *Anal Biochem* 50:399, 1972.

7. Kirton KT, Cornette JC, Barr KL: Characterization of antibody to prostaglandin $F_{2\alpha}$. *Biochem Biophys Res Commun* 47:903, 1972.

8. Dray F, Charbonnel B, Maclouf J: Radioimmunoassay of prostaglandins F_γ, E_1 and E_2. *Eur J Clin Invest* 5:311, 1975.

9. Maclouf J, Andrieu JM, Dray F: Validity of PGE_1 radioimmunoassay by using PGE_1 antisera with differential binding parameters. *FEBS Lett* 56:273, 1975.

10. Maclouf J, Pradel M, Pradelles P, Dray F: (^{125}I) derivatives of prostaglandins; a novel approach in prostaglandins analysis by radioimmunoassay. *Biochem Biophys Acta* 431:139, 1976.

11. Sors H, Maclouf J, Pradelles P, Dray F: The use of iodinated tracers for a sensitive radioimmunoassay of 13,14-dihydro-15-keto-prostaglandin F_α. *Biochem Biophys Acta* 486:553, 1977.

12. Sors H, Pradelles P, Dray F, et al: Analytical methods for thromboxane B_2 measurement and validation of radioimmunoassay by gas liquid chromatography-mass spectrometry. *Prostaglandins* 16:277, 1978.

13. Dray F, Pradelles P, Maclouf J, et al: Radioimmunoassay of 6-keto-$PGF_{1\alpha}$ using an iodinated tracer. *Prostaglandins* 15:715, 1978.

14. Maclouf J, Sors H, Pradelles P, Dray F: Improved sensitivity of iodinated histamine-prostaglandin radioimmunoassay by prostaglandin methyl esters. *Anal Biochem* 87:169, 1978.

15. Eskra JD, Levine L, Carty TJ: Preparation of (^3H)-12-L-hydroxyeidonatetraenoic acid and its use in radioimmunoassay. *Prostaglandins and Medicine* 5:201, 1980.

16. Vaitukaitis JL, Robbins JB, Nieschlag E, Ross GT: A method for producing specific antisera with small doses of immunogen. *J Clin Endocrinol Metab* 33:988, 1971.

17. Hunter WM, Greenwood FC: Preparation of iodine-131 labeled human growth hormone of high specific activity. *Nature* 194:495, 1962.

18. Powell WS: Rapid extraction of oxygenated metabolites of arachidonic acid from biological samples using octadecylsilyl silica. *Prostaglandins* 20:947, 1980.

19. Carr K, Sweetman BJ, Frolich JC: High performance liquid chromatography of prostaglandins: Biological applications. *Prostaglandins* 11:3, 1976.

20. Alam I, Ohuchi K, Levine L: Determination of cyclooxygenase products and prostaglandin metabolites using high-pressure liquid chromatography and radioimmunoassay. *Anal Biochem* 93:339, 1979.

21. Scherer B, Siess W, Weber PC: Radioimmunological and biological measurement of prostaglandins in rabbit urine: Decrease of PGE_2 excretion at high NaCl intake. *Prostaglandins* 13:1127, 1977.

CHAPTER 13

NONCOMPETITIVE VERSUS COMPETITIVE BINDING ASSAYS

Leif Wide

GENERAL CLASSIFICATION OF BINDING ASSAYS

The term *binding assays* (or *ligand assays*) is used for a large group of assays that have had a great impact on biomedical science. It is characteristic of all these binding assays that the substance to be measured, the analyte (P), is bound to a binding reagent (Q) and that the reaction is governed by the law of mass action:

$$P + Q \rightleftharpoons PQ$$

In most binding assays one of the reactants is labeled with a marker. The group of binding assays using a labeled reactant may be subdivided into groups of assays according to a number of different variables. The type of analyte, the type of marker for labeling, the type of binding reagent, and the type of separation technique have all been used as a basis for classification. Terms such as steroid assays, radioassays, immunoassays, charcoal techniques, and different combinations such as radioimmunoassays, enzyme receptor assays, and solid-phase radioimmunoassays, are commonly used. In Figure 1 the methods have been primarily classified according to the nature of the assay into *competitive* or *noncompetitive* assays and, on the basis of which reactant is labeled, into *labeled ligand* or *labeled binding reagent* assays (1,2). The term *ligand* is used in this context for the analyte and for all other compounds that bind to the appropriate binding site on the binding reagent and compete with the analyte. Examples of ligands other than the analyte are labeled ligands and solid-phase ligands. The different ligands do not have to be similar in any other aspect than that they compete for the same binding site on a binding reagent. There are two main groups of competitive binding assays: those using a labeled ligand and those using a labeled binding reagent. The principles of these two groups of assays will be presented first.

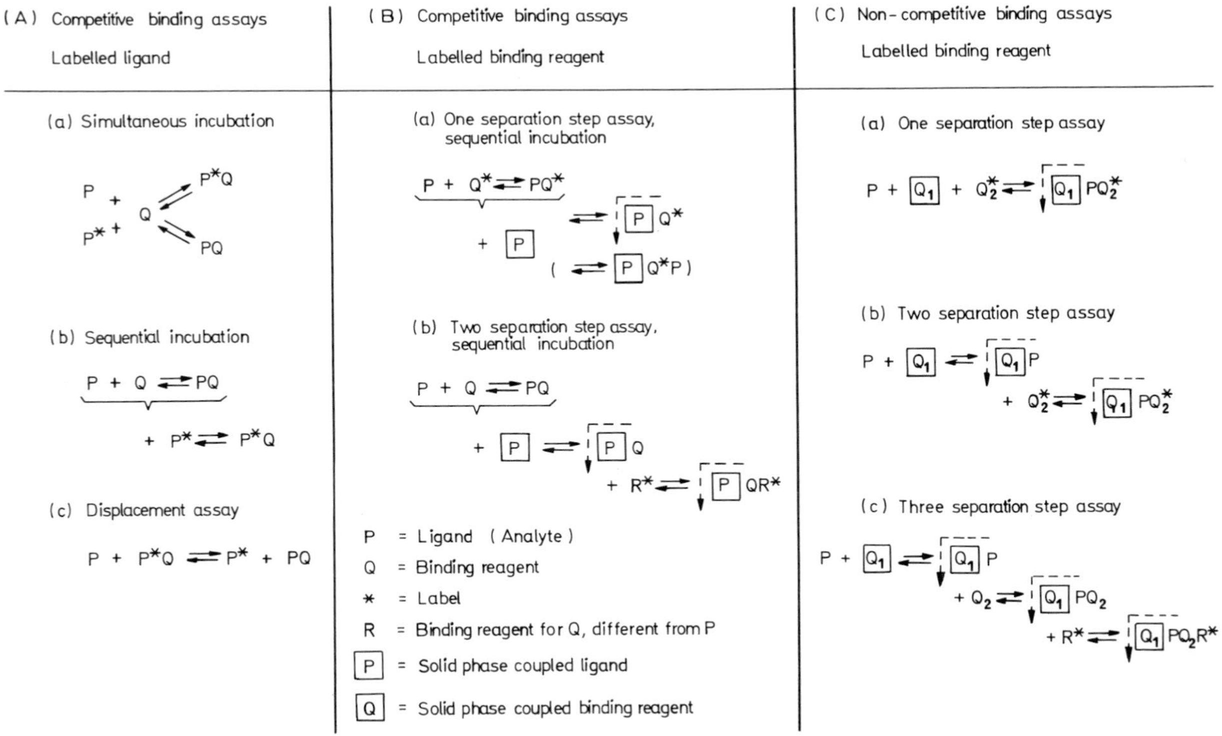

244

Figure 1. Principles of binding assays with a labeled reactant.

COMPETITIVE BINDING ASSAYS

A competitive binding assay method for insulin was developed by Arquilla and Stavitsky in 1956 (3). Insulin was labeled with erythrocytes, and labeled and unlabeled insulin competed for the binding sites on a limited number of antibodies to insulin (Fig. 1*Aa*). The antibody-bound labeled insulin was then detected by the addition of complement which caused a release of hemoglobin from the antibody–insulin–erythrocyte complex. Increasing amounts of unlabeled insulin produced a fall in bound labeled insulin. In this case it was not necessary to remove the bound labeled ligand from the unbound. Such tests were later termed *homogeneous* assays in contrast to *heterogeneous* assays in which a separation step is introduced (4). However, this competitive binding assay for insulin was not sensitive enough for clinical use and was considerably improved by Yalow and Berson (5) who replaced the erythrocytes by a radioactive label, ^{131}I, which increased the sensitivity of the assay. This was the first radioimmunoassay. At about the same time Ekins (6) introduced the use of a ligand labeled with a radioactive isotope in a nonimmunologic competitive binding assay.

If the labeled ligand is added to the incubation mixture of analyte and binding reagent later (sequential incubation in Fig. 1*Ab*), increased sensitivity may be obtained (7). The reaction then must be interrupted before it reaches equilibrium. With a low dissociation rate constant and a long first and short second incubation period the sensitivity may be increased 5 to 10 times when compared to the procedure using simultaneous incubation (8).

A third variant of the labeled ligand competitive binding assay (the displacement assay, Fig. 1*Ac*) was recently described for solid-phase radioimmunoassay of thyroxine and triiodothyronine (9). The labeled ligand was mixed with the binding reagent (solid-phase-coupled antibody) when the reagents were prepared and then stored until used for assay. Only one solution with the reagents then had to be added to the unknown specimen. During the assay dissociation of the immuncomplexes was facilitated by a 2-hour incubation at 60°C, which almost eliminated the disturbing effect on the analysis by thyroxine-binding globulin in the serum specimen.

A radioimmunoassay technique using labeled antibodies (as binding reagent) in combination with solid-phase-coupled antigen (ligand) was developed by Miles and Hales (10). This variant is called an *immunoradiometric* assay and is a one-separation-step assay with sequential incubation (Fig. 1*Ba*). The analyte reacts with a labeled binding reagent. After that a solid-phase-coupled ligand is added to bind the remaining free labeled binding reagent. In the second incubation the analyte and the solid-phase ligand compete for the binding sites on the labeled binding reagent. There is an analogy between this technique and the use of sequential incubation in the labeled ligand assay (Fig. 1Ab). However, there is also an essential difference between the two techniques. When labeled ligands are used, measurement of the analyte is indirect. The binding of labeled ligand to the binding reagent is observed, and it is inversely proportional to the amount of analyte. When labeled binding reagents are used, measurement of the analyte is direct. In this case the binding of labeled binding reagent to the analyte is observed, and it is directly proportional to the amount of analyte. The labeled binding reagent should preferably be univalent to avoid a decrease in sensitivity due to the reaction shown in parentheses in Figure 1Ba.

A similar technique was developed by our group for the assay of allergens (11). The principle is shown in Figure 1Bb in which P is the allergen to be assayed, Q is the reaginic IgE antibody, and R* is a labeled antibody to IgE. In this method binding reagent that has not reacted with the analyte is extracted with a solid-phase ligand and then labeled with R*, which is a binding reagent for Q different from the P in the assay. This method is used both for monitoring the purification of allergens and for standardization of allergen extracts.

NONCOMPETITIVE BINDING ASSAYS

A noncompetitive radioimmunoassay using a labeled binding reagent (labeled antibodies) was introduced by Wide et al. in 1967 (12). It was the first in a series of different "sandwich" radioimmunoassays (13,14). A similar technique was described by Habermann (15) as a *Verknüppfungstest* and by Addison and Hales (16) as a "two-site assay." In sandwich binding assays the labeled binding reagent is used in combination with a solid-phase-coupled binding reagent. The methods are in principle applicable to the measurement of all substances that have at least two binding sites. The two reagents are added to the unknown in excess.

In its simplest form (Fig. 1Ca) both reagents are added simultaneously to the unknown and only one separation step is included in the assay. This is a sensitive assay method provided the binding sites on the analyte for Q1 and Q2 are different and that only a small number of molecules, with binding sites for only one of the two binding reagents, are present in the unknown solution. When these two criteria are not fulfilled, it is advisable to add to the unknown the solid-phase binding reagent first. Then, after incubation, wash away unbound material, incubate again after the addition of labeled binding reagent, and finally wash away unbound labeled material. This is the principle described in Figure 1Cb and exemplified schematically in Figures 2–4.

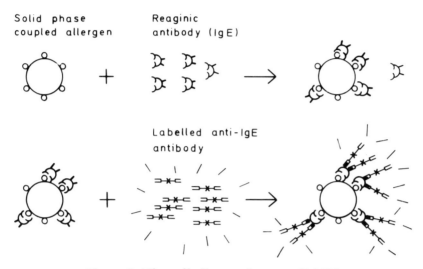

Figure 2. The radioallergosorbent test (RAST).

The noncompetitive radioimmunoassay was first applied to the assay of reagins of the IgE type for specific allergens (Fig. 2). This assay was called the *Radioallergosorbent* test or RAST (12). The sandwich assay was developed because it was not possible to use the conventional radioimmunoassay to obtain the high degree of specificity needed to measure specific reagins. The method should measure only molecules of the IgE class and of these

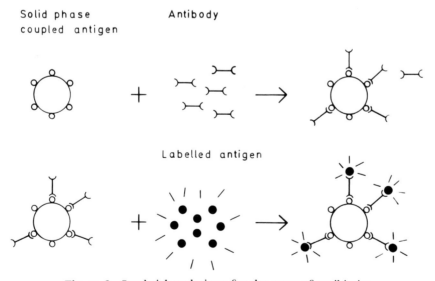

Figure 3. Sandwich technique for the assay of antibiotics.

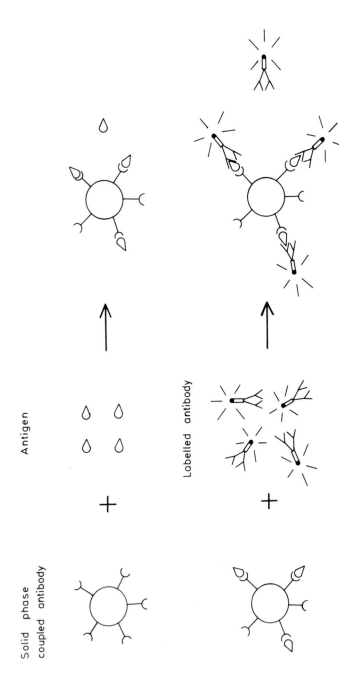

Solid phase coupled antibody

Antigen

Labelled antibody

Figure 4. Sandwich technique for the assay of antigens.

only those directed to a specific allergen. Solid-phase-coupled allergen is added in excess to the reagins in the unknown solution, and after incubation all other IgE molecules are washed away. When labeled anti-IgE is added, these molecules bind only to the solid-phase bound IgE molecules. When after incubation unbound radioactive material is washed away and the remaining radioactivity is measured, a significant uptake of radioactivity on the solid phase indicates the presence of reagins to the particular allergen. This method is now widely used in the diagnosis of atopic allergy, and its clinical significance has become well established (17).

Another sandwich technique (according to Fig. 1Cb) for the assay of antibodies to a particular antigen is shown schematically in Figure 3. In this assay the two binding reagents are the antigen coupled to a solid phase and the same antigen labeled with a marker, for example, a radioactive isotope. The antibodies to be tested are first bound to the solid-phase-coupled antigen. The solid phase is then washed, and when labeled antigen is added it is bound to the free binding site(s) of the antibodies on the immunosorbents. After washing the solid phase the uptake of labeled marker on the solid phase is measured, and it is directly proportional to the number of antibodies in the unknown solution. The antibodies detected may belong to different immunoglobulin classes. However, hitherto we have not been able to detect antibodies of the IgE type with this assay system, indicating that this particular antibody is functionally monovalent in such a system. The assay method is very sensitive and useful in the detection of antibody formation in patients. Rheumatoid factors and complement do not interfere in the assay. Examples of applications are the detection of antibodies to hepatitis antigen and *Aspergillus fumigatus*, to various drugs including hormones, and to various compounds to which an individual might be exposed in his occupation.

Larger molecules have in general a number of different antigenic sites, and most antisera to such large antigens have several populations of antibodies to different structures. Therefore, for the measurement of antigens according to Figure 1Cb the same antiserum may be used both for binding to the solid phase and for labeling. However, it is possible to increase the specificity by coupling antibodies directed to one part of the whole molecule (e.g., the N-terminal) and label antibodies to another part of the molecule (e.g., the C-terminal). If the labeled antibodies are to the C-terminal part, even large amounts of C-terminal fragments will have a negligible effect on the result, as they are removed by the first separation step. This method is illustrated schematically in Figure 4.

The use of two different kinds of binding reagents in a sandwich-like binding assay was reported by Lowenstein et al. (18). Human thyroid-stimulating hormone (TSH) in the unknown specimen was first bound to nuclear receptors in guinea pig thyroid cells. Rabbit antibodies to bovine TSH were then added and bound to the TSH. Finally guinea pig fluorescence-

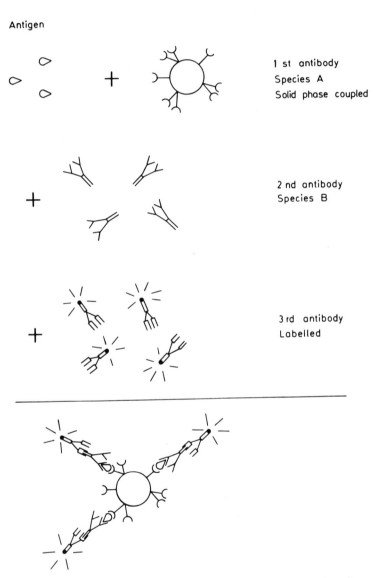

Three step solid phase sandwich RIA

Antigen

1 st antibody
Species A
Solid phase coupled

2 nd antibody
Species B

3 rd antibody
Labelled

Figure 5. A four-layer sandwich technique for the assay of antigens.

labeled antibodies to rabbit γ-globulin were added. Quantitation of TSH was achieved by observing the point of disappearance of nuclear fluorescence with serial dilution of the unknown serum. As little as 10^{-2} mU of TSH per liter of serum could be measured with this sensitive assay.

A similar four-layer sandwich technique, which includes three separation steps, is shown as a formula in Figure 1Cc. An example with three successive immunologic reactions (19) is shown schematically in Figure 5. An antibody from one animal species (A) coupled to a solid phase first binds the antigen. After washing the solid phase, a second antibody from another animal species (B) directed to the same antigen is then bound to the antigen. In the third stage of the assay a labeled antibody directed to the immunoglobulin of species B is added after careful washing of the solid phase. This antibody forms the fourth layer, and after a third washing procedure the presence of the marker on the solid phase is measured. An advantage of this variant is that the same type of labeled antibody can be used for the assay of several different antigens.

NONCOMPETITIVE VERSUS COMPETITIVE BINDING ASSAYS

In the first group of competitive binding assays the amount of binding reagent is fixed and limited. Also, the amount of labeled ligand is fixed and should be in excess vis-à-vis the amount of binding reagent. The distribution of labeled ligand between the bound and free phases is a function of the concentration of the analyte. In the second group of competitive binding assays the amount of labeled binding reagent should exceed that of the analyte. However, the amount of binding reagent also has to be limited in this case, as the amount of solid-phase-coupled ligand added should be in excess vis-à-vis the labeled binding reagent. The analyte and the solid-phase ligand compete for a limited amount of binding reagent. The distribution of labeled binding reagent between the two bound phases is a function of the concentration of the analyte. To obtain a high sensitivity with this method it is essential that almost all the labeled binding reagent be bound when the incubation is interrupted and that the dissociation rate constant be low for the analyte–binding reagent reaction. The dissociation of this complex is influenced by the amount of solid-phase ligand, and the kinetics of all these reactions are of importance in determining the sensitivity of the system.

In the noncompetitive assay, the sandwich method, the solid-phase binding reagent is added in excess vis-à-vis the analyte. When the analyte is present in a low amount, virtually all of it should be bound. In the second step of the assay the labeled binding reagent is added in a large excess and virtually all analyte is "labeled" with this reactant. A low dissociation rate constant is of course also of importance in this method. However, when the solid-phase binding reagent and the labeled binding reagent react with different sites on the analyte, no competition is involved in the assay, which is an advantage for the sandwich technique when compared with the competitive immunoradiometric assay, both of which use a labeled binding reagent.

Ekins (20) has suggested the term *reagent excess* methods for sandwich assays and noncompetitive binding assays, and *limited reagent* methods for labeled ligand competitive binding assays. However, reagents are often in excess over the amount of analyte in limited reagent methods. This drawback of the nomenclature can be avoided if the amount of binding reagent vis-à-vis the total amount of ligand in the assay is taken as a basis for classification. The competitive binding assays would then be *ligand excess* methods and the noncompetitive binding assays would be *binding reagent excess* methods.

It was shown experimentally that the sensitivity of a sandwich technique for the assay of IgE was about 10 times higher than that of the labeled ligand-competitive binding assay (14). In general, labeled binding reagent techniques are potentially more sensitive when compared with labeled ligand techniques. In noncompetitive binding assays the labeled binding reagent (in the sandwich assay also the solid-phase-coupled binding reagent) is added in a large excess, and it is mainly the signal/noise ratio that determines the sensitivity. This ratio is naturally of importance in labeled ligand competitive binding assays also. However, in these assays the amount of binding reagent is very small, and the avidity of the ligand-binding reagent reaction is a most important factor in limiting the sensitivity of the assay.

Antibodies to a molecule may also react with fragments of the molecule. These fragments may have a high activity in a competitive binding assay and give a false high value. If the fragments have only one binding site, they will have an opposite effect on the results in the noncompetitive sandwich assay. Depending on the excess of antibodies in the solid phase, the fragments reacting with these antibodies either have negligible influence or give a false low value. Fragments reacting with labeled antibodies have as a rule no influence on the assay result, as these fragments are removed in the first separation step. Simultaneous assays with competitive and noncompetitive methods can give valuable information about the possible presence of fragments of molecules and about nonspecific inhibition.

A limitation in the use of the noncompetitive sandwich binding assay is that the analyte must have at least two binding sites and be able to bind to the solid-phase binding reagent and the labeled binding reagent simultaneously. It is not possible to use this method for the assay of small compounds, and labeled ligand competitive methods are preferably used in these cases. Large molecules may have a great number of binding sites and may therefore bind a large amount of the binding reagent. The use of labeled binding reagents offers an advantage, particularly with regard to sensitivity, in the assay of such high-molecular-weight compounds.

A complication in the use of sandwich methods is the so-called hook effect in the high concentration range of the analyte. This means that increasing amounts of the analyte will give a lower response and thus a false low result. When assaying substances that may be present in a very wide concentration range, it is usually necessary to assay the unknown in two dilutions. This is a disadvantage of noncompetitive versus competitive binding assays. The precision of the assay is usually good in noncompetitive assays, as the two binding reagents are added in excess and the exact amount added is less critical. This also makes it possible to use various different forms of the solid phase, such as paper disks, the inside surface of test tubes, or small cellulose particles (21).

The labeled binding reagent should preferably be in a purified form. When labeled antibodies are used as labeled binding reagents, they usually are immunosorbent-purified either before or after the labeling. It seems likely that when hybridoma technique-produced purified antibodies become available, this will encourage the use of labeled antibodies for the assay of different antigens. The enhanced structural specificity and the high sensitivity potential of noncompetitive binding assays make it likely that these techniques will be used more in the future and to some extent replace the competitive binding assays in use today.

REFERENCES

1. Schuurs AHWM, van Weemen, BK: Enzyme-immunoassay. *Clin Chim Acta* 81:1, 1977.

2. Wide, L: Principles, technical difficulties and developments of radioimmunoassay procedures, in Turk, JL, Parker D (eds): *Drugs and Immune Responsiveness*. London, Macmillan Press Ltd., 1979, p 223.

3. Arquilla ER, Stavitsky AB: The production and identification of antibodies to insulin and their use in assaying insulin. *J Clin Invest* 35:458, 1956.

4. Rubenstein KE, Schneider RS, Ullman EF: "Homogeneous" enzyme immunoassay. A new immunochemical technique. *Biochem Biophys Res Commun* 47:846, 1972.

5. Yalow RS, Berson SA: Assay of plasma insulin in human subjects by immunological methods. *Nature* 184:1648, 1959.

6. Ekins RP: The estimation of thyroxin in human plasma by an electrophoretic technique. *Clin Chim Acta* 5:453, 1960.

7. Hales CN, Randle PJ: Immunoassay of insulin with insulin-antibody precipitate. *Biochem J* 88:137, 1963.

8. Wide L, Dahlberg PA: Quality requirements of basal S-TSH assays in predicting and S-TSH response to TRH. *Scand J Clin Lab Invest* 40 (suppl 155) 101, 1980.

9. Wide L: Use of particulate immunosorbents in radioimmunoassay, in Van Vanucis H, Langone JJ (eds): *Immunochemical Techniques,* vol B of Colowick SP, Kaplan NO (eds): *Methods in Enzymology.* Vol. 73. New York, Academic Press, in press, 1981, p. 203.

10. Miles LE, Hales CN: Labelled antibodies and immunological assay systems. *Nature* 219:186, 1968.

11. Aronsson T, Wide L: Studies on allergens of horse epithelium with two variants of RAST. *Int Arch Allergy Appl Immunol* 47:224, 1974.

12. Wide L, Bennich H, Johansson SGO: Diagnosis of allergy by an in vitro test for allergen antibodies. *Lancet* II:1105, 1967.

13. Wide L: Radioimmunoassays employing immunosorbents. *Acta Endocrinol* (suppl 142) 207, 1969.

14. Wide L: Solid phase antigen-antibody systems, in Kirkham KE, Hunter WM (eds): *Radioimmunoassay Methods.* Edinburgh, Churchill Livingstone, 1971, p 405.

15. Habermann E: Ein neues Prinzip zur quantitativen Bestimmung hochmolekularer Antigene (Verknüpfungstest) und seine Anwendung auf Tetanustoxin, Serumalbumin und Ovalbumin. *Z Klin Chem Klin Biochem* 8:51, 1970.

16. Addison GM, Hales CN: Two site assay of human growth hormone. *Horm Metab Res* 3: 59–60, 1971.

17. Wide L: Clinical significance of measurement of reaginic (IgE) antibody by RAST. *Clin Allergy* 3 (suppl) 583, 1973.

18. Lowenstein JM, Blum AS, Greenspan FS, Hargandine JR: Immunofluorescent assay of TSH and LATS, in Margoulies M. (ed): *Protein and Polypeptide Hormones,* part 2. Amsterdam, Excerpta Medica Foundation, 1969, p 343.

19. Belanger L, Sylvestre C, Dufour D: Enzyme-linked immunoassay for alpha-fetoprotein by competitive and sandwich procedures. *Clin Chim Acta* 48:15, 1973.

20. Ekins RP: The future development of immunoassay, in *Radioimmunoassay and Related Procedures in Medicine,* vol 1. Vienna, International Atomic Energy Agency, 1978, p 143.

21. Wide L: Solid phase radioimmunoassays, in *Radioimmunoassays and Related Procedures in Medicine,* vol 1. Vienna, International Atomic Energy Agency, 1978, p. 143.

CHAPTER **14**

PRINCIPLES OF
RADIORECEPTORASSAYS

Ian Holdaway

The last decade has seen the widespread introduction of techniques for the measurement of hormone receptors and the use of receptors as binding agents in radioreceptor assay (RRA). Two general categories of receptor assay have been established: first, systems for the assay of receptors in tissues, such as the measurement of estrogen receptors in breast cancer, and second, the use of receptors as binding agents in radioligand assays. The essential difference between RRA and radioimmunoassay (RIA) is that the binding protein used in RRA is itself part of the biologic pathway for hormone action, that is, a receptor rather than an antibody. To this extent, RRA is closer to a true biological assay than RIA. One cannot, however, necessarily equate activity in a RRA with full biologic activity, since hormones may bind to receptors without having further biologic effect. In addition, different hormones may cross-react to a variable extent with the same receptor, so that RRA may on occasion be less specific than RIA. Finally, when employing RRA to measure normal circulating hormone levels in plasma, assay sensitivity may be less than that of RIA. Examples of these differences between RRA and RIA will be given below, and in addition this chapter will outline some of the principles of RRA and discuss several specific examples of assays that are in popular use.

RECEPTOR PREPARATION

Various types of receptor preparation can be used in radioreceptor systems, ranging from crude tissue homogenates, ultrathin tissue slices, and partially purified receptor proteins through to solubilized or highly purified receptors. For RRA purposes, relatively crude receptor preparations are often satisfactory. Tissue either can be processed fresh or in most instances may be stored frozen for later receptor preparation. Definitive processing for the preparation of receptors must, however, be performed rapidly at near-zero temperature to prevent receptor degradation. Once prepared, receptor preparations are usually stable for several months if stored at −70°C or below, and thus batch preparation is possible, allowing aliquots of receptor to be used in serial assays. Repeated freeze-thawing of receptor preparations should be avoided, as loss of potency usually occurs.

LABELED HORMONES

POLYPEPTIDE HORMONES

Polypeptide hormones are usually labeled with ^{125}I by conventional procedures using chloramine-T (1). The concentration of chloramine-T used for iodination should be kept low (2 mM or less), with a final concentration in the reaction mixture of 0.6 mM or less. For peptides such as growth hormone or prolactin this gives a molar ratio of chloramine-T to hormone of 1:150. Because the specific activity and yield of iodination tend to be relatively low at these concentrations of oxidant, ion-exchange chromatography may be necessary to separate labeled from unlabeled hormone before use in RRA (1). Binding of freshly prepared tracer to an excess of receptor of known potency should be performed routinely with each new preparation of label to check binding characteristics. Iodination of peptide hormones by lactoperoxidase (2) has also been used extensively in RRA. Such techniques for "gentler" iodination seem to have a theoretical advantage but in fact usually do not produce labeled material of a quality superior to that produced by chloramine-T iodination.

STEROID HORMONES

Tritiated steroid hormones are used for steroid RRAs. The field has been revolutionized by the synthesis of novel steroids with high specificity for the receptor, for example, promegestone (progesterone receptor assay) and methyltrienolone (androgen receptor assay). These agents bind specifically to receptor proteins and do not bind to the various other steroid-binding proteins such as transcortin which may contaminate receptor preparations.

PURIFICATION OF LABELED HORMONE

Labeled hormone is usually purified after preparation by standard methods, for example, thin-layer chromatography for steroid hormones and

Sephadex column chromatography for purification of iodinated peptides. For some assays additional purification has been found helpful using absorption of labeled hormone to receptor, desorption employing high-molarity solutions, and desalting by column chromatography. Such receptor-purified label may provide assays of enhanced sensitivity, as in RRAs of thyroid-stimulating immunoglobulin (3).

SPECIFICITY OF BINDING TO RECEPTOR

Specific binding of labeled hormones in receptor assays is determined by displacement of label from receptor using excess concentrations of appropriate unlabeled hormone. In steroid receptor systems this may not, however, be an adequate criterion of specificity, since a number of nonreceptor proteins may also bind the ligand specifically. For example, [³H]estradiol binds to sex hormone-binding globulin (SHBG) which frequently contaminates receptor preparations. Similarly, labels such as [³H]progesterone bind to transcortin as well as to the progestin receptor. This problem can be overcome by using an unlabeled competitor hormone that itself does not bind to the contaminating protein, such as the use of stilbestrol in estrogen receptor assay, since this steroid does not bind to SHBG. Alternatively, a labeled steroid analogue with specificity only for the receptor and not for SHBG can be used, for example, moxestrol. In progesterone and androgen receptor systems the labeled hormones may bind to receptor proteins other than the target receptor; for example, labeled progesterone or progesterone analogue may bind to androgen receptor, and vice versa. This problem can be overcome by adding a small amount of unlabeled hormone to saturate the interfering receptor, as in the addition of triamcinolone acetonide to saturate progestin receptors when [³H]methyltrienolone is used as label in androgen RRA.

SEPARATION OF BOUND AND FREE HORMONE

Since receptors are large molecules, separation of free hormone from that bound to receptor is usually straightforward. In steroid receptor assays the absorption of unbound hormone onto dextran-coated charcoal (4) is the favored technique, although separation can also be achieved by a number of other methods. For example, density gradient ultracentrifugation distinguishes labeled hormone bound to different molecular forms of the steroid receptor (5). Polypeptide hormone bound to particulate membrane receptors may be simply separated from unbound hormone by centrifugation at relatively low speed (3,000–5,000g) in the presence of divalent cations (6). Hormone bound to solubilized or highly purified receptors may need to be separated from free hormone by an alternative method of separation such as column chromatography or precipitation with polyethylene glycol (7).

QUALITY CONTROL OF RADIORECEPTORASSAY

Where receptor assays are used regularly for semiroutine purposes, for example, the detection of estrogen receptors in breast cancer and the assay of lactogenic hormones in sequential prolactin RRAs, some form of within-assay and between-assay quality control is essential. For the assay of tissue extracts or plasma samples quality control samples may be included in each assay in a manner analagous to RIA. Where receptor assays are used to detect tissue receptors, for example, estrogen receptors in breast cancer, the problem is more complex. Aliquots of a standard receptor-containing tissue such as rabbit uterine cytosol may be batch-prepared and several aliquots measured in each assay. Alternatively, there are now a number of international quality control programs in which freeze-dried receptor preparations are circulated among laboratories for assay and comparison of between-laboratory differences. Such quality control programs should ultimately lead to much better duplication of receptor results among different laboratories.

EXAMPLES OF RADIORECEPTORASSAYS

ESTROGEN RECEPTOR ASSAYS IN BREAST CANCER

The following procedure, with minor variations, is widely used for estrogen receptor assays in breast cancer (4,5,8). Tumor tissue removed at surgery is transferred on ice to the pathology laboratory. Samples are then taken for histology and as much as possible, preferably 1 g or more, is taken for receptor assay. Tissue is trimmed free of fat and snap-frozen in liquid nitrogen. Thereafter tissue may be stored at −70°C with stability for 1–2 months before assay. For assay, frozen tissue is pulverized with a pestle and mortar at −70°C, and the powdered tissue weighed, thawed, and homogenized in assay buffer (0.01 M Tris–HCl, 0.0015 M EDTA, 0.0025 M dithiothreitol, pH 7.4). Homogenization is best performed using several 10-second bursts of an automatic homogenizer while the tissue is kept at the temperature of melting ice. After homogenization the preparation is centrifuged at 100,000g for 60 minutes, and the supernatant fraction containing the cytosol receptor protein is retained for assay. Assay tubes are prepared in duplicate, with every second pair of tubes receiving 100 μl of 600 nM stilbestrol which is then dried down under nitrogen. To each assay tube is added 200 μl of tumor cytosol, and for each individual sample a series of dilutions of labeled estradiol are added to give final concentrations ranging from 0.4 to 6.0 nM. Thus, for each dilution of label, duplicate tubes receive only label, and a second set of duplicates receive label and excess unlabeled stilbestrol. Samples are incubated for 16 hours at 2°C, and then free hormone is separated from bound by the addition of 1 ml of dextran–charcoal mixture (0.25% charcoal, 0.0025% dextran 80 in 0.01 M Tris–HCl buffer, pH 8). The samples are mixed for 15 minutes at 4°C and then centrifuged for 20 minutes at 1000g. A 1-ml aliquot of supernatant is aspirated and counted in a beta scintillation counter. Total bound/free ra-

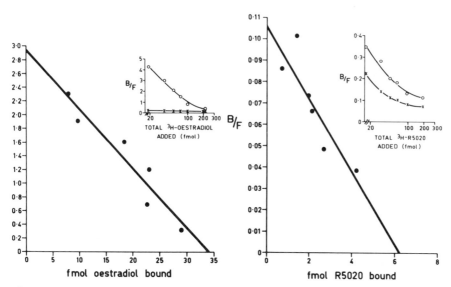

Figure 1. Scatchard plots of binding of [³H]estradiol or [³H]promegestone (R5020) to a cytosol preparation from a human breast tumor. Inserts show total (O) and nonspecific (x) binding. The plots yielded values for estrogen receptor and progesterone receptor of 36 and 7 fmoles/mg cytosol protein, respectively, with affinity values of 4.7×10^{-11} and $2.8 \times^{-10}$ M, respectively.

tios are calculated for each dose of label, and nonspecific binding is subtracted at each dose level. The resulting bound/free ratio is plotted against concentration bound to yield a Scatchard plot (Fig. 1). From such a graph, both the binding site concentration (*x*-axis intercept) and binding affinity (slope) can be obtained for each tumor.

An alternative method employs a single saturating dose of label, usually approximately 6 nM, with excess unlabeled stilbestrol to check specificity as above. From the total amount of label bound an estimation of the binding site concentration may be obtained (9). Results obtained by this simplified technique yield values comparable to those estimated by Scatchard analysis (Fig. 2). Such a system does not, however, allow an independent check of binding affinity. A further method that provides information concerning the molecular characteristics of the binding protein employs sucrose gradi-

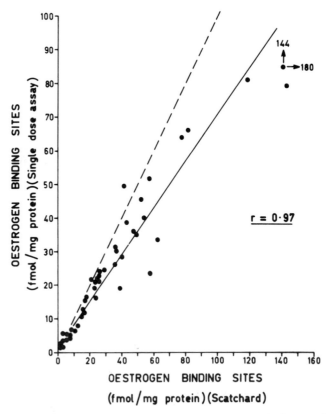

Figure 2. Comparison of results of estrogen receptor assay in human breast cancers measured by Scatchard analysis or by using a single saturating dose of labeled hormone. The dashed line is the line of agreement.

ent centrifugation (5). This procedure has recently been simplified by the availability of vertical tube centrifuge rotors for gradient studies.

The usefulness of estrogen receptor assays in breast cancer has been well established (10,11). In addition to the accepted application of the technique for predicting the response of patients with metastatic disease to endocrine treatment, it also appears that receptor measurements may be used in patients with early breast cancer to identify a group at risk of early recurrence (12). Receptor status in early breast cancer may also provide information on the appropriate type of adjuvant treatment that should be employed in such patients in an effort to delay or prevent recurrence.

RADIORECEPTOR ASSAY OF THYROID-STIMULATING IMMUNOGLOBULINS

The RRA of thyroid-stimulating immunoglobulins is an example of the application of RRA to assay of membrane-bound receptors. RRA of thyroid-stimulating factors has recently gained considerable popularity as an alternative to the earlier and more cumbersome bioassays of long-acting thyroid stimulator (LATS) and LATS protector. The receptor preparation is made from a thyroid gland from a patient with Graves' disease collected at operation and either processed fresh or, if necessary, after storage at −70°C. The tissue is minced and then homogenized in 10 volumes of buffer (10 mmolar Tris, pH 7.5). Either homogenization by hand in glass homogenizers or Polytron homogenization is satisfactory. The homogenate is centrifuged for 5 minutes at $500g$, and the resulting supernatant recentrifuged for 15 minutes at $10,000g$. The sedimented membrane fraction is resuspended in buffer [50 mmolar NaCl, 10 mmolar Tris, pH 7.5, with 1 mg/ml bovine serum albumin (BSA)]. Labeled thyroid-stimulating hormone (TSH) is usually prepared by iodination of highly purified bovine TSH using lactoperoxidase (13). After iodination the label is batch-purified by adsorption to 1 g equivalent of thyroid membranes in 1 ml of Tris–NaCl–BSA buffer. After a 30-minute incubation at 37°C membranes are washed three times with 5-ml aliquots of Tris–NaCl–BSA buffer and recentrifuged. The washed membrane pellet is resuspended in 1 ml of 2 M NaCl containing 1 mg/ml BSA and 10 mmolar Tris, pH 7.5, and after incubation for 30 minutes at 4°C the mixture is diluted in 5 volumes of Tris–NaCl–BSA and centrifuged at $100,000g$ for 15 minutes. The supernatant, containing about 80% of the originally bound TSH, is then purified on a Sephadex G-100 column. Serum samples for assay are prepared by the precipitation of immunoglobulins with ammonium sulfate followed by dialysis (3). Samples of either standard TSH or immunoglobulin extract (200 μl) are then incubated with aliquots of thyroid membrane (approximately 50 τg in 50 μl) for 10 minutes at 37°C. Receptor-purified ^{125}I-labeled TSH

(40 pg in 50 μl of Tris–NaCl–BSA buffer) is then added, and incubation continued for 2 hours at 37°C. The samples are then centrifuged at 25,000g for 15 minutes, and the membrane precipitate is counted after decanting the supernatant. The value of the unknown sample is read from the standard curve (Fig. 3) and is usually expressed as displacement activity compared to that obtained with pooled serum obtained from subjects without thyroid disease (3). This assay has been extensively investigated in patients with Graves' disease (3,4). As currently performed in our unit approximately 75% of patients with Graves' disease have a significant level of thyroid stimulating immunoglobulin. The reason for the lack of identification of stimulating antibodies in approximately 25% of patients with classic Graves' disease is uncertain; it may be related to assay insensitivity or to the transient appearance of the stimulating antibodies which are then undetectable when an assay is carried out at a later stage. The continued presence of thyroid-stimulating immunoglobulin does not appear to predict

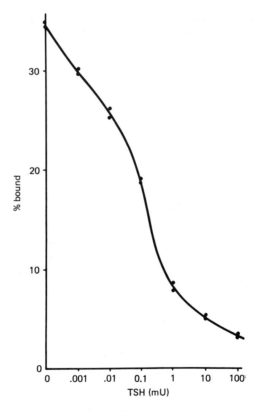

Figure 3. Binding of labeled bovine TSH to human thyroid membranes. For details see text.

which patients will relapse following withdrawal of antithyroid therapy (14). However, some provisional information suggests that the combination of thyroid-stimulating immunoglobulin assay and analysis of HLA haplotype may identify a group of patients with a high likelihood of relapse (15).

RADIORECEPTOR ASSAY OF LACTOGENIC HORMONES

RRA of lactogenic hormones is an example of a classic RRA that has been widely applied to the measurement of lactogenic hormones in plasma and tissue extracts (6). Receptor is prepared from pregnant rabbit mammary tissue. Mammary gland is removed from 31-day pregnant rabbits and rinsed through wet cheesecloth in 0.3 M sucrose. When the washings are clear, the gland fragments are dried, weighed, minced, and homogenized in 0.3 M sucrose. The homogenate is filtered through four and then eight layers of cheesecloth presoaked in 0.3 M sucrose and centrifuged at 15,000g, and the resulting supernatant is then recentrifuged at 100,000g for 60 minutes. The pellet from the high-speed centrifugation contains plasma membrane fractions including the lactogenic receptor (16). Receptor aliquots are stored at a protein concentration of 2–3 mg protein/ml at −70°C. Such receptor preparations are usually potent for up to 2 months. Radiolabeled human prolactin is prepared using chloramine-T or lactoperoxidase. For receptor assay 0.1 ml plasma samples or dilutions of standard hormone are added to 0.1 ml receptor extract containing 2–300 μg protein and diluted to 1.5 ml with assay buffer. Samples are incubated for 6 hours at room temperature, and then a further 1.5 ml of assay buffer is added and the samples centrifuged at 5,000g for 15 minutes. The precipitate containing membrane-bound labeled hormone is then counted, and a standard curve prepared (Fig. 4), from which the hormone concentration in unknown samples may be read.

  The principal difficulty with this form of RRA is interference with tracer binding by protein contained in the extract or plasma samples. Where prolactin concentrations are high and the samples can be diluted in assay buffer this is not a problem; however, in attempting to measure circulating levels of prolactin in plasma from normal individuals there is a considerable problem with assay sensitivity due to this protein effect. In general there is reasonable agreement between the results of plasma assays obtained by RIA and RRA, although on occasion RRA may yield levels different from those obtained by RIA (17). This may be due to the relative nonspecificity of RIA, since plasma from patients with prolactin-secreting pituitary tumors contains high-molecular-weight materials, probably aggregates of prolactin, which are measured by RIA but not by RRA (Fig. 5).

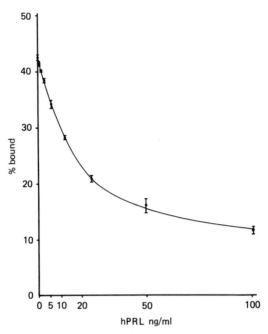

Figure 4. Binding of labeled human prolactin to rabbit mammary gland membranes. For details see text.

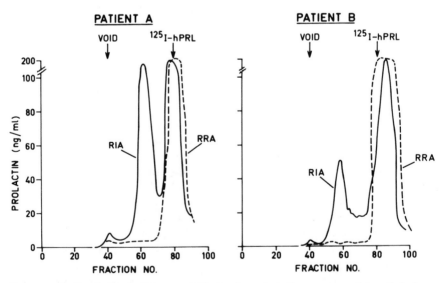

Figure 5. Prolactin levels from serum samples taken from two patients and chromatographed on a Sephadex G-100 column. Both patients had prolactin-producing pituitary adenomas with grossly elevated serum prolactin levels.

ACKNOWLEDGMENTS

The author is supported by grants from the Medical Research Council and the Auckland Medical Research Foundation.

REFERENCES

1. Heber D, Odell WD, Schedewie, H, Wolfsen, AR: Improved iodination of peptides for radioimmunoassay and membrane radioreceptorassay. *Clin Chem* 24:796, 1978.
2. Thorell JI, Johansson BG: Enzymatic iodination of polypeptides with ^{125}I to high specific activity. *Acta Biochem Biophys* 251:363, 1971.
3. Smith BR, Hall R: Thyroid stimulating immunoglobulins in Graves' disease. *Lancet* 2:427, 1974.
4. Korenman SG: Radio-ligand binding assay of specific estrogens using a soluble uterine macromolecule. *J Clin Endocrinol* 28:127, 1968.
5. McGuire WL: Estrogen receptors in human breast cancer. *J Clin Invest* 52:73,1973.
6. Shiu RPC, Kelly PA, Friesen HG: Radioreceptorassay for prolactin and other lactogenic hormones. *Science* 180:968, 1973.
7. Shiu RPC, Friesen HG: Solubilisation and purification of a prolactin receptor from the rabbit mammary gland. *J Biol Chem* 249:7902, 1974.
8. Holdaway IM, Mountjoy KG: Progesterone and oestrogen receptors in human breast cancer. *Aust NZ J Med* 8:630, 1978.
9. McGuire WL, de la Garza M, Chamness GC: Evaluation of estrogen receptor assays in human breast cancer tissue. *Cancer Res* 37:637, 1977.
10. McGuire WL Carbone PP, Vollmer EP: (eds): *Estrogen Receptors in Breast Cancer.* New York, Raven Press, 1975.
11. Holdaway IM, Mountjoy KG, Harvey VJ, et al: Clinical applications of receptor measurements in breast cancer. *Brit J Cancer* 41:136, 1980.
12. Bishop HM, Elston CW, Blamey RW, et al: Relationship of oestrogen-receptor status to survival in breast cancer. *Lancet* 2:282, 1979.
13. Manley SW, Bourke JR, Hawker RW: Reversible binding of labeled and non-labeled thyrotrophin by intact thyroid tissue in vitro. *J Endocrinol* 55:555, 1972.
14. Croxson MS, Lim TMT, Graham FM, Ibbertson HK: Thyrotrophin displacement activity of serum immunoglobulins in health and disease. *Aust NZ J Med* 10:151, 1980.
15. McGregor AM, Rees Smith B, Hall R, et al: Prediction of relapse in hyperthyroid Graves' disease. *Lancet* 1:1101, 1980.
16. Shiu RPC, Friesen HG: Properties of a prolactin receptor from the rabbit mammary gland. *Biochem J* 140:301, 1974.
17. Holdaway IM, Frengley PA, Mountjoy KG, et al: Investigation and management of symptomatic hyperprolactinaemia. *Aust NZJ Obstet Gynaecol* 19:100, 1979.

CHAPTER 15
PRINCIPLES OF IN VITRO BIOASSAYS

William D. Odell

As discussed in Chapter 1, there are four major ways or methods of assessing the relationship between a reference hormone and an unknown sample: *(1)* the in vivo bioassay, *(2)* the radioimmunoassay (or enzymatic assay), *(3)* the in vitro receptor assay, and *(4)* the in vitro bioassay. The most complex of these is the in vivo bioassay, for it involves all the factors concerned in animal use (species, age, sex, housing conditions, diet, genetic heterogeneity, and method of hormone or sample administration), as well as consideration of metabolic clearance rates or metabolism of the hormonal preparations administered and their relative potencies. Frequently, the metabolism or the reference preparation and that of the unknown sample differ, making relative potencies different at various times after administration and in different species of test animals. In attempting to define potencies of unknowns relative to a reference, all these factors are important.

The in vitro bioassay generally does not involve considerations of metabolism or distribution volumes, because during the short incubation times most hormones or other substances under study are not degraded or metabolized. However, some exceptions do exist. The advantages of in vitro bioassays, then, are not only that receptor binding is assessed but also that linkage of receptor binding to subsequent steps in hormone action and final product formation also are assessed.

As for the other in vitro assays (immunoassays and receptor assays), it is essential to maintain constant conditions (pH, osmolality, O_2 tension, protein concentrations, and substrate concentrations) in all tubes or flasks in an in vitro bioassay. Any differences among flasks or tubes can lead to artifactual results. Table 1 lists some of the in vitro bioassays in use today, along with references for methodology. In this chapter, we describe three bioassays as examples of the methods in use; for other assays, the reader is referred to the references cited.

Table 1. Some Examples of In Vitro Bioassays

Tissue or Cell Type	Activity Measured	Product Determined	Source of Cells	Selected References
Dispersed adrenal cells	ACTH	Corticosterone	Rat	Sayers, et al., 1971 (6)
Diaphragm	Insulin	CO_2 production from [^{14}C] glucose or [^{14}C] glucose uptake	Rate	Vallance-Owen and Hurlock, 1954 (8)
Epididymal fat	Insulin	Fatty acid synthesis from glucose or acetate	Rat	Gliemann and Gammeltoft, 1974 (9)
Thyroid cells	TSH	Radioiodine release into medium	Mouse	Brown and Munro, 1967 (10)
Leydig cells	HCG	Testosterone	Rat testes	Moyle and Ramachandran, et al., 1973 (1)
Sertoli cells	FSH	Androgen-binding protein or steroid conversion to testosterone	Rat testes (also Sertoli cell cultures)	Van Damme, et al., 1979 (4); Dufau et al., 1976 (3)
Pituitary cells	GNRH	LH and/or FSH	Rat (also pituitary cell cultures)	Kerdelhue et al., 1970 (11)
Urinary bladder	Antidiuretic hormone	Short-circuit current	Toad	Leaf and Hays, 1961 (12)
Strip of mammary gland	Oxytocin	Contraction	Rabbit	Mendez-Bauer, et al., 1960 (13)

THE LEYDIG CELL–LUTEINIZING HORMONE–
HUMAN CHORIONIC GONADOTROPIN BIOASSAY

This in vitro bioassay uses either cyclic adenomonophosphate (cAMP) or testosterone secretion by dispersed rat Leydig cells as an index of luteinizing hormone (LH) or human chorionic gonadotropin (HCG) activity. For the simplest form of the assay, an enriched Leydig cell suspension is prepared by simply removing spermatic tubules (1). More purified Leydig cell preparations may be prepared by centrifugation in Ficoll. For some purposes, this extra purification step is desirable.

PREPARATION OF LEYDIG CELLS

Sexually mature rats (300 g body weight) were sacrificed, and the testes immediately removed and placed in Krebs–Ringer bicarbonate (KRB) chilled medium. Sufficient testes were collected to supply the number of tubes or flasks required for the assay planned (one testis is sufficient for two to eight flasks). The testes were decapsulated using fine scissors; the testicular masses were added to 50-ml tubes (Falcon, No. 2070) which could be capped securely. Five to 10 testes can be placed in one tube and KRB added in a ratio of 2 to 4 testes per 7 ml of buffer. From Moyle and Ramachandran [1].

Collagenase (Worthington, Freehold, New Jersey) was added to a final concentration of 7 mg/7ml of KRB. The rubes were flushed with 95% O_2–5% CO_2 and placed on their sides parallel to the direction of shaking in a Dubnoff shaker at 37°C. Once the tubules began to disperse (usually in 20 minutes), the tubes were shaken for 10 more minutes. The tubes were removed, and 35 ml 0.9% NaCl was added; the tubes were inverted several times and then allowed to stand at room temperature for 10 minutes, permitting the tubules to settle.

The supernatant, containing suspended Leydig cells, was carefully decanted into clean 50-ml tubes and centrifuged at 100g at 4°C for 10 minutes. The precipitate contained Leydig cells, admixed with red blood cells and other cell types. This precipitate was suspended in KRB containing bovine serum albumin (BSA) (2 mg/ml) and lima bean trypsin inhibitor (0.1 mg/ml) in a volume adequate to add 1 ml of suspended cells to each assay tube or flask. Before addition of the Leydig cell suspension, all tubes were supplied with unknown or reference preparations dissolved in KRB. Just before incubation, the Leydig cell suspension was added rapidly with a 5- or 10-ml pipet. The tube containing the Leydig cell preparation was gently, constantly agitated to maintain homogeneous dispersal of the cells. Next, the tubes or flasks were gassed with 95% O_2–5% CO_2 and incubated 1 or 2 hours at 37°C in a Dubnoff shaker.

At the end of the assay, all tubes or flasks were removed and rapidly chilled or frozen. Aliquots of medium (generally 20–100 μl) were then assayed for testosterone content. A typical dose–response curve is shown in Figure 1*d*.

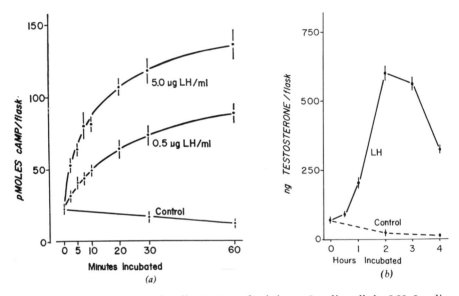

Figure 1. (*a*) Stimulation of cyclic AMP synthesis in rat Leydig cells by LH. Leydig cells (~2.5 × 10⁶) were incubated with LH for varying periods. Vertical bars extend to the limits of the standard error of the mean for four determinations at each point. (*b*) Time course of testosterone synthesis in rat Leydig cell preparations. Leydig cells (~1.4 × 10⁷) were incubated with 1 μg LH/ml for varying periods. Vertical bars extend from the mean to the values found for duplicate incubations. (*c*) Effect of LH and FSH on the stimulation of cyclic AMP synthesis in mouse tumor Leydig cells. Cyclic AMP generated by tumor Leydig cells (7 × 10⁶ per flask) in response to LH and FSH was determined after a 10-minute incubation. Vertical bars extend to the limits of the standard error for four determinations at each point. (*d*) Stimulation of steroidogenesis and cyclic AMP synthesis in rat Leydig cell preparations (A) or in mouse tumor Leydig cells (B). Incubations were terminated at the end of 10 minutes for cyclic AMP measurements and at the end of 2 hours for testosterone determination. (A) 2 × 10⁷ cells were present in each flask used for testosterone estimation and 5 × 10⁶ cells were present in each flask incubated for cyclic AMP measurements. (B) The numbers of cells present in each flask were 6 × 10⁶ for testosterone and cyclic AMP analysis, respectively. In the case of testosterone, the vertical bars extend from the mean to the actual values measured for duplicate incubations. For cyclic AMP, the vertical bars extend to the limits of the standard error for four determinations at each point. [Reproduced from Moyle and Ramachandran, 1973, (1).]

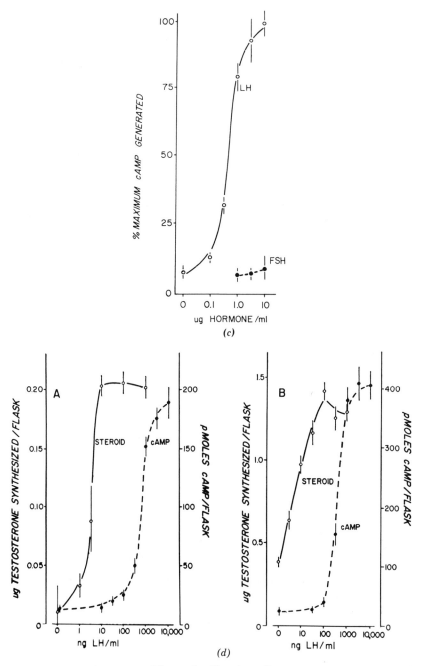

Figure 1. (Continued)

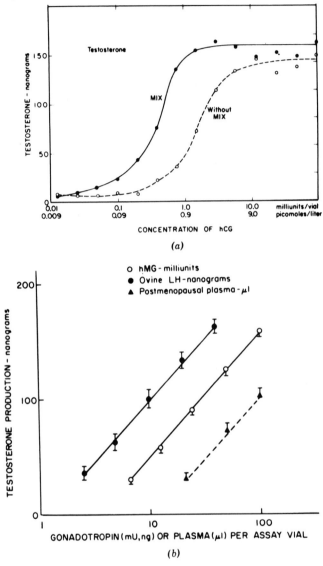

Figure 2. (*a*) Effect of the phosphodiesterase inhibitor MIX upon the testosterone response of dispersed Leydig cells to HCG. (*b*) Dose–response lines for human urinary LH (hMG), ovine LH, and postmenopausal plasma. Incubations were performed without MIX. [Reproduced from Dufau et al., 1974 (2).]

Figure 3. (*a*) Serum LH measured by bioasssy and radioimmunoassay during the normal menstrual cycle. The bio/immuno ratios are indicated at the bottom, and menses are shown by the hatched rectangles. (*b*) Correlation between bioassay and radioimmunoassay determinations of LH during a normal menstrual cycle. [Reproduced from Dufau et at., 1976 (3).]

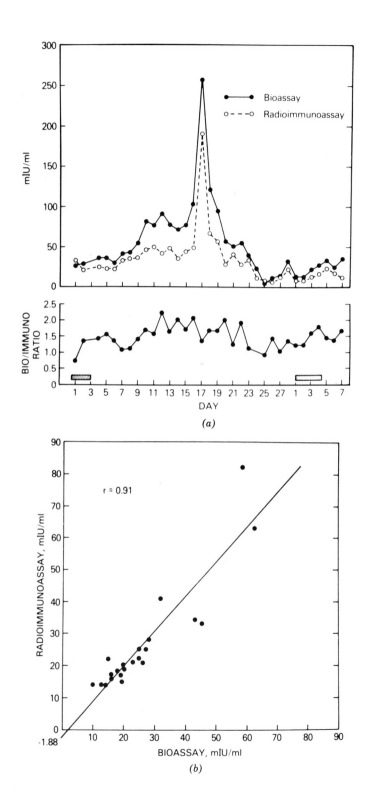

(a)

(b)

273

When cAMP is to be measured, cells and incubation medium are transferred into 1 ml of 1 mM theophylline in a boiling water bath. After 15 minutes, the mixture is allowed to cool and is passed through a 3-cm column of neutral alumina. The eluate is lyophilized and reconstituted in 0.1 M acetate buffer, pH 4. Recovery of cAMP is over 80%. Figure 1a–d depicts data published by Moyle and Ramachandran using this assay (1). Dufau et al. (2) reported that the sensitivity of this assay was improved 6- to 10-fold by the addition of phosphodiesterase inhibitors; 1-methyl 3-isobutylxanthine (MIX) added in a final concentration of 0.1 mM was recommended. Figure 2a and b shows these data, as well as dose–response data for LH in plasma. This assay has been used to quantify LH in the serum of eugonadal subjects. Excellent correlations have been shown between well-performed radioimmuonassays and this in vitro bioassay for LH (Fig. 3a and b) (3).

THE SERTOLI CELL–FOLLICLE-STIMULATING HORMONE BIOASSAY

A second example of an in vitro bioassay is the follicle-stimulating hormone (FSH) bioassay (4,5). This assay depends on the isolation of Sertoli cells from sexually immature male rats. Previous physiologic data demonstrate that Sertoli cells from sexually immature rats show a considerably greater response to FSH than Sertoli cells from sexually mature animals.

Testes from 10-day-old Sprague–Dawley rats were decapsulated and minced before digestion with trypsin and DNase. After the addition of soy bean inhibitor, tubules were enzymatically reacted with collagenase. The cells were then centrifuged and resuspended in Eagle's minimum essential medium (EM-I). Sertoli cells thus obtained from 36 rats were sufficient for 220 tubes (4).

To each tube or chamber, 19-hydroxyandrostenedione was added (200 μl containing 0.5 10^{-6} M). Unknown or known samples were added in EM-11. All tubes or chambers were gassed with 95% O_2–5% CO_2 and incubated with continued gassing for 24–26 hours at 37°C. Production of estradiol from 19-hydroxyandrostenedione was used as an assay response.

In a log–log transformation, Figure 4 shows the dose–response curves for several FSH preparations versus estradiol concentration. Note that the assay is sensitive to ~0.0125–2 MIU FSH, depending on the preparation tested. The assay is specific for FSH. FSHα, FSHβ, HCH, HCG, HTSH, ACTH, HGH, and HPRL were tested, and all reacted at <0.6–0.004% cross-reaction. Such reactions were compatible with known FSH contamination. No FSH activity could be detected in purified ACTH, HGH, HPRL, or GNRH.

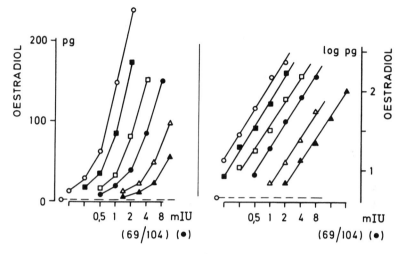

Figure 4. Dose–response curves in the in vitro bioassay for a number of preparations with varying human FSH content. The units of activity presented on the abscissa refer to that of the international reference preparation for FSH (69/104) indicated with solid circles. The remaining preparations have been positioned along the abscissa for illustrative purposes and not in relation to the units indicated on the abscissa. A ratio of 2 between successive doses was used. The amounts of the various preparations used per chamber at the highest level shown were: hFSH-Kabi (O, 1.3 ng), hFSH-NIH (■, 2.5 ng), hFSH β subunit (Δ, 173 ng), hLH (□, 220 ng), and hTSH (▲, 44 ng). The horizontal dotted line represents the amount of estradiol produced in the absence of added human FSH. The same data after a logarithmic transformation are also presented. [Reproduced from Van Damme et al., 1979 (4).]

Other considerations in this and all in vitro bioassays consist of optimizing buffer selection for preparation and incubation; osmolality; time, temperature, and pH of incubation; age and sex of animals from which tissues are obtained; substrate kind and concentration; and product formation. For this assay, 10-day-old animals produced Sertoli cells much more sensitive than older animals, whereas 5-day-old animals were equally sensitive. Since more cells could be obtained from 10-day-old animals, practicality dictated their use.

THE ADRENAL CELL–ACTH BIOASSAY

The adrenal cell–ACTH bioassay (6) uses production of corticosterone by dispersed rat adrenal cells as an index of adrenocorticotropic (ACTH) action. Sixteen adult male rats (300–450 g) were anesthetized with ether and bled by section of the abdominal aorta. The adrenals were removed, freed of fat, quartered, and transferred to a cold (4°C), siliconized 50-ml Erlenmeyer flask which held 20 ml of Krebs–Ringer bicarbonate buffer containing 0.2% glucose (KRBG) and trypsin (Worthington Biochemical Corporation, 0.25 g/100 ml). The flasks were gently agitated and incubated at 37°C in a 95% O_2–5% CO_2 atmosphere. After 20 minutes, the quarters were allowed to settle, and the supernatant containing the freed cells was transferred using a siliconized Pasteur pipet to a cold (4°C), siliconized 250-ml Erlenmeyer flask. Twenty milliliters of fresh trypsin–KRBG solution was added, and the procedure repeated; the process was then repeated three more times. The pool of cell suspensions was distributed between two siliconized 50-ml centrifuge tubes and centrifuged at 100g for 30 minutes at 4°C. The final speed was attained gradually (~10 g/min) over a

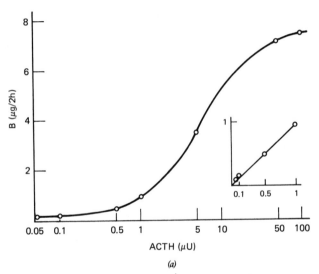

(a)

Figure 5. (a) Dose–response curve of ACTH (log scale) on abscissa versus corticosterone (compound B) production in micrograms per 2 hours on ordinate. The inset illustrates the linear relation between arithmetic values of B production and low concentrations of ACTH. (b) The effects of bovine serum albumin (BSA) in varying concentrations on the in vitro ACTH bioassays. The abscissa shows relative steroidogenic activity (corticosterone production), and the ordinate shows ACTH concentration on a log scale. Four response lines indicate the bioassay response with zero, 2%, 3%, and 0.5% BSA. Individual points are shown except at the 2% BSA, 20 µU ACTH point where the line connects individual points and the mean is shown. (c) The effects of two mechanical procedures of cell preparation on the ACTH steroidogenic dose–response relations. Bar indicates adrenal cells were stirred with a magnetic stirring bar during collagenase dispersal; paddle cells were stirred with a glass paddlelike device. [Constructed from data published by Sayers et al., 1971, (6).]

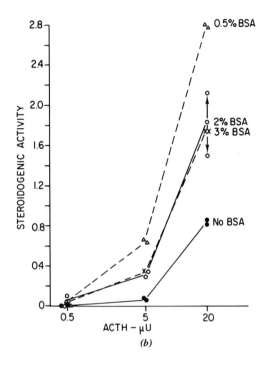

(b)

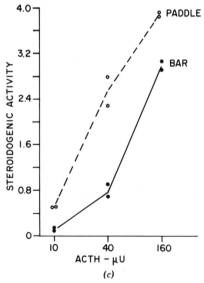

(c)

Figure 5. (Continued)

period of 10 minutes; the total time in the centrifuge was 40 minutes. After centrifugation, the supernatant was decanted and the pellet was resuspended in 34 or 60 ml KRBG containing bovine serum albumin (BSA) (0.5 g/100 ml), lima bean trypsin inhibitor (Worthington Biochemical Corporation, 0.1 g/100 ml), and calcium chloride (final concentration 7.65 mM). Any stringy particles that settled out were removed with a siliconized Pasteur pipet. Aliquots of 0.9 ml of the resuspended cells were added to 36 or 64 Teflon beakers (10-ml capacity). The beakers were gently rocked to ensure uniform distribution. Next, standard or unknown ACTH was added in 0.1-ml volumes. The beakers were placed in a Dubnoff shaker and incubated (66 oscillations per minute) for 2 hours in 95% O_2–5% CO_2 at 37°C. At the end of the incubation, the contents of the beakers were added to centrifuge tubes and the tubes centrifuged at 1000g. The supernatant was decanted, and the quantity of fluorescent steroid measured by the fluorescent method of Silber et al. (7).

As for all in vitro bioassay systems, changes in pH, osmolality, protein, temperature, and oxygen–carbon dioxide tension affect results. For example, Figure 5a shows the effects of differences in protein content (produced by BSA) on the dose responses of ACTH. Figure 5b shows the differences produced by a seemingly minor method change—using a magnetic stirring bar rather than a glass paddle to disperse or prepare the adrenal cells during trypsin incubation. Figure 5c shows the effects of changes in calcium concentration. Each of these studies (Fig. 5a–c) illustrates the great importance of ensuring that the constituents in all flasks are identical, with the exception of the hormonal preparation being tested. (From Sayers et al. [6].)

REFERENCES

1. Moyle WR, Ramachandran J: Effect of LH on steroidogenesis and cyclic AMP accumulation in rat Leydig cell preparations and mouse tumor Leydig cells. *Endocrinology* 93:127, 1973.

2. Dufau ML, Mendelson CR, Catt KJ: A highly sensitive in vitro bioassay for luteinizing hormone and chorionic gonadotropin: Testosterone production by dispersed Leydig cells. *J Clin Endocrinol Metab* 39:610, 1974.

3. Dufau ML, Roch R, Neubauer A, Catt KJ: In vitro bioassay of LH in serum: The rat interstitial cell testosterone assay. *J Clin Endocrinol Metab* 42:958, 1976.

4. Van Damme MP, Robertson, DM, Marana R, et al: A sensitive and specific in vitro bioassay method for the measurement of follicle-stimulating hormone activity. *Acta Endocrinol* 91:224, 1979.

5. Dorrington JH, Roller NF, Fritz LB: Effects of follicle-stimulating hormone on cultures of Sertoli cell preparations. *Mol Cell Endocrinol* 3(1):57, 1975.

6. Sayers G, Swallow RL, Giordano ND: An improved technique for the preparation of isolated rat adrenal cells: A sensitive, accurate and specific method for the assay of ACTH. *Endocrinology* 88:1063, 1971.

7. Silber RH, Busch RD, Oslapas R: Practical procedure for estimation of corticosterone or hydrocortisone. *Clin Chem* 4(4):278, 1958.

8. Vallance-Owen J, Hurlock B: Estimation of plasma-insulin by the rat diaphragm method. *Lancet* 1:68, 1954.

9. Gliemann J, Gammeltoft S: The biological activity and the binding affinity of modified insulins determined on isolated rat fat cells. *Diabetologia* 10:105, 1974.

10. Brown J, Munro DS: A new in vitro assay for thyroid-stimulating hormone. *J Endocrinol* 38:439, 1967.

11. Kerdelhue B, Berault A, Ribot G, Jutisz M: Dosage radioimmunologique de la LH de rat soit dans un milieu d'incubation d'hypophyses soit dans la plasma, après l'administration de LFR et de l'AMP cyclique. *CR Acad Sci* 270:1010, 1970.

12. Leaf A, Hays RM: The effects of neurohypophyseal hormone on permeability and transport in a living membrane. *Recent Prog Horm Res* 17:467, 1961.

13. Mendez-Bauer C, Cabot HM, Caldeyro-Barcia R: New test for the biological assay of oxytocin. *Science* 132:299, 1960.

CHAPTER **16**
ASSAY PERFORMANCE EVALUATIONS FOR QUALITY CONTROL

Jerald C. Nelson

The concept of quality control originated in industrial manufacturing where efforts to ensure uniformity of the products sold led to the generation of specifications for each product line. Individual items were tested for their compliance with these specifications, and those that failed were discarded, thereby ensuring uniformity among the units released. Quality was equated with uniformity. This mechanical approach does not translate readily to the generation of analytic procedure results in a biomedical laboratory. It is not possible to test each individual result for compliance with specifications, but rather an evaluation of the overall performance of an analytic system can be developed that provides an assessment of the constancy or stability of the system. In this situation quality is equated with constancy.

Quality control concepts have been widely applied in clinical chemistry (1–4), especially to automated clinical chemistry procedures. Radioimmunoassay quality control is a newer and still developing area of laboratory science for which there is only a limited literature. There is as yet no general consensus of what constitutes an adequate or acceptable radioimmunoassay quality control program, and yet the importance of quality control in radioimmunoassays is unquestioned. These assays can be readily applied to large numbers of unknown samples, but they are on the whole discontinuous analyses that are labor-intensive and employ sequential and critical handicraft steps. Assay failures are common, and assays are prone to drifts or trends in performance with time. Equipment failures and drifting electronics occur but are less frequent causes of radioimmunoassay failure than operator errors or deterioration in the frequently fragile biochemistry employed. The analytes measured are usually present in far more dilute concentrations than those measured in other clinical chemistry procedures. The standards are often precious or rare, some are not available in pure form, and many, particularly polypeptides, readily absorb to container walls or deteriorate in the dilute working solutions utilized. The radiolabled indicator molecules are themselves inherently unstable. Some radioimmunoassays are sensitive to the nonspecific effects of changes in the chemical or physical composition of the biologic fluid vehicle in which the analytes occur or to seemingly minor changes in the time or temperature of incubation. Consequently, effective quality control procedures are of critical importance in radioimmunoassays, and careful analyses of assay performance are essential to ensure the accuracy, precision, and reproducibility needed to generate reliable results.

A wide variety of quality control parameters and parameter data analyses have been proposed to deal with these problems in radioimmunoassay quality control (5–13). This chapter will approach the topic primarily from the standpoint of the basic concepts involved and will stress the usefulness of the more common quality control parameters.

The performance of a radioimmunoassay requires interpolation of a response variable from a standard curve for the calculation of unknown sample potency. To obtain these elements both standards and unknown samples are processed together with quality control samples in a batch-by-batch fashion. Each batch of assay tubes is often called an *assay run*. On completion of an assay the operator treats the assay data for data reduction and quality control parameter generation and analysis. The first step in analysis is the identification and removal of clearly erroneous data. This is called outlier editing. The second step is to determine whether or not the assay is acceptable for reporting. The third step is to monitor assay performance over the long term to detect significant shifts or trends in assay performance that would indicate early assay failure or systematic error in result reporting. A related activity is troubleshooting an assay that has failed or is approaching failure. Each of these will be discussed in more detail.

OUTLIER EDITING

The possibility exists that in the generation of assay data any single data point may be an aberration. Such errors can occur as a result of equipment failure, changes in line voltage to a counter, operator error, assay tube transposition, biochemical accidents, and radionuclide contamination, to name only a few. These aberrant data points are called outliers and should be deleted, or edited out of the data, before they are used to calculate assay results. Identification of aberrant data sometimes depends solely upon the deviation of these data from the other data points of similar type. Failure to remove outliers can lead to significant errors in assay results.

The crux of the issue is the identification of the data points that are true outliers. Statistical methods exist for outlier identification, such as the tests described by Grubbs (14) and Dixon (15). It is also possible to employ the two-standard-deviation range about the mean to identify outliers. Unfortunately, these statistical methods require a larger number of replicates in each data set than are usually obtained in radioimmunoassay work where both standards and unknowns are run in either duplicate or triplicate. Under these circumstances operator judgment may be the only method of outlier identification.

The following is an example of an outlier among five replicates of the B_0 tube (maximum binding tube) in a radioimmunoassay counting bound radioactivity and employing a B/B_0 response variable. Obviously, inaccuracy in the calculation of B_0 introduces errors throughout the assay, since each standard and each unknown employs this common element in its individual response variable. The counts per minute in this example were:

$$10,157 \qquad 17,245 \qquad 10,040 \qquad 9,981 \qquad 10,343$$

The data point 17,245 stands out as a possible outlier. It is, however, within the two-standard-deviation range of the mean which is 5,182 to 17,923. Had the set of data points consisted of only the first two, namely, 10,157 and 17,245, as would have occurred if B_0 had been run only in duplicate, identification of the outlier would be impossible from the data at hand. In both instances, however, an experienced operator fully familiar with the procedure might know that the B_0 counts with this assay were commonly in the 10,100 to 10,200 range and thereby would have additional information that would help to identify 17,245 as an aberrant data point.

Requiring an acceptable level of agreement between members of a data set is one useful way of indicating the likelihood that an outlier is present. The coefficient of variation (CV)* is frequently used as a standard measure of variance for this purpose. In the five-member example the CV is 27.6%. After deletion of the outlier it becomes 1.6%. In the two-member example the CV is 35.5%. The selection of a limit of acceptability for the CV of any data set is arbitrary, but a limit in the range 5–20% is useful in clinical laboratory assays.

Operator judgment is clearly susceptible to bias and is hazardous in the hands of inexperienced operators. Although measurement of the CV helps to identify areas where difficulty exists, it is useless in identifying which member of the data set is an outlier. At present the best method of outlier identification remains the considered judgment of an experienced and knowledgeable chemist fully familiar with the analytic procedure.

$$*CV = \frac{SD}{mean} \times 100.$$

INDIVIDUAL ASSAY AND RESULT APPROVAL

After outlier editing, assay data are processed and unknown sample results calculated. Before these results are recorded a responsible operator is required to render a judgment regarding the quality of the assay run. In making this judgment he or she compares certain parameters of assay performance for the present assay run and previous assay runs. If the assay is judged to be acceptable, the results will be reported; if not, the results will be discarded and the assay repeated. It is at this point in radioimmunoassay work that quality control activities approach most closely those of manufacturing, yet two important differences remain. In radioimmunoassay work the entire assay run, including its standard curve, quality control samples, and unknowns must be considered together rather than considering each unknown sample as a separate item. Second, specifications for assay approval are only partly objective. Heavy reliance still must be placed on operator judgment. This becomes critical when the quality control parameters studied are in part within acceptable limits but partially outside acceptable limits or when all parameters are within limits but there is nonetheless evidence of systematic error such as a shift or trend in assay performance. The fundamental issue is the question of whether or not the analytic process behaves in an acceptably constant and reproducible manner. Such constancy is equated with quality and is essential if the current results are to bear the same relationship to assay standards and to physsiologically important reference ranges such as the normal range existing in preceding runs of the same assay. The quality control parameters used in making this comparison include (1) the results of quality control samples, (2) the standard points and standard curve, and (3) the precision of unknown sample replicates.

QUALITY CONTROL POOLS

When a single sample is analyzed repeatedly, the results can be expected to be similar, varying only within a narrow range reflecting the irreducible random errors of the method. If such is not the case, something is wrong with the performance of the assay. Samples designed specifically to make these observations are called *quality control samples.* Typically they combine specimens from several individuals and are therefore called *quality control pools.* If the concentration of analyte in the quality control pool has been determined independently by an appropriate reference method, the pool

can be called an *accuracy pool,* since it not only provides a measure of reproducibility but also a measure of closeness to the true value. If the true value
is unknown, the pool is referred to as a *fixed-level pool* or a *precision pool.*
Quality control pools prepared within the laboratory are called *internal
quality control pools,* whereas those prepared by an outside agency are called
external quality control pools. A program of monitoring the results from internal quality control pool samples is referred to as an *internal quality control
program,* whereas one using external quality control pools is called an *external quality control program* or a *proficiency testing program.* Several large reagent vendors, regulatory agencies, and scientific societies make available a
variety of external quality control materials for proficiency testing. Their
use provides the additional advantage of laboratory-to-laboratory comparison of assay performance in which both the results and the precision of
repeated determinations can be compared (16). Such programs are carried
out by the College of American Pathologists (17), the World Health
Organization (7) and the Supraregional Assay Service of the United Kingdom (9).

The design and utilization of quality control pool samples is of practical
importance. Three or more quality control pools with different analyte
concentrations should be used in each assay. The concentrations selected
should cover the range of reportability of the assay and also be located near
significant decision-making cutoff points such as the limits of the normal
range. When assay runs are long and have a large number of tubes, the
quality control samples should be placed at several points in the sequence
of tubes. This allows monitoring for the detection of significant front-to-
back variation or an end-of-the-run effect, such as may occur in lengthy
nonequilibrium assays or assays with significant incubation damage to the
tracer where incubation times vary from the beginning to end of the tube
sequence. Repetition of quality control samples should be more frequent,
that is, after every 10 to 20 unknowns, in "loose" assays of less precision,
and less frequent, that is, every 20 to 50 unknowns in "tight" assays of
greater precision. The volume of quality control pools should be sufficient
to last for long-term monitoring. They should be stored in multiple
aliquots so that all aliquots will have undergone the same number of
thawing and freezing steps. Ideally they should be stored separately from
assay standards to lessen the likelihood of simultaneous and parallel deterioration.

Quality control sample data are treated in the same way as unknown
sample data, and the results are reported as the mean of duplicates or
triplicates. When samples from the same pool are introduced at several
points in the assay sequence, the same number of replicates is used at each
point and one result generated from each set. The analysis of these results
begins with inspection of a linear graph on which the analyte concentration
is plotted on the *y* axis against time on the *x* axis. An example is shown in

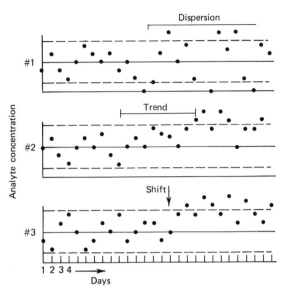

Figure 1. A Levey–Jennings-type graph of a quality control parameter showing three types of changes: (1) loss of precision with increased random error, (2) an upward trend, (3) and upward shift. [From Grannis and Carageher (2).]

Figure 1. These are called Levey–Jennings graphs or Sheward charts and usually include the mean and the two-SD range about the mean of pool results from prior assays taken from a time period in which the assay was judged to be performing optimally. The mean becomes the expected or target value, and the range about the mean becomes the limits of acceptable variance for this parameter. A separate graph is prepared for each quality control pool or quality control parameter. The setting of limits of acceptability is arbitrary and should be based on the best judgment of the laboratory director. For some applications or some assay systems the two-SD range may not be the most appropriate range.

When all quality control sample results are within the limits of acceptability, there is strong evidence that the assay is "in control." There are certain circumstances, however, when this may not be true, as will be discussed later.

Intra-assay variance is a measure of assay precision and can be measured by the CV among replicates of each quality control pool. This is an additional advantage of the inclusion of more than one set of each quality control pool sample in each assay run. A target value should be set for the upper limit of allowable variance. Though this upper limit is to a large extent arbitrary, it is usually between 5 and 10% CV in most radioimmunoassays. In addition to measuring the variance among replicate quality control pool samples, results should be examined for the possibility of systematic error introduced at some point midway in a single assay's performance. This is manifested as a shift or trend in pool results, which is often best detected by inspecting a graphic display of the Levey–Jennings type in which results for each replicate set are plotted individually. Any front-to-back shift increases the variance among replicate sets within the entire assay run, and when such is suspected, increasing the number of quality control samples included throughout the assay allows the generation of sufficient data to test for the significance of the difference between the quality control pool samples in the front of the assay run and those in the back of the assay run. The mean of quality control pool results from the entire assay may be within limits of acceptability even when an assay has unacceptable intra-assay variance or clear front-to-back shifts. This underscores the importance of separately assessing mean values and precision.

STANDARDS AND STANDARD CURVE

The first radioimmunoassays developed used ^{131}I-labeled polypeptide hormones. The harshness of the iodination reaction, the rapid decay of ^{131}I, and radiation damage to the hormones all lead to rapid deterioration of each lot of tracer prepared. At times, marked variations occurred in assay performance from one iodination lot to the next. The inclusion of one or more standard curves in each assay run was essential to achieve acceptable assay reproducibility, and the standard curve was not necessarily expected to remain constant from run to run. Changes in standard curve position and even standard curve shape were observed especially when the response variable B/T was employed, since the amount of radioactivity bound progressively decreased in all tubes in subsequent runs with deterioration of the label. As the state of the art has improved, ^{125}I has replaced ^{131}I, iodination procedures have become more gentle, and some ligands are labeled with longer-acting radionuclides such as ^{3}H and ^{57}Co. Small haptens such as steroids, iodothyronines, and drugs, are resistant to radiation damage. As a result, stability of standard curve position and shape have come to be the rule rather than the exception. This is especially true with assays that do not use total radioactivity in their response variables but use response variables such as B/B_0 and F/F_0 in which the common element of the response variable varies with changes in immunoreactivity. With high-quality reagents, careful handicraft, and scrupulously controlled reaction conditions, standard curves in many assays remain constant over long periods of time (18), and it is useful to monitor the reproducibility of the standard curve as part of the quality control program.

The simplest and most informative method of monitoring the standard curve position for bias is to follow the interpolated value of fixed response variables. When response variables are fixed, any variation in their interpo-

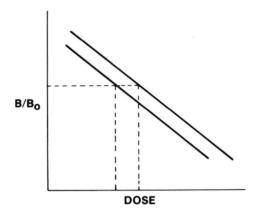

Figure 2. The effect of a standard curve shift on the interpolated value of a constant response variable (B/B_0).

lated values reflects variations arising solely in the standard curve position, as illustrated in Figure 2. The most widely used response variables for this purpose are those representing 20, 50, and 80% displacement of the label. It is also helpful to select fixed response variables that coincide with the expected response variables for each quality control pool. This allows an analysis of the contribution of standard curve variability to the overall variability seen in quality control pool results.

Many laboratories employ linearized transformation of the standard curve such as a logit–log plot. Under these circumstances the standard curves can be described by their slopes and intercepts. Monitoring these parameters also gives a measure of standard curve stability, but interpretation of these data is more difficult. These standard curve quality control parameters are easily plotted on Levey–Jennings graphs for analysis by inspection in the same manner as described for quality control sample results. It is important to remember that constancy of the standard curve is not a requisite for an acceptable assay. Variability in the standard curve position or shape, however, that exceeds that expected from prior experience can be an important indication of assay failure.

It is important to evaluate assay standards for precision as well as bias. The simplest assessment of standard curve precision is inspection of the standard curve points and their variance around the standard curve drawn from them. This assessment cannot be made if standard curve data are plotted solely as the mean of replicates for each standard point. It is important that each singlicate be graphed separately. Simple inspection can be supplemented by objective measures of standard curve precision by using either the coefficient of correlation for linearized standard curves or alternatively the standard error of fit. These measures of variance can also be monitored on Levey–Jennings graphs.

Standard precision is most critical in determining the common element of the response variable (e.g., the B_0 in assays using B/B_0). Many laboratories use a larger number of replicate tubes for this common element (usually 5 to 10 replicates) even when unknowns are run in duplicate or triplicate in order to increase the precision and reproducibility of this standard point. In assays prone to front-to-back shifts repetition of this point throughout the assay, like the repetition of quality control pools, provides an important evaluation for front-to-back variations. Variance among these replicates can be measured by the CV and analyzed graphically.

INDIVIDUAL UNKNOWN RESULTS APPROVAL

Quality control samples and standard points can be assessed for both bias and precision, but unknown samples can be assessed only for precision. This assessment is possible only when unknown samples are run in two or more replicates, and most assays employ either duplicates or triplicates. Though no prediction of the level of potency is possible in an unknown sample, a prediction of the expected agreement among replicates is possible from prior experience. Precision among these replicates is commonly monitored as the CV, and maximum limits of variation are set for acceptable unknown performance. These limits usually vary from 5 to 15%, and unknown sample replicates that fail to achieve this level of precision disqualify the unknown for reporting even though the assay as a whole has been approved. Such unknowns are "failed for precision" and run in a subsequent assay.

In summary, individual assay approval involves an analysis of assay constancy as reflected by the absence of bias and the presence of acceptable precision in quality control sample results and assay standards. In addition, precision among replicates of each unknown sample must be acceptable before an individual result is reported.

LONG-TERM MONITORING

Many radioimmunoassays are susceptible to change with time. This may be due to a variety of factors including biochemical or immunochemical deterioration of a critical reagent during storage, to a change in assay conditions such as the temperature or timing of incubation, or to a change in a critical reagent such as the standard lot or antibody. Any laboratory with long-term experience in radioimmunoassay performance analysis has encountered unexpected bias in assay results introduced by such shifts or trends in assay performance. Long-term monitoring for their detection includes monitoring quality control sample results, monitoring standard curve stability, and following the pattern and precision of certain unknown sample result data. There are two aspects of this long-term monitoring. The first examines the data for shifts or trends that would introduce bias into assay results. The second examines for shift or trends in precision. Both types of changes can occur separately or concurrently.

QUALITY CONTROL SAMPLE RESULTS

The first step in long-term monitoring is to analyze quality control pool results from the approved and reported assays for the detection of shifts or trends in assay performance. Although simple inspection of Levey–Jennings graphs may identify such changes, as demonstrated in Figure 1, statistical or mathematical methods of analysis are needed. Three methods have been described. They are window-to-window comparisons, the CUSUM technique, and Trigg's technique. In window-to-window comparisons the quality control pool data from one time period are compared to those of another similar time period. These time periods are called *time windows*. The data from one window are compared to those from another time window for a significant difference using appropriate statistical tests such as Student's *t* test. In this type of analysis it is important to bear in mind that the two sets of data may differ not only in means but also in variance and that an apparent difference in mean values may be meaningless if there is a significant difference in variance. The presence of a significant difference in variance can be tested for with standard statistical tests

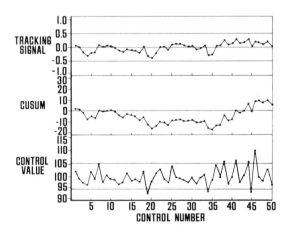

Figure 3. Control chart of the quality control parameter value with random variation about a mean of 100 and a standard deviation of 3, the corresponding CUSUM value and the corresponding Trigg's tracking signal. [From Cembrowski et al. (21).]

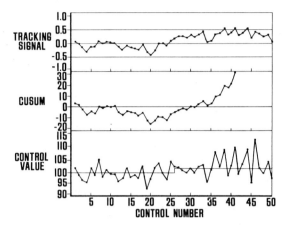

Figure 4. Control chart with the same data as in Figure 3 except for the introduction of a stepwise increase of 2% in results 26 through 50. [From Cembrowski et al. (21).]

for variance such as the *F* test. The window-to-window comparison approach suffers from the fact that it is retrospective and that the operator must define the periods of suspicion in order to select the window limits. It is, however, especially useful for routine comparisons of assay performance from month to month, quarter to quarter, or year to year. An example of this is discussed later and is shown in Table 2.

The CUSUM technique uses the cumulative sum of the differences between the observed quality-controlled parameter and its expected or target value for detecting changes in the average of a series of quality control results. It is similar to the method of moving averages used in financial

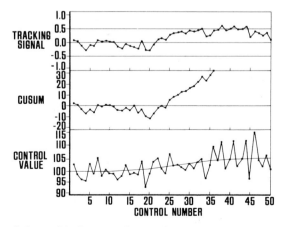

Figure 5. Control chart with the same data as shown in Figure 3 except with the introduction of a progressive trend between results 16 and 36 leading to a total increase of 4%. [From Cembrowski et al. (21).]

analysis. The expected value is determined from a prior time window selected as a reference period representing optimal assay performance. Subsequent variations from this mean are added in a cumulative fashion. If the variances about this mean are random, the positive variances will offset the negative variances as the data are accumulated. If, however, a systematic error is introduced, the cumulative sum will gradually rise (or fall) as shown in Figures 3–5. The graph of the cumulative sum can be monitored with a geometric device known as a V mask (Fig. 6) which can be constructed in such a way as to detect errors at different levels of significance or within different numbers of assay runs after the introduction of the change in assay performance. When the assay is in control, all previously plotted points lie inside the limits of the V mask. When points lie outside the V mask, as shown in Figure 6, the assay is out of control. Kemp et al. (6) have reported a nomogram for simplifying calculations of the vertex angle (2ϕ) and the lead distance (d). For details of its application the reader is referred to Kemp et al. (6), Lewis (19), and Undrill and Frazer (4). An alternative method of monitoring CUSUM data is to establish upper and lower limits of acceptability, as described by Westgard et al. (20). The CUSUM method has the advantage of indicating the time of onset of the change in assay performance and has been reported to be more sensitive than conventional quality control-monitoring methods for the detection of systematic changes in radioimmunoassays (8).

Trigg's technique makes the assumption that the next quality control parameter observation can be predicted from an exponentially weighted average of prior observations. The difference between the prediction and the actual value is called the *forecast error*. This forecast error is averaged by

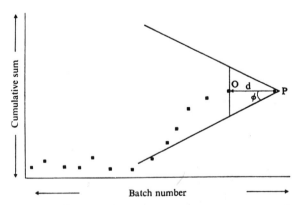

Figure 6. Application of the V mask to CUSUM quality control data for the detection of shifts or trends. ϕ is one half the vertex angle and d is the lead distance, both derived from a nomogram. 0 is the point coincident with the last plotted CUSUM point. [From Kemp et al. (8).]

exponential smoothing and dividing by a function of the variance in the data called the *mean absolute deviation* which is related to the standard deviation. The result is a tracking signal which varies around zero when the process is under control but approaches either plus one or minus one if significant systematic error is introduced. An example is shown in Figures 3–5 which compare Trigg's technique and the CUSUM technique with a graph of the raw data. Trigg's technique is suitable for computerization but does not indicate the time of introduction of the change and is more complex in both concept and calculation. The reader is referred to Cembrowski et al. (21) for a full description of Trigg's tracking signal, its calculation, and its analysis. Trigg's technique has been said to be more sensitive in the detection of trends, whereas the CUSUM technique is more sensitive in the detection of shifts, but more experimental data are needed regarding this point.

Quality control pool replicates also provide important information regarding the presence or absence of deterioration in assay precision. These data can be examined for a change in variance by monitoring the CV in a manner similar to the monitoring of quality control sample results. The data are first plotted on a Levey–Jennings graph and may be analyzed for shifts or trends by the CUSUM technique, as described by Wilson et al. (12) for radioimmunoassay quality control data.

STANDARD CURVE DATA

Reproducibility of quality control sample results is essential evidence of assay reproducibility, but assay deterioration may occur although quality control pool results remain within limits. An example of this is shown in Figures 7 and 8 which present data from a human growth hormone (HGH)

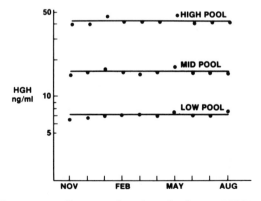

Figure 7. Monthly mean quality control pool results from a HGH radioimmunoassay over a 9-month period. Note the logarithmic scale on the vertical axis.

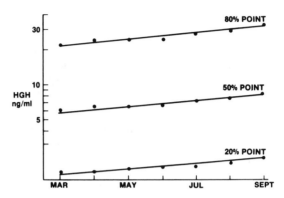

Figure 8. Monthly mean interpolated values for the fixed displacement points (i.e., fixed response variables) from the standard curve of the same HGH radioimmunoassay as in Figure 7. Note the progressive rise indicating assay deterioration over a 6-month period despite constant quality control pool results.

radioimmunoassay that progressively deteriorated over a period of 6 months although quality control pool results remained constant. In this figure quality control pool results are shown as the mean for each month, and the period of deterioration extended from March to September. As can be seen from Figure 7, quality control pool values (represented here on a logarithmic scale) remained constant during this time period as during the preceding months of acceptable performance. However, assay deterioration was suspected by the responsible chemist who felt that unknown sample results seemed to be rising. A retrospective analysis of standard curve stability included an analysis of the interpolated values for the fixed

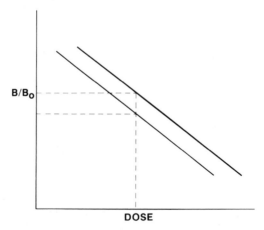

Figure 9. Illustration of offsetting shifts in both the response variable (B/B_0) and the standard curve leading to a constant interpolated value.

response variables at the 20, 50, and 80% displacement points. As can be seen from Figure 8 in which monthly means of these values are reported, the interpolated values rose progressively, indicating a shift in the standard curve upward and to the right. The problem was traced to concurrent deterioration of frozen aliquots of the control pools and of assay standard solutions, both of which had been stored in the same freezer. These combined effects on assay performance are represented in Figure 9. When fresh standards were prepared with a new lot of HGH reference preparation and the normal range redetermined, the assay returned to control concurrent with a return of the standard curve to its expected position. It is clear that comprehensive quality control programs must monitor more than just quality control pool results to guard against this type of error and that monitoring the constancy of the standard curve is also important.

A second example of the value of monitoring both standard curve reproducibility and quality control sample results is shown in Figures 10 and 11. These data were taken from a serum cortisol assay over a period of 4 months. Here the quality control pool values drifted progressively downward. Concern about assay failure arose because one member of the laboratory team felt that unknown sample results seemed to be running lower than previously. At first the responsible operator ascribed this to deterioration of stored control sera. Retrospective analysis of standard curve stability clearly showed a shift in the standard curve position. The data in Figure 11 are from the 50% displacement point. Concurrent downward trends in both quality control sample results and fixed response variable interpolated values clearly indicate that the problem was a shift in the standard curve downward and to the left rather than the deterioration of quality control pool aliquots as initially thought. The problem was traced to progressive

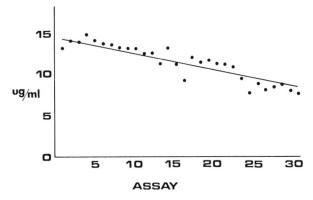

Figure 10. A downward trend in results for a quality control pool in a cortisol radioimmunoassay occurring over a period of 4 months, due to progressive evaporation of standard solutions in ethanol.

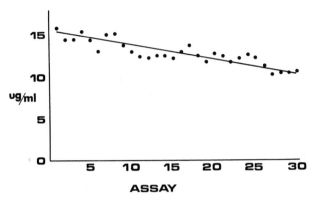

Figure 11. Interpolated values for the 50% displacement point ($B/B_0 = 50\%$) from the assay shown in Figure 10. The parallel decline in both quality control pool results and fixed response variable interpolated values indicates clearly a shift in the standard curve downward and to the left.

evaporation of the ethanol standard solutions which, although stored in a common laboratory freezer, remained unfrozen because the temperature was above the freezing point of ethanol. The preparation of new standards and redetermination of the normal range returned the assay to control, parallel with the return of the standard curve to its expected position.

Not only the position of the standard curve but also the shape of the standard curve may change with time. This is a serious problem when calculated standard curves or computer-generated standard curves are used employing a fixed mathematical model of the standard curve data. Changes in antibody lot, incubation temperature, or incubation time or other modifications in assay biochemistry or assay performance can lead to subtle changes in the standard curve shape. Simple inspection of the standard curve along with the data point for each singlicate of assay standards is a minimum requisite for detecting this problem. This observation cannot be made when a mathematical formula is substituted for a standard curve display. An example is shown in Figure 12. In this case a total estrogen assay that had previously been validated and for which a logit–log linearization of the appropriately truncated standard curve had been shown to be valid was modified by a reduction in the incubation time when the responsible technician responded to physician pressure to reduce the turnaround time. The shortening of the incubation, however, led to a slight change in the shape of the standard curve, and the highest portion of the standard curve no longer fit the previously selected linear model. As a consequence, the highest points on the standard curve consistently were above and to the right of the computer-generated straight line, and values in this region were consistently interpolated with low values.

The best analysis for detecting a change in standard curve shape from a

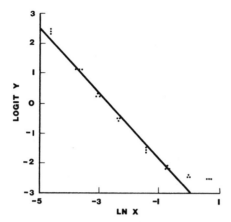

Figure 12. Computer-generated linear logit–log standard curve for a total estrogen assay which no longer fits the linear model previously selected.

previously adopted model is to monitor the interpolated value of each standard curve point from its own standard curve. When the standard curve shape remain constant, the interpolated values remain similar to the expected values. An example of this type of analysis is shown for the total estrogen assay in Table 1.

Standard curve precision as well as standard curve position and shape remain constant with acceptable assay reproducibility. Quality control measurements of standard curve precision, like the coefficient of correlation or

Table 1. Total Estrogen Assay[a]

Standard (ng/tube)	Interpolated Value of the Standard Point (ng/tube)
0.01	0.01
0.03	0.02
0.05	0.05
0.10	0.10
0.25	0.27
0.50	0.45
1.00	0.59
2.00	0.64

[a]Comparison of the known standard concentration with the reported concentration when assay standards were read from their own standard curve as unknowns. These data are from the total estrogen assay shown in Figure 11. The error introduced by nonlinearity at the high end of the standard curve is apparent at the 1.00 and 2.00 points.

standard error of fit, can be monitored for long-term trends by both a Levey–Jennings graph and CUSUM analysis.

UNKNOWN SAMPLE RESULTS

Though each unknown sample result is truly unknown, the pattern of unknown sample results considered together may be an indicator of assay performance, and important information regarding assay reproducibility may be obtained from their analysis. The usefulness of these observations varies from laboratory to laboratory depending upon the nature and constancy of the population of patients or subjects being studied and the volume of unknowns processed.

When the volume of samples processed is relatively large or the population of subjects from which they are taken is a large, healthy one, it may be assumed that the unknown sample results within the normal range closely approximate those for the normal population. Analysis of these results as a quality control parameter has been proposed by Hoffman et al. as the "average of normals" method (22). Monitoring the mean of these unknown sample results allows a testing of these assumptions. If this mean remains constant with acceptable assay performance, long-term monitoring of the value in subsequent assays may provide additional certainty of assay constancy.

For some analytic systems in some laboratories, monitoring the proportion of unknown results that lie within the normal range or the proportion of results that lie within some other physiologically relevant range may also be of value in monitoring long-term assay performance. There are no published data on this aspect, but anecdotal reports of laboratory experiences, including some of the examples cited above, suggest that assay failures may be detected more readily if such observations are used.

A measure of assay reproducibility can be obtained if a fixed portion of previously assayed unknown samples are reanalyzed. This method of generating quality control data has been called the *random duplicates* method (23). Variance among repeated measurements is a measure of assay reproducibility. There are, however, no data on the relative usefulness of this quality control parameter in comparison to other quality control parameters in radioimmunoassay work.

Theoretically, the most valuable utilization of unknown sample results in generating quality control data is obtained from the blind submission of known normal samples randomly distributed among other unknowns in a single-blind fashion. These known normal samples would provide important data regarding assay shifts or trends. When assay shifts were unavoidable, as occurs in clinical laboratories relying on vendor kits after vendor substitutions of new lots or reagents, these data would also provide an immediate estimate of the "new" normal range.

MISCELLANEOUS

There are some assay performance parameters that, though not essential to assay approval or long-term monitoring, are nonetheless easy to generate and frequently helpful in understanding assay failures. These include the total counts, nonspecific binding, initial binding, that is, binding in the zero standards (B_0 in assays counting bound radioactivity and F_0 in assays counting free radioactivity), and extraction recoveries.

Precision in the pipetting of radioactivity is a critical factor in detemining assay precision and reproducibility. This precision can be monitored as the CV among multiple replicates of the total counts. This is best done by including total count tubes at various positions in the assay sequence and graphing the resulting CV on a Levey–Jennings plot. Any significant change in the precision of pipetting total radioactivity may influence assay results adversely and certainly indicates deterioration in either operator performance or equipment performance.

Nonspecific binding should be determined in each assay run to correct raw counts during data reduction and also to provide a crude measure of radiochemical purity and immunoreactivity among different tracer lots. It rises when the tracer preparation is contaminated with increased free radionuclide and also rises with damage to radiolabeled ligand. Along with the initial binding it provides a useful indicator of change in tracer performance.

The maximum binding of label to antibody in the absence of unlabeled analyte is represented in the response variable B/B_0 for assays counting bound radioactivity and F/F_0 for assays counting free radioactivity. Any fall in the former or rise in the latter may be a sign of deteriorating immunoreactivity.

In assays that employ extraction of the biologic fluid to be analyzed before the quantification of analyte concentration, knowledge regarding the efficiency of the extraction or extraction recovery is essential in the calculation of results. In some systems recoveries vary sufficiently from sample to sample, so that a recovery calculation is required of each individual unknown and quality control sample. In others, extraction recovery remains relatively constant among unknowns, and parallel extraction of standards may introduce the appropriate correction in the assay result reporting. In either case more information about assay performance is provided by monitoring extraction recoveries directly. The extraction recoveries may vary with different lots of extracting solvents and, on occasion, may be so poor as to prevent assay reportability, an event that can be identified early in the course of assay analysis when extraction recoveries are monitored.

All performance evaluations for quality control begin with a reference period during which assay performance is judged to have been optimal. This reference period is the time when an expected or target value for each quality control parameter is established and during which clinical correlations of physiologic correlations data are obtained. This initial reference period provides the time window with which future time windows will be compared. In analogy to the moving averages method of financial analysis, some clinical laboratories have introduced moving windows as opposed to fixed windows for providing the reference data to which current assay performance parameters are compared. The assumption underlining this approach holds that assays run in the recent past are more valid for comparison to current assays than assays run in the distant past. This moving window approach has serious limitations in radioimmunoassay work, since the extent of the initial assay evaluation is rarely repeated routinely, especially as it relates to redetermining physiologic ranges such as the normal range. Table 2 presents data from a parathormone (PTH) radioimmunoassay monitored over a period of 18 months. Mean data are shown for a single representative quality control pool. When each quarter was compared with the preceding quarter in a moving window fashion, the assay value was judged to be in control (despite the step-up in values between the second quarter and the third quarter). However, long-term evaluation shows a slow but progressive rise in quality control pool results with each succeeding quarter, which became highly significant when the first quarter window was retained and compared to the sixth quarter, with a rise of 39% from 75 μl equivalents to 104 μl equivalents. This was associated with a 10% misclassification error when samples from normal subjects were run

Table 2. Quality Control Pool 1[a]

Quarter		Significance	
First, $N = 37$	75 ± 32 ⎫	NS	⎫
Second, $N = 33$	85 ± 27 ⎬	$p < 0.02$	⎪
Third, $N = 51$	94 ± 34 ⎭	NS	⎬ $p < 0.001$
Fourth, $N = 49$	96 ± 25 ⎫	NS	⎪
Fifth, $N = 85$	101 ± 44 ⎬	NS	⎭
Sixth, $N = 106$	104 ± 40 ⎭		

[a]Comparison of a fixed window to a moving window method of assessing reproducibility in a PTH radioimmunoassay quality control pool monitored over 18 months and 361 assay runs. Values are means ± SD (microliter equivalents/milliliter). When the current quarter is compared with only the preceding quarter, no significant change is demonstrated despite the continual and gradual deterioration in assay performance. Comparison of the last quarter with the initial quarter properly indicates the highly significant trend.

during the sixth quarter, and results were interpreted against the normal range determined during the first quarter. Any laboratory director electing to use moving window averages for radioimmunoassay quality control purposes must be aware of the limitations of this method in detecting gradual long-term trends.

Assay performance parameters may also be used in assay troubleshooting. An example of this is shown in Table 3. These data were taken from a PTH radioimmunoassay found to have unacceptable variance. A study for determining the source of variance was designed to look at the stepwise increase in variance introduced by each succeeding step in assay performance. The parameters measured included:

1. Replicate counting of a single total count tube to determine the variance introduced by counter performance.
2. Replicates of total count tubes to determine the additional variance introduced by tracer pipetting.
3. Replicates of the initial binding (B_0) tubes to measure the additional variance added in the pipetting of antibody plus the separation of free from bound.
4. Replicates of the sample response variable to measure any additional variance introduced in the pipetting of unknowns.
5. The variance among the interpolated results for the sample to detect magnification or minification of variance introduced by interpolation.

The CV was used as the measure of variance. Since the CV is sensitive not only to variance but also to the number of observations made, 30 replicates of each observation were measured. As can be seen in Table 3, there is increasing variance with the increasing number of steps, but the greatest

Table 3. Analysis of the Source of Variance in a Radioimmunoassay[a]

Source	CV
Repeated counting of a single total count tube	1.07
All total count tubes	1.43
B_0 tubes	1.64
Sample response variable (B/B_0)	1.70
Sample interpolation results	4.40

[a]An analysis of the contribution of each successive step to overall assay variability. Thirty replicates of each count or tube were used to calculate the CV. The magnitude of the stepwise increase in the CV provides a measure of the increased variance introduced at each step in the procedure.

increase in variance is introduced by interpolation. This was the result of a shallow slope for the standard curve. The greatest opportunity for improving precision in this assay could be afforded by introducing a new antibody with a higher affinity which gave a steeper standard curve. After the substitution of a new antiserum, precision was acceptable.

CONCLUSION

From the foregoing it is clear that radioimmunoassay quality control programs are complex and that the state of the art is still developing. The selection of an appropriate quality control program for each laboratory and each assay involved depends in part upon the application for which the assay is intended, the number of samples and the size of assay runs, the availability of computerization for data reduction and quality control parameter data analysis, and the level of sophistication of the laboratory staff. An example of a listing of the quality control parameters available in a contemporary computerized radioimmunoassay laboratory is shown in Table 4. The extent and complexity of the program selected is a matter of judgment for the laboratory director. There is considerable anecdotal clinical experience suggesting that many current clinical laboratory quality control programs for radioimmunoassays err on the side of oversimplicity. Further studies should help to identify the most useful parameters and the

Table 4. Quality Control Parameter Menu[a]

1. Total counts, mean	13. Control pool 2, mean
2. Total counts, CV	14. Control pool 3, mean
3. B_0/T (or F_0/T), mean	15. Control pool 4, mean
4. B_0/T (or F_0/T), CV	16. Control pool 1, CV
5. Nonspecific binding, mean	17. Control pool 2, CV
6. Standard curve slope	18. Control pool 3, CV
7. Standard curve intercept	19. Control pool 4, CV
8. Standard curve coefficient of correlation	20. Mean of unknown results within normal range
9. 20% displacement point value	21. Percentage of unknowns in normal range
10. 50% displacement point value	
11. 80% displacement point value	22. Extraction recovery, mean
12. Control pool 1, mean	23. Extraction recovery, CV

[a]An example of the quality control parameters available for monitoring in a contemporary computerized radioimmunoassay laboratory.

most effective parameter analysis and allow simplifications with elimination of all but the essential observations. The basic concepts will, however, remain unchanged.

REFERENCES

1. Buttner J, Borth R, Boutwell JH, et al: International Federation of Clinical Chemistry: Approved recommendation on quality control in clinical chemistry. *Clin Chim Acta* 98:129F, 1979.

2. Grannis GF, Carragher TE: Quality control programs in clinical chemistry. *CRC Crit Rev Clin Lab Sci* 7:327, (June) 1977.

3. Russell CD, DeBlank HJ Jr, Wagner HN Jr: Components of variance in laboratory quality control. *Johns Hopkins Med J* 135:344, 1977.

4. Undrill PE, Frazer SC: An approach to quality and performance control in a computer-assisted clinical chemistry laboratory. *J Clin Patho* 32:100, 1979.

5. Challand GS, Cox L: Identification of an unusual gamma counter fault using Trigg's technique for trend detection. *Ann Clin Biochem* 15:117, 1978.

6. Cernosek SF Jr, Gutierrez-Cernosek RM: Use of a programmable desk-top calculator for the statistical quality control of radioimmunoassays. *Clin Chem* 24:1121, 1978.

7. Hall PE: The World Health Organization's programme for the standardization and quality control of radioimmunoassay of hormones in reproductive physiology. *Horm Res* 9:440, 1978.

8. Kemp KW, Nix ABJ, Wilson DW, Griffiths K: Internal quality control of radioimmunoassays. *J Endocrinol* 76:203, 1978.

9. Hunter WM, McKenzie I: Quality control of radioimmunoassays for proteins. *Ann Clin Biochem* 16:131, 1979.

10. McDonagh BF, Munson PJ, Rodbard D: A computerized approach to statistical quality control for radioimmunoassays in the clinical chemistry laboratory. *Comput Programs Biomed* 7:179, 1977.

11. Spierto FW, Shaw W: Problems affecting radioimmunoassay procedures. CRC *Crit Rev Clin Lab Sci* 7:365, 1977.

12. Wilson DW, Griffiths K, Kemp KW, et al: Internal quality control of radioimmunoassays: Monitoring of error. *J Endocrinol* 80:365, 1979.

13. Woo J, Cannon DC: A quality control program for the radioimmunoassay laboratory. *Am J Clin Pathol* 66:854, 1976.

14. Grubbs FE: Sample criteria for testing outlying observations. *Ann Mathemat Stat* 21:27, 1950.

15. Dixon WJ: Processing data for outliers. *Biometrics* 9:74, 1953.

16. DeLeenheer AP, De Ruyter MG M, Steyaert HLC: A method for the statistical evaluation of results in external quality control surveys. *Clin Chim Acta* 71:229, 1976.

17. Hansel JR, Haven GT: Changes in level of precision of common ligand assays during a seven-year interval. *Am J Clin Pathol* 72:32, 1979.

18. Berk LS, Nelson JC, Lewis JE, Hillock, RH: Use of theoretical standard curves in STAT ^{125}I radioimmunoassays. *Clin Chem* 22:1186, 1976.

19. Lewis CD: Statistical monitoring techniques. *Med Biol Eng* 9:315, 1971.

20. Westgard JO, Gorth T, Aronsson T, de Verdier C: Combine shewhard CUSUM controlled chart for improved quality control in clinical chemistry. *Clin Chem* 23:1881, 1977.

21. Cembrowski, GS, Westgard JO, Eggert AA, Toren EC Jr: Trend detection in control data: Optimization and interpretation of Trigg's technique for trend analysis. *Clin Chem* 21:1396, 1975.

22. Hoffman RG, Waid NE: "The average of normals" method of quality control. *Am J Clin Pathol* 43:134, 1965.

23. Carstairs KC, Peters E, Kuzin EJ: Development and description of the "random duplicates" method of quality control for a hematology laboratory. *Am J Clin Pathol* 67:379, 1977.

INDEX

ACTH, 3, 33, 50, 155, 156, 274-275, 278
Adjuvants, 35-36
  in immune response, 26
Adrenal cell-ACTH bioassay, 275-278
Adsorbent techniques, 117-121
Albumin, 43, 205
Aldosterone, 164, 166, 190, 191, 196
Allergens, 246
Analyte heterogeneity, 89
Animals for antibody production, 5, 34-35
  inbred animals, 35
  random-bred animals, 35
ANS, 208, 209, 213, 215
Antibody, 17-19
  affinity, 33, 41
  assessment, 38-48
  preparation, 34
Antibody binding site, 18-19
  constant regions in, 16
  hinge region in, 18
Antibody-bound label, 5
Antibody-polymerization separation
      method, 122
Antibody specificity, 33, 42
  specific interference, 42
Anti-carcinoembryonic antigen, 38
Anti-α-fetoprotein, 38
Antigen-antibody precipitation, 24, 155
Antigen-antibody reaction, 4, 23, 125-147
  association constant, 23
  reversibility, 23
Antigens, 16-17
  active site, 23, 48
  multiple binding sites and specificity,
      249, 253
  stability, 36
  stereochemistry, 56-57
Anti-prostatic alkaline phosphatase, 38
Antiserum (antisera):
  affinity, 7
  from animals, 27-28
  antibodies, 6-7

hybridomas for preparation of, 28-29, 253
  preparation, 5-7
  selection, 43
  specificity, 6
Anti-β-subunit serum, 45
Arrhenius equation, 192
Aspergillus fumigatus, 249
Assay kinetics, 125, 126
Assay performance criteria, 131
Assay reproducibility, 85
Assay run, 282
Assay sensitivity, 33, 41, 143-145
  peptide purity in, 76
  protein purity in, 76
  radiolabel amount in, 71
  radiolabel counting rate in, 71
Assay specificity, 88, 90
Assay standardization, 85-86, 89
  unitage in, 94
Association rate constant, 125, 126, 146-147
Average association constant, 142

B cells, 19, 30-31
Benzamidine chlorhydrate, 151
Binding assays classification, 243
Binding reaction, 88
Binding reagent, see Labeled binding
      reagent
Bioassays:
  in vitro:
    advantages, 267
    principles, 267-278
  in vivo, 1-3, 86
    complexity, 267
Bisdiazotized benzidine, 56, 58
Blood iodothyronines, 205
Blood thyroid hormones, 205-207
Bolton-Hunter method, 70, 73-74
Bound and free antigen, 9, 24, 107-123,
      199-200, 211-212, 257-258
Bovine serum albumin, 55, 59-65, 169, 172,
      209-210, 227

305

Calcitonin, 33-35, 40, 50, 150
c-AMP, *see* Cyclic adenomonophosphate
Carbodiimide, 55, 57, 59-62, 65, 210
Carriers, 26, 35
Charcoal, 117, 155, 179, 211
Chemical equations, 125-147
Chemical separation method, 114-117
Chloramine-T method, 70, 71, 75, 210, 256, 263
Chromatoelectrophoresis, 108, 155
C1q molecules, 23
Coated tube method, 200
Coefficient of correlation, 133, 288, 297-298
Coefficient of variation, 131, 283, 286, 293, 301
College of American Pathologists, 285
Column chromatography, 161, 210, 258
Competitive binding, 125-147
    optimization, 141, 146
Competitive binding assays, 243-246
    displacement assay, 245
    history of, 245
    incubation methods, 245
    reactant concentrations in, 251
    sensitivity, 245, 251
Cooperative binding, 138
Correlation, coefficient of, *see* Coefficient of correlation
Corticosterone, 275
Cortisol, 11, 164, 189, 190, 198, 295
Cross-reactivity, 43-48
CUSUM technique, 290-292
    advantages, 292
CV, *see* Coefficient of variation
Cyclic adenomonophosphate, 269

Damaged hormone, 112-113
DASP, 155
Data representation, 128-131
    B/B_o *vs.* log dose, 130
    B/F *vs.* log dose, 130
    B/T *vs.* log dose, 130, 287
    F/B *vs.* log dose, 130
    F/T *vs.* log dose, 130
    $H*R$ *vs.* log dose, 130
    logit B/B_o *vs.* log dose, 130
DCC, 179, 181, 188-189, 191, 198
Degoxin, 65, 198
Density gradient centrifugation, 257
Dextran, 17, 122
Dihydrotestosterone, 33, 116, 165-166, 169
Diiodothyronine, 205, 209
Diiodothyropropionic acid, 210

Diiodotyrosine, 205, 207
Dinitrobenzene, 17
Dissociation rate constant, 125, 126, 146-147
DIT, *see* Diiodotyrosine
Dose-response curve, 121
Double-antibody method, *see* Immuno-precipitation

ECBS standards, 91, 94, 95-97
EDTA, 151
Eicosanoids, 225, 227
Endoporoxides, 241
β-Endorphin, 34-35, 41, 43, 150, 157, 212
P-Endorphin, 33
Equilibrium assay, 126
Equilibrium constant, 141
Erythropoietin, 96
Estradiol, 165, 177, 182, 191-192, 198, 257
Estriol, 168, 180, 198
Estrogens, in breast cancer, 258-261

Farr technique, 23
Fc receptors, 19-23
α-Fetoprotein, 43
Fibrinogen, 55
First-order mass action, 126
Follicle stimulating hormone, 43, 45, 48, 73, 77, 82, 157, 212, 274
Forecast error, 291
Four-layer sandwich radioimmunoassay, 251
Freund's adjuvant, 5, 26-27, 36, 209, 228
FSHα, 274
FSHβ, 274
F-test, 291

Gastrin, 35, 96, 156
Gel filtration, 110, 161, 210-211, 257
Glucagon, 4, 35, 120, 150, 155-156
Gluteraldehyde, 55
Glycoprotein hormones, 43, 48, 70, 96
GNRH, 274
Gonadotrophins, 34, 48
Grave's disease, 261-262
Growth hormone, 34, 70, 74, 82, 89, 256

Half-maximal dose, 131
Haloperidol, 63
Haptens, 16, 35, 56
HCG, *see* Human chorionic gonadotrophin
HCH, 274
Hemocyanin, 209
Heparins, 89, 153

Hepatitis antigen, 249
Heterogeneous radioimmunoassay, 245
Heterologous radioimmunoassay, 45, 191-193, 196
Heteroscedasticity, 131
High pressure liquid chromatography, 236-237
Histocompatibility complex, 31
Homologous radioimmunoassay, 191, 193, 198
Hook effect, 253
Hormones, *see specific hormones*
HPRL, 274
Human chorionic gonodotrophin, 33, 38, 43, 45, 70, 73, 77, 82, 93, 155, 157, 269, 274
Human growth hormone, 96, 274, 293, 295
Human judgment, in radioimmunoassay, 303
Human placental lactogen, 33
Hybridomas for antisera preparation, 28-29, 253
Hydroperoxyeicosanoic acid, 228

Ia proteins, 31
Idiotype, 31
Immune complexes, 24
Immune response, 15
  adjuvants in, 26
  antigen administration route in, 26, 30, 36
  antigen dose in, 30, 37
  genes, 31
  genetic predisposition in, 30
  heterogeneity, 15, 28
  hypersensitivity, 15
  immunization schedule in, 37
Immunoadsorption, 188
Immunogenicity, 16
  chemical structure and, 16
  molecular size and, 16
Immunogens, 16
Immunoglobulin, 17, 89
  molecular chain structure, 17-19
Immunoglobulin A (IgA), 17, 18, 19, 20, 25
Immunoglobulin D (IgD), 17, 19, 20
Immunoglobulin E (IgE), 17, 18, 19, 20, 25, 247, 249, 252
Immunoglobulin G (IgG), 17, 18, 19, 20, 23, 24, 25, 26, 172, 182, 184
Immunoglobulin M (IgM), 17, 19, 20, 25, 26
Immunoprecipitation, 110-114, 189
  amount of carrier γ-globulin in, 111
  effect of temperature on, 111, 112

first antibody in, 110
  second antibody in, 110, 111
Immunoradiometric assay, 87, 245, 252
Immunoreceptor assay, 87
Immunoregulation, 30-31
Immunospecificity, 15
Insulin, 3-4, 36, 69, 93, 108, 110, 150, 155-156, 245
Insulinase, 3
In vitro assay, sources of error, 267
In vitro bioassay:
  advantages, 267
  principles, 267-278
In vivo bioassay, 1-3, 86
  complexity, 267
Iodinatated iodothyronines, 210-211
Idothyronines, 205-207, 208
Iodothyronine thyroxine, 205, 207, 209, 210, 212, 213, 214, 215
Ion-exchange chromatography, 256

Jerne's network hypothesis, 31

Label, *see* Radiolabeling
Labeled binding reagent, 243, 246, 251-252
Labeled ligand, 243, 252
Lactogenic hormones, 263
Lactoperoxidase method, 70, 73-74, 256, 261
LATS, *see* Long-acting thyroid stimulator
Law of mass action, 243
Least detectable dose, 131, 133, 143
Leucine-enkephalin, 33
Leukotriene A, 228
Levey-Jennings graphs, 286-288, 290, 293
Leydig cell-luteinizing hormone, human chorionic gonadotropin bioassay, 269
  sensitivity, 274
Leydig cells, 269
LH, *see* Luteinizing hormone
Ligand, 243
  labeled, 243, 252
Ligand assays, 243
Ligand excess method, 252
Limited reagent method, 252
Linear regression, 132
Lineweaver-Burke analysis, 141, 142
β-Lipotrophin, 34, 43, 50, 157
Long-acting thyroid stimulator, 261
Low speed centrifugation, 122, 258
Luteinizing hormone, 43, 45, 48, 70, 73, 75, 77, 82, 89, 116, 157, 212, 269, 274
Lymphocytes, 19
Lysergic acid, 56, 65

α_2-Macroglobulin, 154
Macrophage, 22
Mannich reaction, 56
Marcholanis, J. J., 73
Mass action, law of, 243
Mass spectrometry-gas chromatography, 225
Mathematical analyses, 125-147
Mean absolute deviation, 292
Membrane-bound receptors, 261
Memory cells, 26
Methionine-enkephalin, 33
Methyltrienolone, 256-257
γ-M globulin, 154
Michaelis-Menten analysis, 141-142
MIT, see Monoiodotyrosine
Molecular weight and immunogenicity, 16,
     35, 55
Monoclonal antibodies, 28-30, 38
Monocytes, 25
Monoiodothyronine, 205, 209
Monoidotyrosine, 205, 207
Morphine, 65
Moxestrol, 257
Multibinding site, 139
Multicomponent-antigen behavior, 138
Murphy-Pattee method, 207
Mycobacterium tuberculosis, 36
Myeloma cells, 5, 17, 28-29, 38

Nitrous acid, 56
Noncompetitive binding assays, 243, 246-251
     advantages, 253
     vs. competitive binding assays, 251-253
     limitations, 252-253
     precision, 253
     reactant concentrations in, 251
Nonequilibrium assays, 140-141
Nonideal behavior, 138-141
Noniodinated tyrosine, 205
Nuclear fluorescence, 251

Optimal concentrations, 145
Outlier editing, 282-283
Outlier identification, 282-283
     operator bias in, 283-284
     by operator judgment, 283-284
Outliers, 282
Ovalbumin, 55, 59

Paper chromatography, 214
Parathormone, 34, 50, 170, 150, 155-157,
     300-301
Parathyroid hormone, 96

Peptide radioiodination, 69
Peyer's patches, 20
Phagocytes, 25
Picryl chloride, 17
Polyethylene glycol, 29, 115, 168, 198
Polypeptide hormones, 34, 256
Prealbumin, 205
Premixing of reagents, in steroid assay,
     174-175
Primary immunologic reactions, 23
Proadrenocorticotrophin, 89
Progesterone, 164, 166, 191, 198, 257
Prohormones, 160
Prolactin, 10, 34, 40, 70, 76, 96, 156, 212,
     256, 263
Promegestone, 256
Prostacyclin, 227, 241
Prostaglandin, 229
Prostaglandin endoperoxides, 227
Prostanoid antibody specificity, 237
Prostanoid antiserum:
     affinity, 229
     animal immunization, 228
     dose reponse, 229
     preparation, 227-229
     specificity, 229
Prostanoid assay:
     sensitivity, 225, 229, 241
          iodinated tracers and, 229, 231
     specificity, 225, 241
Prostanoid biologic concentrations, 225
Prostanoid purification, 235
Prostanoid radioimmunoassay, 225-241
     limitations, 241
     reliability, 225
     reproducibility, 225
     specificity, 238-240
          blank value in, 238
Prostanoids half-life, 225
Protein A, 212
Protein assay methods, 1-3
     history of, 3-4
Protein bioassay, 1-2
Protein immunoassay, 2
     artifacts, 10-11
     contaminants in, 8
     reproducibility, 11
     sources of error in, 9-11
Protein morphology-structure assay, 3
Protein radioiodination, 69-70
Protein receptor assay, 2
Purification:
     of radioiodinated hormones, 77

of radioiodinated peptides, 77, 78
of radioiodinated proteins, 77, 81

Radial immunodiffusion, 216-217
Radioallergosorbent test, 247
Radioimmunoassay:
  approval criteria, 284
  complexity, 303
  deterioration, 293-294
  failure causes, 299
    bound and free estimation errors, 299
    counting errors, 299, 301
    equipment performance, 299
    extraction recovery errors, 299
    interpolation errors, 301
    nonspecific binding, 299
    operator performance errors, 299
    pipetting precision errors, 299, 301
    radiochemical contamination, 299
    radiochemical impurity, 299
    time factors, 300
  human judgment in, 303
  influencing factors, 149-160
    bound and free antigen separation, 154
    controls, 150
    enzyme inhibitors, 150
    molecular size, 156, 157-160
    nonspecific interference, 151
    osmolality, 153
    pH, 151
    polymorphism, 155
    protein heterogeneity, 155-156
    serum proteins, 150, 154
    temperature, 150
    tracer damage, 149-150
  long-term monitoring, 289-290
  performance evaluation, 281-303
  quality control, 281-303
    basic concepts, 282
    parameters, 282, 284
    reasons for, 281
  quality control pools, 284-287
    accuracy pool, 285
    design, 285
    external quality control pools, 285
    external quality control program, 285
    fixed-level pool, 285
    incubation time, 285, 296
    interval, 285
    interval quality control program, 285
    nonequilibrium assays, 285
    precision, 285, 286
    proficiency testing program, 285

    reactant concentrations, 285, 296
    repetition requirements, 285
    systematic errors, 286-287
  quality control samples, 284
    reproducibility of results, 293, 295
    results, 299-293
  reproducibility, 284, 287
  run size, 303
  see also Sandwich radioimmunoassays
  simultaneous, of multiple hormones, 215
  standard curve, 287-289
    bias, 288
    linearized transformation, 288
    position, 287, 296-297
    precision, 288-289, 297
    reproducibility, 293
    shape, 287, 296-297
    stability, 288
    variability, 288
  unknown sample results, 289, 298
    assay failures, 298
    assay reproducibility, 298
    assay shifts, 298
    assay variability, 298
  see also Protein, immunoassay
Radioinsulin, 3
Radioiodinated peptides, storage of, 82
Radioiodinated proteins, storage of, 82
Radioiodination methods, 69-70, 191-199
  label purity in, 69-70
  optimization, 70
Radioisotopes in immunoassays, 71
  C-3, 8
  C-4, 8
  C-14, 7, 8, 71
  H-3, 8, 71, 162, 169, 172, 182, 188-189,
    191-192, 198-200, 256, 287
  I-125, 7, 71, 72, 73, 74, 75, 168, 191, 192,
    194-196, 198-200, 229, 231, 256, 261,
    287
  I-131, 7, 71-72, 245, 287
  S-35, 7, 71
Radiolabeling, 4, 7-8
Radioreceptor:
  preparation, 255-256
  specificity, 257
Radioreceptor assay:
  categories, 255
  examples, 258-265
  principles, 255-265
  quality control, 258
  vs. radioimmunoassay, 255
  reproducibility, 258

see also Protein, receptor assay
Random duplicates, 298
RAST, *see* Radioallergosorbent test
Rate constants, 125
Reagent method, 252
  excess, 252
  limited, 252
Reference materials, 85, 90-91, 99-103
  availability, 95
  preparation, 4, 8-9, 91
  stability, 92-93
Residual sum of squares, 132
Reticuloendothelial cells, 25
Reverse triiodothyronine, 205, 209, 212
RIA, *see* Radioimmunoassay
Rosettes, 20
RRA, *see* Radioreceptor assay

Sandwich radioimmunoassays, 246-247
  sensitivity, 249, 252
Scatchard plot, 41, 69, 129, 141, 260
Sebacoyl dichloride, 56
Secretin, 96
Sendai virus, 29
Sephadex chromatography, *see* Gel filtration
Sepharose, 122
Sertoli cell-follicle stimulating hormone
      bioassay, 274-275
  optimizing experimental conditions, 275
  sensitivity, 274
Sertoli cells, 274-275
Serum albumin, 55, 209, 227
Sex hormone-binding globulin, 257
SHBG, *see* Sex hormone-binding globulin
Silicic acid chromatography, 235
Sip's relationship, 172
Slope steepness, 131
Sodium metaperiodate, 56
Solid-phase-coupled antigen, 245-246, 249
Solid-phase-coupled binding reagent, 252
Solid-phase-coupled ligands, 243, 253
Solid-phase separation methods, 121-122,
      184
Soybean trypsin inhibitor, 151
Standard charts, 286
Standard deviation, 133
Statistical analyses, 131
Steady state, 127
Steric inhibition, 154
Steroid-antibody bond, 171-174
  electrostatic forces, 172
  hydrophobic nature, 172
  lipoprotein extract effects, 172-174

pH effects, 172
solvent blank effects, 172-174
temperature effects, 172
Steroid antiserum:
  affinity, 181-184, 191, 194-195
    equilibrium constants, 181
  sensitivity, 198
  specificity, 163-171, 190, 191, 198
Steroid assay kinetics, 174-180
Steroid assay sensitivity, 174, 177, 181,
      194-195, 196
Steroid purification, 161
Steroid radioimmunoassay, 161-201
  antibody physical form and, 184-187
  dissociative agents, effect of, 174-180
  elimination of extraction in, 187
  exchange reactions in, 174-175
  optimization, 201
  reaction rates and, 174-180
  separation methods, effect of, 174-180, 191
  steroid dose, effect of, 181-189, 200
Storage:
  of radioiodinated peptides, 82
  of radioiodinated proteins, 82
Structure-function assay, *see* Protein
      morphology-structure assay
Students t test, 290
  sensitivity, 292
17 β-Succinyl estradiol, 59
Succinyl poly-L-lysine, 209
17 β-Succinyl testosterone, 60
Sucrose gradient centrifugation, 260-261
Supraregional Assay Service of the United
      Kingdom, 285

TBG, *see* Thyroid hormone, binding
      inter-α-globulin
TCDPG method, 70, 75
T cells, 20, 30-31
Testosterone, 33, 56, 116, 164, 169, 191-192,
      198
Tetraiodothyroacetic acid, 207, 210
Thin layer chromatography, 229, 231,
      235-236, 256
7 α-Thiocarboxyalkyl steroid, 63
1 α-Thiocarboxymethyl-5α-dihydro-
      testosterone, 60
6 α-Thiocarboxymethyltestosterone, 62
Thromboxane A, 241
Thyrocalcitonin, 156
Thyroglobulin, 55, 205, 207, 209, 210, 216,
      227
Thyroid hormone antisera, 209-210

Thyroid hormone binding inter-α-globulin,
    205, 208, 209, 212-213, 215-216
Thyroid hormone formation, 205
Thyroid hormone radioimmunoassay,
    205-217
  autoimmune iodothyronine in, 212
  counting errors in, 212-213
    via enzyme radioimmunoassay, 215-216
    free hormone concentration measure-
      ments in, 214-215
    genetic factors in, 213
    for human tissues and nonhuman
      species, 213-214
    mass screening for hypothyroidism by,
      215
    plasma protein interference in, 208-209
    principles and special problems, 207
    sources of error, 212-213
    species differences, 213
    standard curves, 211
    standards variability in, 212
    variations in serum proteins in, 212
Thyroid stimulating hormone, 3, 43, 45, 48,
    70, 74-75, 77, 82, 115, 155-157, 212,
    249, 251, 261, 274
Thyroid stimulating immunoglobulins,
    261-263
Thyrotropin, 93, 96
Thyrotropin releasing hormone, 58
Thyroxine, 4
Thyroxine-binding globulin, 4

Time-windows, 290-291
Titer, 5, 39
  final, 5
  initial, 5
Titration curves, 41
Toluene 2,4-diisocyanate, 56
Tracer, see Radiolabeling
Trasylol, 150
Trigg's technique, 290-292
Triiodothyroacetic acid, 207, 210
Triiodothyronine, 205, 207, 209, 210, 212,
    213, 214, 215
Triioidothyropropionic acid, 207, 210
TSH, see Thyroid stimulating hormone
Two-site assay, 246
Two-standard-deviation range about mean,
    283

Unweighted regression, 131, 137

Variation, coefficient of, see Coefficient
    of variation
Vasopressin, 33-34, 50, 75
Verknüppfungstest, 246
V-mask, 291

Weighted regression, 131, 137
WHO, see World Health Organization
Window-to-window comparisons, 290-291
World Health Organization, 285
    standards, 91, 94, 95-97